MEDICAL MICROBIOLOGY

A Laboratory Study

Third Edition

Revised Printing

William G. Wu

San Francisco State University

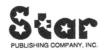

Star

PUBLISHING COMPANY, INC.

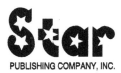

PUBLISHING COMPANY, INC.

Star Publishing Company, Inc.
Belmont, CA 94002

www.starpublishing.com

Copyright © 1995 by William G. Wu

Revised Printing 1999, 2009

(10 digit) ISBN 0-89863-180-7 — (13 digit) ISBN 978-0-89863-180-7

All rights reserved. No part of this publication may be reproduced, stored in a
retrieval system, or transmitted, in any form or by any means, electronic,
digital, mechanical, photocopying, recording, or otherwise, without the prior
written permission of the publisher.

Printed in the U.S.A.

0 9 8 7 6 5 4 3 2

i, ii , v 1- 09

TABLE OF CONTENTS

PREFACE TO THE THIRD EDITION

Modern medical microbiology, like other disciplines, continues to become more complex, both at the academic and the practical level. Microbial diseases common today were uncommon or nonexistent in the recent past, as exemplified by Lyme disease, legionellosis, and Acquired Immunodeficiency Disease Syndrome (AIDS). Some of these have forced us to revise our views on what we should consider as clinically important agents of disease. Current applications of evolving technology are also causing taxonomists to review existing schemes and relations of microorganisms to each other. New and modified types of assays to differentiate and identify these continue to be introduced into the laboratory. These reasons and more have prompted this Third Edition *of Medical Microbiology: A Laboratory Study.*

This edition of the Manual has again been enlarged, primarily in areas of background, so as to allow its use without reference to other textbooks. The application of computers (Exercise 2) and the use of a commercially-available DNA probe (Exercise 3) for microbial identification have also been incorporated to provide users with laboratory experience in these techniques. Also, miniaturized and rapid assays have received special emphasis through added descriptive materials. However, as in previous editions, in laboratory work, the still widely-used standard methods, while updated, will continue to receive primary emphasis for two reasons: namely (i) they display all the usual principles of identification that are commonly found in miniaturized assays; and (ii) it is less costly when media can be prepared on site. Expanded referencing allows the user to further investigate topics of interest (which is always strongly encouraged), and serves to explain further methods not completely covered in this manual.

Other changes have been included in this Third Edition hopefully to make the Manual easier to use. Procedural flow diagrams, for example, have been included in many of the more complex exercises, as have photographs to permit visualization of organisms, growth patterns, and aspects of laboratory techniques.

Many individuals have contributed to this edition of *Medical Microbiology: A Laboratory Study* and I wish to acknowledge their assistance. They are Dr. Remo Morelli, San Francisco State University, for his reviews of previous editions of the manuscript; Dr. James C. McLaughlin, Director of Microbiology at the University of New Mexico Hospital, Albuquerque, who critically reviewed the manuscript of the Manual; Dr. Rick Bernstein, Professor of Biology at San Francisco State University, who freely volunteered his considerable expertise concerning computer-assisted identification and application of nucleic acids probes to microbial identification; and Dr. S. T. Kellogg, Assistant Professor in the Department of Bacteriology and Biochemistry, University of Idaho, Moscow who has generously allowed the use of MICRID and MICRIDX and gave helpful comments on the use of these computer-assisted identification programs. Furthermore, Dr. Russel K. Enns, Director of Technical Affairs of Gen-Probe, San Diego, CA provided invaluable assistance in arranging to use the Gen-Probe DNA probe system in this Manual, and lastly, Dr. David Cox, Chief, Treponemal Immunobiology Section, Centers for Disease Control, Atlanta, GA, who agreed to serve as a source of treponemal cultures for Exercise 14, and provided valuable advice on the culture and storage of *Treponema pallidum.* To each I extend my grateful appreciation and thanks.

I welcome suggestions, comments, and recommendations. Please write to me c/o Star Publishing Co., Inc., Belmont, CA 94002

William Wu

GENERAL INSTRUCTIONS

This course deals with the nature and effects of microorganisms pathogenic for man and animals. Many diseases caused by these organisms may be adequately treated with antibiotics and other drugs; however, others may lead to illnesses which are difficult to treat by any means.

To avoid the possibility of infecting yourself or other people, strict rules must be observed. Anyone who chooses to disregard these rules or exhibits carelessness which endangers others will be subject to immediate dismissal from the course. If any doubt arises as to the procedure involved in handling infectious material consult the instructor. The following ruled must be observed:

1. Wear a laboratory coat when working in the classroom. Keep all clothing and unnecessary books off the benches, chairs, and floor within the room.
2. Do not place anything in your mouth that has come into contact with infectious material This includes pencils, food, and fingers. Do not eat, drink, or smoke in the laboratory.
3. Clean bench tops with disinfectant before and after each period of use.
4. Flame wire loops and needles before and immediately *after* transfer of cultures. *Do not* migrate through the laboratory with loop or pipette containing infectious material.
5. Properly label all cultures including name, initials, or group number, section, specimen, and date.
6. Dispose of unwanted material in the proper containers. Markings should be removed from all glassware, but not from disposable plastic material. *Do not let your unwanted and unneeded materials accumulate.*
7. Containers with viable cultures and used microscope slides must be sterilized before washing.

These rules are not designed to restrict you, but rather to encourage the use of proper techniques in handling all microoorganisms.

The laboratory work will be done more effectively and efficiently if the subject matter is understood before coming to class. To accomplish this, read appropriate laboratory directions prior to the actual class. Also, consult your text or other references for detailed information concerning the organisms you will be studying. Using these methods you can avoid confusion in the laboratory as well as save time and effort.

Much of the work in the laboratory is designed to be carried out in partnerships. This is to facilitate coverage of the subject matter and encourage discussion of data and results. This does not, however, release you from collecting your own data, making your own interpretations, and drawing your own conclusions.

INTRODUCTION

The goal of *Medical Microbiology, A Laboratory Study* is to give insight and understanding of many microorganisms that cause human disease. Although primary emphasis is placed on methods of laboratory isolation and identification of these organisms, one must not lose sight that a deeper understanding than just technique is intended. There is a need to understand each step and how it contributes to the final goal. Furthermore, by using various assays, we must grasp not only the mechanism of the test itself, but also gain insight into the organism being studied. Indeed, in some cases, assays have been included primarily to demonstrate some important biological facet rather than to differentiate between organisms. It is only through such an understanding that a full appreciation of microbial interaction with its environment (including within the human host) can be gained.

A. APPROACHES TO IDENTIFICATION

The usual sequence of events in identification of a microorganism implicated in disease include several steps. Whether all steps are needed depends on the type and size of the specimen, the extent of microbial invasion, and the type of microorganism(s) suspected to be present. The steps may include enrichment to selectively increase the relative numbers of the desired organism(s); isolation, usually on agar plates or tissue culture containers; and identification. The latter employs microscopic, physiologic, detection of cytotoxic or other cell altering properties, and/ or serological techniques.

Standard Methods: The basic approach in isolation and identification used in this manual will be those considered as "standard methods." These are techniques that have been developed and used over many years, and have become established as reliable for their purpose. When variations to these are developed, as rapid tests, they are generally compared to these standard methods to assess sensitivity, specificity, and other aspects of reliability.

The standard approach makes use of common laboratory containers as petri dishes and test tubes. In the context of miniaturized rapid assays it can be considered to be the "macroassay." Although these have the obvious advantage of having been time-tested with respect to standardization and accuracy (which does not necessarily mean that they are always completely standardized or accurate in their end result) they are not without their disadvantages. For example, isolation and pure cultures are usually required, a problem suffered by many methods despite technical advances. They are also generally slower in obtaining final results than microassays, especially in steps following isolation which usually require at least one or more days. Of course, by their very nature, macroassays also require larger quantities of media and chemical reagents, and more incubation and storage space.

2. Alternative Tests: In a continuing effort to reduce the time and effort to complete laboratory diagnosis of microbial disease agents without reduced accuracy, methods that vary from standard procedures have and are being developed. The general thrust of these has been to miniaturize, simplify, and streamline the standard macroassays, to develop new approaches to identification, and to incorporate automation while attempting to maintain high levels of specificity and sensitivity. Such alternative assays have become known by various names including rapid tests, miniaturized or micromethods, and non-traditional assays. The method employed in most cases take advantage of one or more of the following:

   a. Antibody specificity and sensitivity, especially monoclonal antibodies (see Exercise 2, for a further discussion concerning antigens and antibodies, and their applications to rapid assays);

   b. Physiological characterization of the microorganisms, especially by use of microassays; and

   c. Genetic analysis.

The last of these, discussed in more detail in Exercise 3, is in its infancy in terms of application for routine laboratory identification of pathogenic microorganisms. However, there is little doubt that it will eventually have a major impact on our capacity to truly accomplish "rapid" identification, probably without primary isolation of pure cultures that is currently required by most methods.

It is not the intent of this manual to provide a comprehensive description of various alternative methods that are available. However, examples will be provided in most of the exercises. Furthermore, expanded information can be found in many references, some of which are provided (1, 2, 8) at the end of this and other sections.

B. LABORATORY SAFETY

Studying potentially pathogenic microorganisms necessitates a constant awareness and attention to not only your own actions, but also to your surroundings. Laboratory safety is more than a set of rules and proper methods that must be adhered to; it is a manner of thinking and acceptance by all participants in an environment containing hazardous agents that such agents can and do cause infections, and not always to the "other person." Although strains of organisms used in this manual are selected to reduce this possibility, carelessness and failure of techniques by a single individual in a class can clearly have undesirable consequences to themselves and to others. To recognize and emphasize some of these possibilities it is instructive to read Collins (5), Pike (9), and Wedum (11).

As the scientific community has become more aware of laboratory-associated hazards, recommended safety procedures are becoming increasingly emphasized and standardized (e.g. references 6, 7). For instance, "biosafety levels" have been established for microorganisms (10). Level 1 (least hazardous) to 4 (most hazardous) are based upon a combination of factors including the level of hazard posed by the microorganism, the type of activity being done with it, the laboratory facilities and safety equipment available, and laboratory techniques and practices being carried out. Furthermore, the Centers for Disease Control (3, 4) have established a set of "universal precautions" for the handling of blood, body fluids (as vaginal secretions; semen; and cerebrospinal, peritoneal, amniotic, pericardial, synovial, pleural fluids; and saliva, but the latter only in a dental setting) or any body fluid contaminated with blood from all patients. These guidelines arose primarily over the prevention of transmission of Human Immunodeficiency Virus (HIV) and hepatitis B virus, but has come to encompass any pathogenic microorganism that may be transmitted by blood and other body fluids. Although specimens from these sources are generally not used in work covered in this manual, and HIV and HBV are not included for study, all should be aware of these guidelines given in pertinent references.

Although a basic set of laboratory rules appropriate to the work outlined in this manual are given below, you should also be aware of the contents of the "safety manual" within your laboratory facility. This contains the guidelines referred to above (4, 10) concerning "Update: Universal precautions for Prevention of Transmission of Human Immunodeficiency Virus, Hepatitis B Virus, and Other Bloodborne Pathogens in Health Care Settings," and "Safety in Microbiological and Biomedical Laboratories," or equivalent documents. Furthermore, it may hold other safety documents covering hazardous chemicals.

General Safety Instructions

To avoid the possibility of infecting yourself or other people, strict rules must be observed. Anyone who chooses to disregard these rules or exhibits carelessness which endangers others will be subject to immediate dismissal from the course. If any doubt arises as to the procedure involved in handling infectious material consult with the instructor. The following rules must be observed.

1. Wear a laboratory coat when handling infectious and other hazardous materials including viable cultures and toxic materials. Keep your work area clear and free of unneeded clutter. Keep all clothing and unnecessary books off the benches, chairs, and floor within the classroom.
2. Do not place anything in your mouth that may have come into contact with infectious material. This includes pencils, food, and fingers. Wear protective gloves when handling patient specimens or in other appropriate situations. No mouth pipetting is permitted. Always use pipetting devices.
3. Clean bench tops with disinfectant before and after each period of use. Also, disinfect

fomites *immediately* when suspected microbial contamination has occurred.

4. The wearing of contact lenses in a laboratory environment should be avoided. Chemical vapors as well as direct exposure to liquids containing hazardous microorganisms and chemicals are quickly drawn under the lens possibly resulting in eye damage.

5. All procedures involving potentially infectious materials should be performed to minimize the creation of droplets and aerosols. Use a biological safety cabinet or other containment devices for procedures where there is potential for these to occur.

6. Flame wire loops and needles before and immediately *after* transfer of cultures. *Do not migrate through the laboratory with a loop or pipette containing infectious material.*

7. Properly label all cultures with name, initials, or group number, section, specimen, and date.

8. Dispose of unwanted material in the proper containers. Markings should be removed from all glassware, but not from disposable plastic material. *Do not let your unwanted and unneeded materials accumulate.*

9. Containers with viable cultures and used microscope slides must be sterilized before washing.

10. Review the Safety Manual in the laboratory.

11. Become informed concerning procedures and action to be taken in the event of a laboratory accident or other emergency. *Immediately* inform your instructor of *any* laboratory accident.

The laboratory work will be done more effectively and efficiently if the subject matter is understood before coming to class. To accomplish this, read appropriate laboratory directions prior to the actual class. Also, consult your text or other references for detailed information concerning the organisms you will be studying. Using these methods you can avoid confusion in the laboratory as well as save time and effort.

Much of the work in the laboratory is designed to be carried out in partnerships. This is to facilitate coverage of the subject matter and encourage discussion of data and results. This does not, however, release you from making your own interpretations, and drawing your own conclusions.

REFERENCES

1. Balows, A., W. J. Hausler, Jr., K. L. Herrmann, H. D. Isenberg, and H. J. Shadomy (ed.). 1991. Laboratory safety in clinical microbiology. Manual of clinical microbiology, 5th ed. American Society for Microbiology, Washington, D. C. p. 59-136.

2. Baron, E. J., L. R. Peterson, and S. M. Finegold. 1994. Bailey & Scott's diagnostic microbiology, 9th ed. Mosby-Year Book, Inc., St. Louis. p. 97-167.

3. Centers for Disease Control. 1989. Guidelines for prevention of transmission of human immunodeficiency virus and hepatitis B virus to health-care and public-safety workers. Morbid. Mort. Weekly Rep. 38 (Suppl. 6):3-37.

4. Centers for Disease Control. 1988. Update: Universal precautions for prevention of transmission of human immunodeficiency virus, hepatitis B virus, and other bloodborne pathogens in health-care settings. Morbid. Mort. Weekly Rep. 37:377-382; 387-388.

5. Collins, C. H. 1983. Laboratory-acquired infections: History, incidence, causes, and prevention. Butterworths, London. 227 p.

6. Committee on Hazardous Biological Substances in the Laboratory, Board on Chemical Sciences and Technology, and Commission on Physical Sciences, Mathematics, and Resources, National Research Council. 1989. Biosafety in the laboratory. National Academy Press, Washington, D. C. 222 p.

7. Miller, B. M., D. H. M. Gröschel, J. H. Richardson, D. Vesley, J. R. Songer, R. D. Housewright, and W. E. Barkley (ed.). 1986. Laboratory safety: Principles and practices. American Society for Microbiology, Washington, D. C. 372 p.

8. Peter, J. B. 1990. Use and interpretation of tests in medical microbiology, 2nd ed. Specialty Laboratories, Inc., Santa Monica, CA. 177 p.

9. Pike, R. M. 1979. Laboratory-associated infections: Incidence, fatalities, causes, and prevention. Ann. Rev. Microbiol. 33:41-66.

10. U. S. Department of Health and Human Services, Public Health Service, Centers for Disease Control and Prevention, and National Institutes of Health. 1993. Biosafety in microbiological and biomedical laboratories, 3rd ed. HHS Publication No. (CDC) 93-8395. U. S. Government Printing Office, Washington, DC 20402. 177 p.

11. Wedum, A. G. 1964. II. Airborne infection in the laboratory. Am. J. Pub. Hlth 54:1669-1673.

SECTION I
PATHOGENIC BACTERIOLOGY

A. THE GRAM-POSITIVE BACTERIA

INTRODUCTION

1. General comments.

The organization of this laboratory manual is such that the Gram-positive bacteria are studied in two separate sections. Most of the cocci are covered in Exercises 1 and 2. The remainder of the Gram-positive bacteria are included in Exercises 16 through 22. A general introduction to all is given here.

The major groups of medically important Gram-positive bacteria are shown in Table 1-1. However, this fails to draw together some of their relationships which, in turn, influences their sequence of study in this manual. For example, based on sequence homology of 16S-rRNA oligonucleotides of Gram-positive, nonsporeforming bacteria with a G + C ratio of less than 55 mol% belong to the *Clostridium-Lactobacillus-Bacillus* branch. This includes *Streptococcus, Staphylococcus,* and *Listeria. Erysipelothrix,* based on this type of analysis, relates more closely to the mycoplasmas (7). Interestingly, both *Erysipelothrix* and *Listeria* were formerly in the family *Corynebacteriaceae* (2) based on phenotypic characteristics.

It is useful to note at this point the changing perceptions of what taxonomic relationships are between groups of bacteria. You will find many examples in this manual of families, tribes, genera, and species that have been de-emphasized, deleted, renamed, or reorganized. A major reason for this is that such categories were established using morphologic and other phenotypic characteristics. In the earlier editions of *Bergey's Manual of Determinative Bacteriology* (e.g. 2) this led to the establishment of a phylogenetic classification. In recent years, additional data, especially on genetic relatedness, has shown that many of these rela-

tionships are not as close as was once supposed. Therefore, an artificial form of classification has developed, and is generally followed today in, for example, all four volumes of the current *Bergey's Manual of Systematic Bacteriology* (e.g. 9). In this type of scheme, taxonomic levels above that of genus are de-emphasized, leading to a kind of situation described above where *Erysipelothrix* and *Listeria* were removed from the *Corynebacteriaceae.* However, as even more data become available, natural relationships are again becoming prominent, and with this, the arrival of new phylogenetic groups, along with the reestablishment of already familiar ones (17).

In medical microbiology, the Gram-positive cocci are, logically, studied together, as done in this manual (Exercises 1 and 2). Also, though differing markedly in the oxygen relationships, both *Bacillus* and *Clostridium* form endospores. This has led to their being in sequential exercises (Exercises 17 and 18) for study. Despite the development of genotypic unrelatedness of *Listeria* and *Erysipelothrix,* phenotypic characteristics will continue to hold sway. Both are covered in a single exercise (Exercise 19). *Actinomyces* and *Nocardia,* and to a certain extent, *Mycobacterium,* also form a natural group. They are generally slower growing bacteria, and especially *Nocardia* and *Actinomyces* can have a highly filamentous and branched organization. These growth characteristics have led to the consideration that they may be "higher bacteria." Indeed, the colony characteristics and diseases associated with these genera have historically closely allied them to the true fungi by the medical mycologists. It can be added that *Mycobacterium* and *Nocardia* are acid-fast, the only two among all the medically important bacteria. Generally, all the anaerobic species except some *Clostridium* (as discussed in the

Table 1-1
Major Groups of Gram-positive Bacteria of Medical Importance (8, 15)

Genus	Morphology	Oxygen Relationship	Catalase Reaction	Benzidine Reaction	Comments
Staphylococcus	Coccus	Fᵃ	+ᵇ	+	Arranged in clusters
Streptococcus	Coccus	F	−	−	Arranged in chains
Enterococcus	Coccus	F	−	−	Arranged in chains
Peptostreptococcus	Coccus	Ana	−		Arranged in chains or clusters
Gardnerella	Rod	F	−		Stains Gram-negative, variable
Listeria	Rod	F	+		
Erysipelothrix	Rod	F	−		
Corynebacterium	Rod	A, F	+		Diphtheroid arrangementᶜ
Mycobacterium	Rod	A	+		Branched rods, high lipid amounts
Nocardia	Rods and coccoid	A	+		Branched forms; aerial hyphae produced
Bacillus	Rod	A, F	+		Forms endospores
Clostridium	Rod	Ana	−		Forms endospores
Propionibacterium	Rod	Ana	+		
Eubacterium	Rod	Ana	−		
Lactobacillus	Rod	Ana, M	−		
Bifidobacterium	Rod	Ana	−		
Actinomyces	Rod	Ana	−		Forms branches, diphtheroid

ᵃ A = strictly aerobic, Ana = anaerobic, F = facultatively anaerobic, and M = microaerophilic.
ᵇ + = usually positive, − = usually negative.
ᶜ Diphtheroid arrangement means having a microscopic arrangement similar to *Corynebacterium* spp. See Exercise 20.

introduction to anaerobic bacteria, Section E), are found as part of the normal human flora and produce disease only under certain circumstances. Other types of associations will become apparent as we study these and other genera.

Not all the groups given in Table 1-1 will be studied in this manual. Therefore, a brief comment here concerning these may be useful. *Gardnerella vaginalis*, for instance, is an agent of bacterial vaginosis. Interestingly, this organism stains Gram-negative to Gram-variable (Table 1-1), but has a cell wall similar to Gram-positive bacteria (11). Its presence in infection is best detected on the basis of Gram-stained vaginal smears (10, 16) and clinical grounds, rather than culture identification. Key indicators are foul smelling vaginal secretions and the presence of small Gram-negative to Gram-variable bacteria (as opposed to the larger Gram-positive lactobacilli, common inhabitants of the vagina as normal flora) surrounding epithelial cells (called "clue cells"). A drop of 10% KOH to the vaginal fluid also produces a "fishy" odor (1).

Lactobacillus, Eubacterium, and *Bifidobacterium* also will be relatively neglected in subsequent exercises. These being anaerobic organisms, they are generally studied with others in this group (Exercises 16 and 17). They are isolated from a variety of infections, as discussed in Section E. However, none are frequent isolates as pathogens. In any case, identification procedures for these follow those generally described for anaerobes in that Section.

2. The Gram-positive Cocci.

The pathogenic Gram-positive cocci are primarily members of the families *Micrococcaceae* and *Streptococcaceae*. (Note: Although reference to the family *Streptococcaceae* has virtually been eliminated from the current Bergey's Manual of Systematic Bacteriology (15) it will continue to be used here.) Some characteristics of these two families are shown in Table 1-2. From this it is clear they have overlapping types of morphology and oxygen relationships. However, catalase production and the presence of a cytochrome system detected with the modified benzidine test (3) generally can separate the *Micrococcaceae*. It is positive, while the *Streptococcaceae* is not. Also, DNA homology between these families is disparate being 64-75% (expressed as mole percent content of guanine and cytosine (Mol% G + C) in DNA; further information on this topic is found in Exercise 3, page 72) for *Micrococcaceae* and 34-46% for *Streptococcaceae* (14).

Table 1-2
Some Characteristics of the Families *Micrococcaceae* and *Streptococcaceae*[a]

Characteristic	Micrococcaceae (15)	Streptococcaceae (5)
Morphology	Cocci	Cocci
Arrangement	Clusters, tetrads, pairs	Single, pairs, short to long chains
Oxygen Relationships	Strictly aerobic to facultatively anaerobic	Facultatively anaerobic
Mol % G + C in DNA	64 - 75	34 - 46 (8)
Catalase reaction	Positive[b]	Negative
Has Cytochrome System	Positive	Negative[b]

[a] The family *Micrococcaceae* include *Micrococcus, Staphylococcus, Stomatococcus,* and *Planococcus.*
The family *Streptococcaceae* includes *Streptococcus, Leuconostoc, Pediococcus, Aerococcus,* and *Gemella* (4), *Lactococcus* (14) and *Enterococcus* (6, 13).
[b] Rare exceptions.

In terms of disease agents the genera of Gram-positive cocci of greatest interest are *Staphylococcus* of the family *Micrococcaceae,* and *Streptococcus* and *Enterococcus* of the family *Streptococcaceae. Micrococcus* spp., though rare disease agents, are of most significance because of their ubiquitous nature, including being found on humans. Because of their similarity in morphology and catalase reaction to *Staphylococcus,* they may easily be confused with the latter during early stages of identification. However, they are readily distinguishable because *Staphylococcus* spp. are facultatively anaerobic and therefore fermentive; *Micrococcus* are oxidative. Furthermore, both genera can be separated from *Streptococcus* and *Enterococcus* because the latter tends to form chains of cocci while staphylococci and micrococci usually do not, forming clusters and tetrads. Too, the latter are catalase-positive while the members of the *Streptococcus* and *Enterococcus* catalase-negative (Table 1-1).

Pathogenic Gram-positive cocci are also grouped within the anaerobic bacteria. These genera, the *Peptococcus* and *Peptostreptococcus* will be addressed in Section E and Exercise 16 where the anaerobic bacteria are discussed.

REFERENCES

1. Baron, E. J., L. R. Peterson, and S. M. Finegold. 1994. Bailey & Scott's diagnostic microbiology, 9th ed. Mosby-Year Book, Inc., St. Louis. p. 258-273.
2. Breed, R. S., E. G. D. Murray, and N. R. Smith (ed.). 1957. Bergey's manual of determinative bacteriology, 7th ed. Williams & Wilkins, Baltimore.
3. Deibel, R. H., and J. B. Evans. 1960. Modified benzidine test for the detection of cytochrome-containing respiratory systems in microorganisms. J. Bacteriol. **79**:356-360.
4. Deibel, R. H., and H. W. Seeley, Jr. 1974. *Streptococcaceae* fam. nov., p. 490. *In* R. E. Buchanan, and N. E. Gibbons (ed.), Bergey's manual of determinative bacteriology, 8th ed. The Williams & Wilkins Co., Baltimore.
5. Facklam, R. R., and J. A. Washington II. 1991. *Streptococcus* and related catalase-negative Gram-positive cocci, p. 238-257. *In* A. Balows, W. J. Hausler, Jr., K. L. Herrmann, H. D. Isenberg, and H. J. Shadomy (ed.), Manual of clinical microbiology, 5th ed. American Society for Microbiology, Washington, D. C.
6. Hardie, J. M. 1986. Genus *Streptococcus* Rosenbach 1884, p. 1043-1047. *In* P. H. A. Sneath, N. S. Mair, M. E. Sharpe, and J. G. Holt (ed.), Bergey's manual of systematic bacteriology, Vol. 2. Williams & Wilkins, Baltimore.
7. Kandler, O., and N. Weiss. 1986. Regular, nonsporing Gram-positive rods, p. 1208-1209. *In* P. H. A. Sneath, N. S. Mair, M. E. Sharpe, and J. G. Holt (ed.), Bergey's manual of systematic bacteriology, Vol. 2. Williams & Wilkins, Baltimore.
8. Kloos, W. E., and D. W. Lambe, Jr. 1991. *Staphylococcus,* p. 222-237. *In* A. Balows, W. J. Hausler, Jr., K. L. Herrmann, H. D. Isenberg, and H. J. Shadomy (ed.), Manual of clinical microbiology, 5th ed. American Society for Microbiology, Washington, D. C.
9. Krieg, N. R., and J. G. Holt (ed.). 1974. Bergey's manual of systematic bacteriology, V. 1. Williams & Wilkins, Baltimore.
10. Nugent, R. P., M. A. Krohn, and S. L. Hillier. 1991. Reliability of diagnosing bacterial vaginosis is improved by a standardized method of Gram stain interpretation. J. Clin. Microbiol. **29**:297-301.
11. Piot, P. 1991. *Gardnerella, Streptobacillus, Spirillum,* and *Calymmatobacterium,* p. 483-487. *In* A. Balows, W. J. Hausler, Jr., K. L. Herrmann, H. D. Isenberg, and H. J. Shadomy (ed.), Manual of clinical microbiology, 5th ed. American Society for Microbiology, Washington, D. C.
12. Schleifer, K. H. 1986. Gram-positive cocci, p. 999-1002. *In* P. H. A. Sneath, N. S. Mair, M. E. Sharpe, and J. G. Holt (ed.), Bergey's manual of systematic bacteriology, Vol. 2. Williams & Wilkins, Baltimore.
13. Schleifer, K. H., and R. Kilpper-Bälz. 1984. Transfer of *Streptococcus faecalis* and *Streptococcus faecium* to the genus *Enterococcus* nom. rev. as *Enterococcus faecalis* comb. nov. and *Enterococcus faecium* comb. nov. Int. J. Syst. Bacteriol. **34**:31-34.
14. Schleifer, K. H., J. Kraus, C. Dvorak, R. Kilpper-Bälz, M. D. Collins, and W. Fischer. 1985. Transfer of *Streptococcus lactis* and related streptococci to the genus *Lactococcus* gen. nov. System. Appl. Microbiol. **6**:183-195.
15. Sneath, P. H. A., N. S. Mair, M. E. Sharpe, and J. G. Holt (ed.). 1986. Bergey's manual of systematic bacteriology, Vol. 2. Williams & Wilkins, Baltimore. 1599 p.
16. Spiegel, C. A., R. Amsel, and K. K. Holmes. 1983. Diagnosis of bacterial vaginosis by direct Gram stain of vaginal fluid. J. Clin. Microbiol. **18**:170-177.
17. Staley, J. T., and N. R. Krieg. 1974. Classification of procaryotic organisms: an overview, p. 1-4. *In* N. R. Krieg, and J. G. Holt (ed.), Bergey's manual of systematic bacteriology, V. 1. Williams & Wilkins, Baltimore.

EXERCISE 1
Staphylococcus

INTRODUCTION

The genus *Staphylococcus* consists of Gram-positive cocci that are catalase-positive, facultatively anaerobic and fermentive in nature. Microscopically they are characteristically seen in grape-like clusters (*staphyle* = Gr. n. for "bunch of grapes"), though other arrangements also can be found (see Photo 1-1). There are 27 member species and 7 subspecies (13, 14) as compared to the 3 species, *S. aureus*, *S. epidermidis*, and *S. saprophyticus* recognized in 1974 (2). This trend of increase in species will be seen within several genera as you progress through this manual. It exemplifies expanded methods defining phenotypic characteristics and genetic analysis. These include colony characteristics, enzymes produced, fermentation patterns, antimicrobial sensitivity patterns, and measuring genetic relatedness, especially by DNA homology. In the classification of bacteria, 60-70% homology is arbitrarily taken to represent inclusion at the species level, assuming a reasonable fit with other characteristics (10).

Diagnostically *Staphylococcus* spp. are commonly grouped as coagulase-positive or coagulase negative. This reflects their capacity to produce clumping factor and/or free coagulase, which in turn, indicates their capacity to produce infection. Clumping factor, once thought to represent a form of coagulase, is made up of staphylococcal surface receptors that bind fibrinogen causing self-clumping (5, 20). Free coagulase is a 64,000 M_r protein excreted from the *S. aureus* cell that can initiate fibrin clot formation (6, 12). Genetic studies verify that clumping factor and free coagulase are unrelated (17). Most importantly, the significant human pathogen of the genus is *S. aureus*, the only coagulase-positive organism in humans. This organism may be isolated from the skin or mucous membranes of the nasopharynx, present as a parasite. However, it does cause infections being isolated from boils (i.e. furuncles), carbuncles, abscesses, pneumonia, bacteremia, endocarditis, food poisoning, scalded skin syndrome, toxic shock syndrome, etc. These conditions may arise from organisms that are endogenously being temporarily or chronically carried on the host (usually on the skin, nasopharynx, and less commonly in the vagina), and entering a susceptible site or agreeable habitat to cause disease. Alternately, it may be spread from carriers to susceptible individuals by aerosols, direct contact, or by other means (21). *S. aureus* is also found in lower animals, as are the other coagulase-positive species, *S. intermedius*, *S. delphini*, and *S. hyicus* (14). The remainder of species are coagulase-negative staphylococci (CNS). The most common of these in humans is *S. epidermidis*, long considered normal flora and generally non-pathogenic bacteria found especially on the skin. However, urinary tract infections, nosocomial bacteremia, catheter-related infections, prosthetic joint infections, vascular graft infections, and others associated with this organism now make it more than just a passive resident. Rather it is an opportunistic pathogen, the most frequent among the CNS. Others include *S. saprophyticus* (associated with urinary tract infections, especially among females) (1), *S. haemolyticus*, *S. schleiferi*, and *S. lugdunensis* (14).

Patient specimens suspected of harboring a pathogenic *Staphylococcus* sp., as with all samples potentially harboring pathogens, should be transported to the laboratory for culture. The basic goal is to provide a specimen at the laboratory that has not changed in its microbial flora or concentration over that present at the time the specimen was taken (3, 9). Methods of transport will depend on the type of specimen, time required between collection and specimen culture, and the types of analysis to be done on the specimen other than microbial culture. However, it may include refrigeration if the sample cannot be processed in 1-2 hours, and use of a transport medium, especially if the sample is contained on a swab. Non-nutritive buffering semi-solid agar as Stuart's, Amies, or Cary and Blair medium (Note: See Appendix 5 for product sources, and Appendix 6 for address of suppliers) are commonly used (3, 8). These prevent drying while maintaining microbial viability, yet do not allow overgrowth.

Blood specimens are usually placed directly into a bottle containing growth medium as trypticase soy broth (TSB) or TSB containing agar (biphasic culture bottle), brain heart infusion (BHI), or Columbia broth. Sodium polyanethol-sulfonate (SPS), an anticoagulant, may be added. It also inactivates components of complement, neutrophils, and certain antimicrobial compounds (15).

Other types of samples such as urine and tissue biopsies will generally be transported in the form collected without alteration, but should be refrigerated if a delay is to be encountered. Stool specimens should additionally be placed in a glycerol-0.033M phosphate buffer (equal parts) solution. With cerebrospinal fluid (CSF), it is urgent that these are processed quickly because of the rapidly fatal course of bacterial meningitis (9).

Primary isolation of *Staphylococcus* spp. is generally straight forward, but isolated colonies are critical, not only for isolation of pure cultures, but also for observing characteristic colony traits. These include colony size, color, morphology, and other features. Staphylococci are not fastidious (they will grow, for example, on nutrient agar), and being facultative, readily multiply in ambient air at 35°C. To aid in early identification, isolation media commonly used are sheep blood agar (SBA, Photo 1-2, 1-3) and mannitol salt agar (MSA, Photo 1-4). Additionally, enrichment to increase the numbers of wanted microorganisms may be done with a part of the specimen. Here, thiogly-collate broth may be used, allowing growth both aerobically near the surface and anaerobically at the bottom of the tube (14). However, note that this medium is not selective, thus unwanted contaminates may become predominant.

Finally, it must not be forgotten that Gram-stained smears are to be prepared from the original specimen and microscopically observed. The importance of this cannot be over empha-sized. With experience, microscopic examination frequently will immediately suggest the genus of organism present, perhaps providing an aid for early confirmation of a tentative diagnosis by the physician. At the very least it will inform which kinds and the relative numbers to expect from culture. Of course, other forms of microscopy as dark field and phase contrast also can be quickly done and frequently provide invaluable information.

Identifying tests for staphylococci are directed toward: (i) separation of the genus *Staphylococcus* from other Gram-positive cocci, such as *Micro-*

coccus, Streptococcus, or *Enterococcus* discussed earlier and presented in Tables 1-1 and 1-2; and (ii) separation of species within the genus *Staphylo-coccus*. Table 1-3 provides information that will differentiate between species of *Staphylococcus* isolated from humans. Many assays given in Table 1-3 will be carried out and explained in the exercise. However, some of those not included are the heat-stable nuclease and alkaline phosphatase tests. *S. aureus* and *S. schleiferi* both produce nuclease, an enzyme that can degrade both DNA and RNA, and is stable to boiling for 15 minutes. It is detectable by placing a suspension of boiled organisms in wells of a commercially available thermonuclease test agar or by other means (3, 14). Alkaline phosphatase can be detected using phosphate-containing substrates such as phe-nolphthalein diphosphate or *p*-nitrophenylphos-phate. In the former, a red color follows addition of developing reagents; in the latter a yellow color is produced from the colorless substrate due to the formation of *p*-nitrophenol (14).

Alternative Methods

Early diagnosis of disease is always important for the welfare of the patient. Obviously patient signs and symptoms have a key role in this. Laboratory diagnosis serves to provide clinicians with confirmatory data or important information that might not be available in any other way. In the recent past, more emphasis has been placed on reducing the time from initial patient contact to diagnosis by the microbiology laboratory. This has in part been possible through technological advancements and in part through miniaturization of standard assays (and their commercial avail-ability) so results can be obtained more rapidly. The following discussion concerns aspects of these, and some reasons for their use.

Commercial miniaturized assays are available for biochemical identification of staphylococci. The Staph-Ident® System and API® Staph-Trac™ (see Photo 1-5) are two examples of these. These consist of trays with cupules (10 for Staph-Ident; 20 for Staph-Trac) containing a variety of dried substrates. The suspect isolate is suspended in an appropriate liquid medium, then dispensed into the cupules, the liquid dissolving the substrate. The Staph-Ident system is incubated at 35-37°C for five hours, then the chromogenic reactions read and species determination made. From the brief incubation period, you may correctly assume

Table 1-3
Cultural Differentiation of Species of *Staphylococcus* (3, 14)

Species	Free Coagulase	Clumping Factor	Lysis on Blood agar[b]	Heat-Stable Nuclease	Nitrate Reduction	Alkaline Phosphatase	Acid Produced From				Novobiocin Resistance[c]
							D-Mannitol	D-Trehalose	Sucrose	D-Mannose	
Clinically important species:											
S. aureus	+[a]	+	+	+	+	+	+	+	+	+	−
S. epidermidis	−	−	−	−	+	+	−	−	+	(+)	−
S. haemolyticus	−	−	(+)	−	+	−	V	+	+	−	−
S. lugdunensis	−	(+)	(+)	−	+	−	−	+	+	+	−
S. saprophyticus	−	−	−	−	−[a]	−	+	+	+	−	+
Clinically important species of low incidence:											
S. capitis	−	−	(−)	−	V	−	+	−	(+)	+	−
S. cohnii	−	−	(−)	−	−	−	V	+	−	(V)	+
S. hominis	−	−	−	−	V	−	−	(+)	(+)	−	−
S. saccharolyticus	−	−	−	−	+	V	−	−	−	(+)	(+)
S. schleiferi	−	+	(+)	+	+	+	−	(+)	−	+	−
S. simulans	−	−	(−)	−	+	±	+	(+)	+	V	−
S. warneri	−	−	(−)	−	V	−	V	+	+	−	−
S. xylosus	−	−	−	−	V	V	+	+	+	+	+

[a] Symbols: + = 90 - 100% positive; ± = weak positive; − = 10% of less positive; V = 11 - 89% positive; ( ) = Delayed reaction.
[b] Bovine blood agar. Production of incomplete lysis (green or brown color) is considered negative.
[c] Novobiocin resistance with ≤16 mm diameter inhibition zone using 5μg concentration disk.

that microbial growth is not a key factor. The reactions are largely dependent on *in situ* enzymes contained in the heavy inoculating suspension (3). Conversely, Staph-Trac, while requiring a less dense inoculum, requires 24 hours of incubation. The 19 biochemical tests allow speciation of *Staphylococcus* and differentiation from *Micro-coccus*. Probable identification can be made in several ways, all using data bases established by the manufacturer. The first is by use of differential charts in which the user matches their data with that most closely corresponding to species on the chart. The second is by use of the Staph-Ident Analytical Profile Index or List, a data base derived from reference strains and clinical isolates. This allows data from the isolate to be converted to numerical values or profiles. These are then compared to those in the Profile Index to yield a probable identification. Finally, the third method is to handle the data by semi-automation using the Uniscept® dezine-er™ System. Data can be digitally entered into a computer through an automatic plate reader or by manual entry. The computer then analyzes the data, compares it with its own data bases, and renders a probable identification. The manufacturer also has avail-able semi-automated identification systems for Gram-negative and other bacteria, and yeasts, as well as for antimicrobial susceptibility tests.

Vitek Systems represents one of the automated systems available for staphylococcal (and many other microorganisms) identification and antimicrobial susceptibility testing (see Photo 1-6). Briefly, it consists of a small plastic card (in this instance, a "Gram-positive Card" would be used). Channels within the card lead from the outside to small wells inside containing different substrates. The card is filled with a suspension of the suspect organism and placed into an incubator-reader. It can then be automatically read for changes in optical density (OD) in each well, the OD being dependent on physiologically-based color changes. Preliminary results can be viewed on a video monitor, and a computer-assisted final report, which includes identification possibilities and probabilities, is generated. Testing is usually completed in 4 to 24 hours. Jorgensen (11) provides insight into advantages (such as being a highly automated system) and disadvantages (as limitation of fixed format of cards, and past weakness in accuracy in antimicrobial assays) of this system. Stager and Davis (18) also compares features and accuracy of this and many other types of automated systems including many of those useful in staphylococcal identification. These include the Aladin™ System, AutoSCAN®, and the MIDI Microbial Identification System.

In contrast to Vitek and other automated systems that depend on chromogenic changes, the MIDI Microbial Identification System (MIS) is unique in using fatty acid analysis of pure culture isolates to establish identification. This is accomplished by extraction and methylation of fatty acids from a culture, then analyzing the types and amounts of each fatty acid by high resolution gas chromatography. Data are matched to MIDI-MIS Libraries of chromatographic data, and identification probabilities established for the isolate.

A genetic probe system is also commercially available for identification of *S. aureus* from culture (Accuprobe™). While it is reported by the manufacturer to be 100% specific and sensitive compared to standard culture identification methods, further evaluation through published literature is not yet available. Experimental systems using the polymerase chain reaction (PCR) are also being investigated. For example, amplification of the *nuc* gene, which encodes for thermostable nuclease, is capable of detecting *S. aureus*. While highly sensitive and specific for organisms in saline (detects 6 colony-forming units), cerebrospinal fluid (10-20 CFU), and from swabs, its sensitivity for those in blood and urine was reduced (1000 and 100 CFU, respectively) (4). However, the potential for PCR for use in identifying these organisms directly in patient specimen where its sensitivity is acceptable makes it a candidate for a truly rapid assay. (Further information on genetic probes, PCR, and the Gen-Probe system is given in Exercise 3, **page 75.**)

MATERIALS
(See Appendices 2, 3, and 4 for staining, reagent, and media formulation, respectively):

Part 1
A. Per pair of students:
   1 culture each of *S. aureus*, *S. epidermidis*, and *S. saprophyticus*
   1 mannitol salt agar (MSA) "Y" plate (i.e. Petri dish divided into 3 parts)
   1 sheep blood agar (SBA) "Y" plate
   3 tubes D-trehalose broth
   3 tubes nitrate broth
   3 Novobiocin disks, 5 μg concentration

B. Per student:
   4 sterile swabs
   1 tube with 1 ml trypticase soy broth (TSB)
   1 MSA "X" plate (i.e. one divided into quarters)
   1 tongue depressor

Part 2
A. Per pair of students:
   Catalase reagent (3% H_2O_2)
   Nitrate test reagents
   (Note: Staining and test reagents stored in the laboratory. Temperature-stable materials will be located in the reagent cabinet; those unstable at room temperature are located in the refrigerator.)
B. Per student:
   1 tube D-trehalose
   1 Novobiocin disk, 5 μg
   ½ Mueller-Hinton agar plate
   ½ MSA plate
   1 tube nitrate broth
C. Per pair of students:
   2 β-lactamase detection disks
   1 Pasteur pipette
   1 Petri dish
   Per bench:
   1 culture of β-lactamase producing *S. aureus*
   1 dropper bottle with sterile distilled water

Part 3
Per pair of students:
   1 tube containing 0.25 ml rabbit plasma (for clumping test)
   5 Wassermann tubes (13 x 100 mm) containing 0.5 ml rabbit plasma/tube (for free coagulase test)

LABORATORY PROCEDURES
Part 1
(Refer to Figures 1-1 and 1-2 for procedural diagrams of steps given below.)
A. Each pair of students will be provided with stock cultures of *S. aureus*, *S. epidermidis*, and *S. saprophyticus*. Note the culture ages (if unmarked, you may assume that they are approximately 24-hours old), then carry out the following with each culture.
   1. Prepare a Gram's stain using the following steps.
      a. Gently heat-fix a dried smear of bacteria.

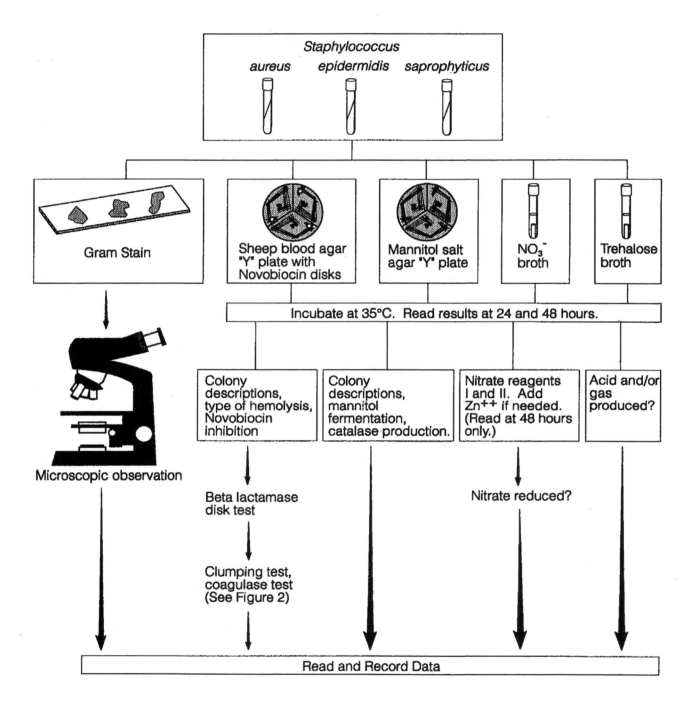

Figure 1-1: Overview of procedure for stock *Staphylococcus aureus, S. epidermidis,* and *S. saprophyticus.*

b. Flood smear with solution of crystal violet for one minute.

c. Briefly wash off crystal violet with *gentle* stream of tap water, then drain off excess.

d. Apply Gram's iodine for one minute and repeat washing procedure.

e. Decolorize with acetone. (This reagent quickly removes crystal violet, therefore use care not to overdecolorize.) Briefly wash in tap water as in Step c.

f. Counterstain with safranine for 10 seconds, then wash in tap water, blot dry, and observe. Gram-positive organisms will appear blue, Gram-negative red. Microscopically observe under the oil immersion objective. Draw and/or describe your observations.

(Note: Procedures for proper use and care of the microscope are given in Appendix 7; terminology for description of bacterial colony forms is given in Appendix 1.)

2. Transfer each species to the media listed below, attempting to obtain isolated colonies as demonstrated. (Note: In this and future exercises many types of tests and media will be used to identify microorganisms. However, they may not all be required to accomplish identification. Therefore, attempt to distinguish those media or tests that are most significant as each group of organisms is studied.)

a. One-third plate of mannitol salt agar (MSA).

b. One third plate of sheep blood agar (SBA).

Place a 5 μg novobiocin disk into the heavily streaked area of each organism of one of the above plates. To do so, use sterile forceps, dropping the disk onto the desired area, then gently pressing it into place. Resterilize the forceps after all disks are in place. (Note: Forceps may be sterilized by dipping the tips into 95% ethanol, draining off the excess, then igniting with a flame to burn off the remainder. Repeat procedure, then allow to cool before use. *Caution:* Keep flame away from flammable materials, including the stock ethanol bottle. You should never place surgical instruments,

as forceps and scissors, directly in the flame of a Bunsen burner to sterilize.)

3. Inoculate each organism into:

a. 1 tube nitrate broth.

b. 1 tube D-trehalose fermentation broth.

4. Label your tubes and plates with at least the name or code used for each species, your laboratory section and group number, and date of inoculation. *Always* place these into a container, which also should be completely labeled. Incubate at 35°C for 18-24 hours, then observe and record your findings. (Blank data sheets are given at the end of each exercise for your use.) Reincubate at 35°C for an additional 24 hours and again observe cultures. Record differences, if any, noted between the 24-hour and 48-hour readings. Generally, how long should potential pathogens be incubated before observing their cultural characteristics?

B. Each student attempt to isolate a *Staphylococcus* sp. from his or her (i) throat; (ii) nares of the nose; (iii) anterior bend of elbow; and (iv) forehead by the following procedures:

1. Moisten a sterile swab in a tube containing trypticase soy broth (TSB). Remove excess liquid from the swab by pressing and turning against the inner surface of the tube.

2. Ask your partner to swab the required parts of the body. The throat swab is done with the oral cavity well-lighted. Press on the tongue with a tongue depressor and carefully insert the swab so as not to touch the tongue or uvula that are heavily laden with indigenous flora. Rub the swab over the tonsils and pharynx, then withdraw it, again using care to avoid contact with other tissue. Nose samples can be obtained by insertion of the swab into the anterior nares. Forehead and anterior elbow samples can be swabbed by a wiping motion over a small area. Use a separate swab for each sampling.

3. Roll each swab across the surface of one quadrant of an MSA "X" plate so as to receive a heavy inoculum, after which it may be discarded. Do not streak for isolation.

4. Properly label each plate and incubate at 35°C in an inverted position in a container for 24-48 hours.

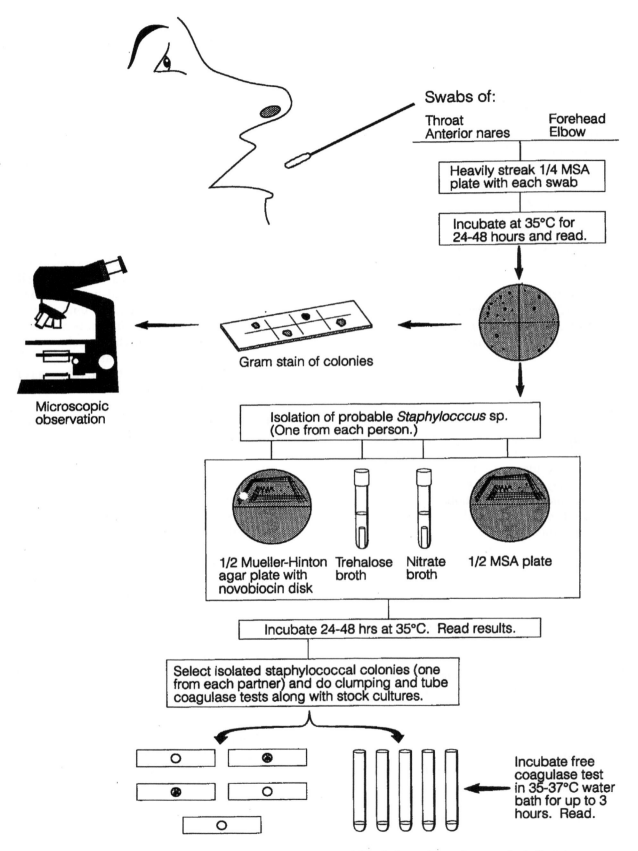

Figure 1-2: Isolation and characterization of *Staphylococcus* sp. from each student.

Part 2

A. Observe cultures from *Part I-A.*

   1. All plates with known cultures: Macroscopically observe and compare colony characteristics of *S. aureus, S. epidermidis,* and *S. saprophyticus.* Use a dissecting microscope or magnifying lens to observe the pattern of the colony margins. Describe your findings using proper terminology (e.g. convex elevation, optically translucent, entire margin, butyrous consistency, color, etc.; a description of these and other terms is found in Appendix 1). Always remember to record the culture age.

   2. Mannitol salt agar: Besides colony characteristics, observe for the presence of mannitol fermentation (is there a yellow zone around the colony?). Because the medium has a high NaCl (7.5%) content, it is selective for organisms that can withstand this environment. (What are the names of some other Gram-positive cocci that can grow at this NaCl concentration other than *Staphylococcus*?) Also, it is helpful as an identifying medium since any organism that can grow and ferment mannitol will also produce a yellow zone. (What causes the yellow color?).

   3. Sheep blood agar: Observe the type of hemolysis produced in SBA, if any. Alpha (α) hemolysis is typified by a narrow zone of partially lysed red cells around the colony. The zone may be green to brown in color. Beta (β) hemolysis is seen as a zone of complete red cell lysis characterized by transparency of the medium in that area. A lack of hemolysis when no visible red cell lysis has occurred is also a possibility. These are best characterized as non-hemolytic or ahemolytic. Although a misnomer, such colonies are frequently called gamma (γ) hemolytic.

   4. D-trehalose tubes: After 24 hours, observe for the presence of acid and gas production. Reexamine after 48 hours if negative at 24 hours. Fermentation is typified by a yellow color in phenol red broths containing sugars. This indicates a pH of 6.8 or less (acid). If a cerise color is seen, a shift to a more alkaline pH is shown. If no color change is noted, and growth is present, the sugar is not fermented, and shows the pH is unchanged at 7.3-7.4 (16). Gas evolution is seen by the collection of a bubble in the Durham tube. Generally, about 10% of the tube volume or more must be filled before it is considered positive.

   5. Nitrate test: After 48 hours incubation test each culture for nitrate reduction. Do this by placing 10 drops nitrate reagent I and 10 drops nitrate reagent II (see Appendix 3 for reagent formulae and Appendix 4 for composition of medium) into each tube. Appearance of a red color shows the presence of **nitrite**. If this color does not appear within 30 seconds, a pinch (about 20 mg) of metallic zinc is added to the tubes. This will reduce nitrate, if still present, to nitrite. Appearance of color now means the organism did not reduce nitrate; if a color still does not appear, complete reduction of nitrate occurred and neither it nor nitrite is present. An uninoculated nitrate broth tube should be included in this test to assure that reagents are giving proper results (16).

   6. Novobiocin inhibition test: The novobiocin test is an example of an antimicrobial *differentiation* assay (see Photo 1-7). This assay is to be distinguished from antimicrobial susceptibility or sensitivity tests. The latter is used to determine the effectiveness of different antimicrobial compounds against particular microorganisms, especially for therapeutic applications. Measure the diameter of the zone of non-growth (zone of inhibition) around each novobiocin disk, if any, with a millimeter ruler. The presence of a zone of $\leq$ 16 mm is considered positive for resistance to it (See Table 1-3).

   7. The catalase test: Place a drop of 3% H_2O_2 (catalase reagent) on top of colonies on mannitol salt agar. Replace petri dish lid quickly to eliminate the possibility of aerosol dissemination of the organisms due to gas bubble formation. (This test should not be used directly on blood agar plates. Why?) Alternately, a filter paper strip can be use placed in an empty petri dish, colony material rubbed on to the strip with a loop or needle, then wet the strip with 1-2 drops of catalase reagent. Quickly replace the petri dish cover. It is always useful and

appropriate to include control cultures in any assay using labile reagents, such as that used here. In this instance, since known stocks of *Staphylococcus* are being used, these act as positive controls. Any *Streptococcus* sp. can be employed as a negative control.

Are the three species of *Staphylococcus* catalase positive as exhibited by gas evolution? What reaction is taking place to cause bubble formation? (Note: Hydrogen peroxide is unstable at room temperature, therefore should be stored in the refrigerator when not in use.)

B. Staphylococcal isolates:

Observe cultures obtained from the throat, nose, bend of the elbow, and forehead. Describe the appearance of the colonies on the data sheets provided. Select one isolated colony that appears to be a typical *Staphylococcus* sp. for further examination. (Is it catalase-positive? Does it have a butyrous colony consistency? A yellow, white or grey color? Entire margin? And convex elevation? Does it ferment mannitol on MSA?) If staphylococci are found, carry out the following steps (Figure 1-2):

1. Do a Gram's stain and observe.
2. Streak for isolation onto ½ Mueller-Hinton (M-H) agar and ½ MSA plate. The other part of these plates are to be used by your partner.
3. Place a 5 μg novobiocin disk onto the heavily streaked area of the M-H plate. (Why is Mueller-Hinton rather than MSA used for this purpose?)
4. Inoculate a tube each of nitrate and trehalose broths. Incubate all cultures for 24-48 hours, then read as described in *Part 2*-A above.

C. Detection of Beta Lactamase:

Many clinically important bacteria, such as *S. aureus, Neisseria gonorrhoeae* (agent of gonorrhea), and *Haemophilus influenzae* (associated with meningitis) can be capable of producing β-lactamase (or penicillinase). By doing so, they are refractory (i. e. resistant) to the effects of penicillin G and several other beta lactam ring-containing compounds susceptible to this enzyme. This has obvious implications in treatment of infection caused by these organisms. If the enzyme is produced, one of the most powerful and eco-

nomical forms of chemotherapeutic treatment against bacterial disease agents becomes useless. Furthermore, it is important for the physician to be aware of the problem so proper chemotherapy can be given.

Several chromogenic assays can be used to detect the presence of β-lactamase. Methodology for the rapid acidometric, rapid iodometric, and rapid chromogenic cephalosporin methods, and their advantages and disadvantages may be found in Howard, et al. (7) and Stratton (19). In the acidometric- and chromogenic cephalosporin-type assays, the presence of the enzyme causes development of colored compounds due to the breakdown of penicillin G (acidometric assay) or cephalosporin (chromogenic cephalosporin assay). In the iodometric assay iodine reagent reacts with starch to produce a purple color unless products of β-lactamase action on penicillin G are present. The presence of the enzyme is therefore seen as a decrease in the usual purple of the iodine-starch mixture (7).

Here, each pair of students will do a modified chromogenic cephalosporin assay using commercially available filter-paper disks impregnated with that reagent (Cefinase™ discs). Do so by using a culture of β-lactamase producing *S. aureus* provided for this assay, along with either the *S. epidermidis* or *S. aureus* (β-lactamase negative) stock cultures used earlier on SBA or MSA plates inoculated for *Part 1*-A. Aseptically place two disks into an empty petri dish and wet each with two drops of sterile distilled water. Transfer a large inoculum with a sterile loop from each culture to separate disks and rub onto the surface. Does a red color develop in the presence of the enzyme (Photo 1-8)? When you are finished with the assay, discard the entire petri dish containing the disks into the appropriate container. Also, dispose of the culture that is β-lactamase positive.

Part 3

The Coagulase and Clumping Tests (14):

A key test for the determination of *Staphylococcus* pathogenicity is the coagulase test. As discussed earlier species that elaborate clumping factor and/or free coagulase are considered coagulase positive and generally can cause infection. Rabbit, human, or other types of blood plasma can be used.

1. Test for Clumping Factor by the Slide Test (3) (Figure 1-2):
   a. In separate drops of distilled water contained on clean slides, carefully prepare a heavy, **homogenous** suspension of known *S. aureus, S. epidermidis,* and *S. saprophyticus,* as well as the staphylococcal isolate from an area of the body of each person. Do not use MSA or other inhibitory medium as a source of the organisms. To avoid droplet contamination of the bench, place your slide on top of a paper towel wet with disinfectant before starting.
   b. Place one large drop of rabbit plasma next to each drop containing the homogenous suspension of organisms. Quickly stir each preparation of bacteria and plasma with the end of separate toothpicks.
   c. Macroscopically observe for *immediate* clumping of organisms (within 10 seconds) that shows a positive clumping test.
2. Coagulase Tube Test (3):
   a. Working in pairs, select isolated colonies of known *S. aureus, S. epidermidis,* and *S. saprophyticus* from your SBA plate, and remove with a loop. Transfer to separate 13 x 100 mm tubes containing 0.5 ml "coagulase plasma." Homogenize the organisms well on the side of the tube just above the surface of the plasma. Slant the tube to immerse the homogenized organism and rub them off the side of the tube with your loop. Repeat with isolates from yourself and your partner.
   b. Incubate all tubes in a 35-37°C *water bath.* Observe for coagulation of the plasma at the end of one and three hours as demonstrated by your instructor. Any degree of clotting is considered a positive test. Record your results. (Note: Don't forget to label properly your tubes. Don't forget to discard your tubes after incubation.)
3. Compare the results obtained with the clumping test with the tube test. Discuss the advantages and disadvantages of each method. It is generally accepted that a positive test for clumping factor by *S. aureus* also will be positive for free coagulase in the tube test. However, the reverse may not be true. A suspected *S. aureus* that gives a negative slide test should therefore be confirmed with the tube test (14).

There are several commercially-available forms of the tests for clumping factor and free coagulase. An example is Staphase® III that combines them into a single procedure. The principle and the running of the test is similar to that given above. Its advantage is that a negative clumping test can proceed directly to the gelation assay merely by lengthening incubation. Also, the clumping test appears to be more sensitive than the standard test as described above. BBL® Staphyloslide 100™ detects clumping factor only using red cells coated with fibrinogen (Photo 1-9). The presence of clumping factor-containing bacteria leads to a macroscopically visible red cell clumping within 15 seconds. Latex particles are used in the Bacto™ Staph Latex Test, the Remel Staph Latex kit, Sero Stat Staph Latex slide test, Staph Latex Slide Test, and ImmunoSCAN™ Staphlatex Latex Agglutination Test. The latex particles are coated with plasma that contains both fibrinogen and IgG. The former is bound by clumping factor, the latter *nonspecifically* binds to Protein A, also a surface component of *S. aureus.* In all these, a positive test is noted by the clumping ("agglutination") of latex particle-bacteria complexes within 60 seconds. You should note that none of these tests use specific antibody, thus none are based upon antigen-antibody reactions. They are therefore not serological tests.

Part 4

1. Read results obtained from your body isolate (*Part 2*-B). Does novobiocin inhibit growth to ≤16 mm in diameter? Can it reduce nitrate? Ferment mannitol (MSA) and trehalose?
2. Review the data you have collected from this exercise. Do the results of known *S. aureus, S. epidermidis,* or *S. saprophyticus* correspond to those given in Tables 1-1, 1-2 and 1-3? With the limited information available from your body isolate, is it likely to be *S. aureus*? Or a coagulase-negative staphylococci? What further assays should be done to identify the species if it is a CNS?

QUESTIONS

1. Outline the probable mechanism involved in the coagulation of plasma due to free coagulase. (Hint: See Reference 6.)
2. What are some of the other types of laboratory tests not given in Table 1-3 available for the identification of *Staphylococcus* spp.? For those you give, tell what species for which these are most useful?
3. The capacity to cause infection by microorganisms, including *S. aureus*, is frequently related to their capacity to produce harmful end products. Name two of those demonstrated in this exercise, and their known or hypothesized effect in humans to contribute to the disease-causing process.
4. Examination of Table 1-1 indicates that results of the modified benzidine test demonstrating the presence of a cytochrome system, at least in as far as given, and the catalase test are similar. Is there ever a situation where they would not be similar? Why?

REFERENCES

1. Archer, G. L. 1990. Staphylococcus epidermidis and other coagulase-negative staphylococci, p. 1511-1518. *In* G. L. Mandell, R. G. Douglas, Jr., and J. E. Bennett (ed.), Principles and practices of infectious diseases, 3rd. ed. Churchill Livingstone New York.
2. Baird-Parker, A. C. 1974. Genus II. *Staphylococcus* Rosenbach 1884, p. 483-489. *In* R. E. Buchanan, and N. E. Gibbons (ed.). Bergey's manual of determinative bacteriology, 8th ed. The Williams & Wilkins Co., Baltimore.
3. Baron, E. J., L. R. Peterson, and S. M. Finegold. 1994. Bailey & Scott's diagnostic microbiology, 9th ed. Mosby-Year Book, Inc., St. Louis. p. 53-64; 97-122; 321-332.
4. Brakstad, O. G., K. Aasbakk, and J. A. Maeland. 1992. Detection of *Staphylococcus aureus* by polymerase chain reaction amplification of the *nuc* gene. J. Clin. Microbiol. **30**:1654-1660.
5. Hawiger, J., S. Timmons, D. D. Strong, B. A. Cottrell, M. Riley, and R. F. Doolittle. 1982. Identification of a region of human fibrinogen interacting with staphylococcal clumping factor. Biochemistry **21**:1407-1413.
6. Hemker, H. C., B. M. Bas, and A. D. Muller. 1975. Activation of a pro-enzyme by a stoichiometric reaction with another protein. The reaction between prothrombin an staphylocoagulase. Biochim. Biophys. Acta **379**:180-188.
7. Howard, B. J., J. Klaas II, S. J. Rubin, A. S. Weissfeld, and R. C. Tilton. 1987. Clinical and pathogenic microbiology. The C. V. Mosby Co., St. Louis. p. 853-854.
8. Isenberg, H. D., F. D. Schoenknecht, and A. von Graevenitz. 1979. Cumitech 9, collection and processing of bacteriological specimens. Coordinating editor S. J. Rubin, American Society for Microbiology, Washington, D. C. 22 p.
9. Isenberg, H. D., J. A. Washington II, G. V. Doern, and D. Amsterdam. 1991. Specimen collecting and handling, p. 15-28. *In* A. Balows, W. J. Hausler, Jr., K. L. Herrmann, H. D. Isenberg, and H. J. Shadomy (ed.). Manual of clinical microbiology, 5th ed. American Society for Microbiology, Washington, D. C.
10. Johnson, J. L. 1986. Nucleic acids in bacterial classification, p. 972-975. *In* P. H. A. Sneath, N. S. Mair, M. E. Sharpe, and J. G. Holt (ed.). Bergey's manual of systematic bacteriology, Vol. 2. Williams & Wilkins, Baltimore.
11. Jorgensen, J. H. 1991. Antibacterial susceptibility tests: automated or instrument based methods, p. 1166-1172. *In* A. Balows, W. J. Hausler, Jr., K. L. Herrmann, H. D. Isenberg, and H. J. Shadomy (ed.), Manual of clinical microbiology, 5th ed. American Society for Microbiology, Washington, D. C.
12. Kawabata, S., T. Morita, S. Iwanaga, and H. Igarashi. 1985. Enzymatic properties of staphylothrombin, an active molecular complex formed between staphylocoagulase and human prothrombin. J. Biochem. **98**:1603-1614.
13. Kloos, W. E. 1990. Systematics and the natural history of staphylococci. 1. J. Appl. Bacteriol. Symp. Suppl. 25S-37S.
14. Kloos, W. E., and D. W. Lambe, Jr. 1991. *Staphylococcus*, p. 222-237. *In* A. Balows, W. J. Hausler, Jr., K. L. Herrmann, H. D. Isenberg, and H. J. Shadomy (ed.), Manual of clinical microbiology, 5th ed. American Society for Microbiology, Washington, D. C.
15. Koneman, E. W., S. D. Allen, W. M. Janda, P. C. Schreckenberger, and W. C. Winn, Jr. 1992. Color atlas and textbook of diagnostic microbiology, 4th ed. J. B. Lippincott Co., Philadelphia. p. 94-104.
16. MacFaddin, J. F. 1980. Biochemical tests for identification of medical bacteria, 2nd ed. Williams & Wilkins, Baltimore. p. 36-50; 249-260.
17. McDevitt, D., P. Vaudaux, and T. J. Foster. 1992. Genetic evidence that bound coagulase of *Staphylococcus aureus* is not clumping factor. Infect. Immun. **60**:1514-1523.
18. Stager, C. E., and J. R. Davis. 1992. Automated systems for identification of microorganisms. Clin. Microbiol. Rev. **5**:302-327.
19. Stratton, C. W., and R. C. Cooksey. 1991. Susceptibility tests: special tests, p. 1153-1165. *In* A. Balows, W. J. Hausler, Jr., K. L. Herrmann, H. D. Isenberg, and H. J. Shadomy (ed.), Manual of clinical microbiology, 5th ed. American Society for Microbiology, Washington, D. C.
20. Strong, D. D., A. P. Laudano, J. Hawiger, and R. F. Doolittle 1982. Isolation, characterization, and synthesis of peptides from human fibrinogen that block the staphylococcal clumping reaction and construction of a synthetic clumping particle Biochemistry **21**:1414-1420.
21. Waldvogel, F. A. 1990. Staphylococcus aureus (including toxic shock syndrome), p. 1489-1510. *In* G. L. Mandell, R. G. Douglas, Jr., and J. E. Bennett (ed.), Principles and practices of infectious diseases, 3rd. ed. Churchill Livingstone, New York.

Exercise 1
Data Table 1: *Staphylococcus* Known Culture Readings for Day 1

		Culture	S. aureus			S. epidermidis			S. saprophyticus		
		Age	MSA[a]	SBA	Other	MSA	SBA	Other	MSA	SBA	Other
Colony size and Colony Form[b]	mm										
	Punctiform										
	Irregular										
	Circular										
	Rhizoid										
	Filamentous										
	Other										
Colony Surface	Flat										
	Raised										
	Convex										
	Pulvinate										
	Other										
Colony Margin	Entire										
	Undulate										
	Lobate										
	Erose										
	Other										
Colony Consistency	Butyrous										
	Viscid										
	Membranous										
	Brittle										
	Other										
Colony Optical Character	Opaque										
	Translucent										
	Glistening										
	Other										
Colony Surface	Smooth										
	Rough										
	Other										
Colony Color Hemolysis											
	Type										
Other											

[a] MSA = Mannitol salt agar, SBA = Sheep blood agar. [b] See Appendix 1 for description of colony terminology.

Exercise 1
Data Table 2: *Staphylococcus* Known Culture Readings for Day 2

		Culture	S. aureus			S. epidermidis			S. saprophyticus		
		Age	MSA[a]	SBA	Other	MSA	SBA	Other	MSA	SBA	Other
Colony size and Colony Form[b]	mm										
	Punctiform										
	Irregular										
	Circular										
	Rhizoid										
	Filamentous										
	Other										
Colony Surface	Flat										
	Raised										
	Convex										
	Pulvinate										
	Other										
Colony Margin	Entire										
	Undulate										
	Lobate										
	Erose										
	Other										
Colony Consistency	Butyrous										
	Viscid										
	Membranous										
	Brittle										
	Other										
Colony Optical Character	Opaque										
	Translucent										
	Glistening										
	Other										
Colony Surface	Smooth										
	Rough										
	Other										
Colony Color Hemolysis											
	Type										
Other											

[a] MSA = Mannitol salt agar, SBA = Sheep blood agar. [b] See Appendix 1 for description of colony terminology.

Exercise 1
Data Table 3: *Staphylococcus* Isolates Readings for Day 1

		Culture	Isolate 1			Isolate 2			Isolate 3			Isolate 4		
			MSA[a]	SBA	Other	MSA	SBA	Other	MSA	SBA	Other	MSA	SBA	Other
Colony size and Colony Form[b]	mm													
	Punctiform													
	Irregular													
	Circular													
	Rhizoid													
	Filamentous													
	Other													
Colony Surface	Flat													
	Raised													
	Convex													
	Pulvinate													
	Other													
Colony Margin	Entire													
	Undulate													
	Lobate													
	Erose													
	Other													
Colony Consistency	Butyrous													
	Viscid													
	Membranous													
	Brittle													
	Other													
Colony Optical Character	Opaque													
	Translucent													
	Dull													
	Glistening													
	Other													
Colony Surface	Smooth													
	Rough													
	Other													
Colony Color Hemolysis														
	Type													
Other														

[a] MSA = Mannitol salt agar, SBA = Sheep blood agar. [b] See Appendix 1 for description of colony terminology.

Exercise 1
Data Table 4: *Staphylococcus* Isolates Readings for Day 2

		Culture	Isolate 1			Isolate 2			Isolate 3			Isolate 4		
			MSA[a]	SBA	Other	MSA	SBA	Other	MSA	SBA	Other	MSA	SBA	Other
Colony size and Colony Form[b]	mm													
	Punctiform													
	Irregular													
	Circular													
	Rhizoid													
	Filamentous													
	Other													
Colony Surface	Flat													
	Raised													
	Convex													
	Pulvinate													
	Other													
Colony Margin	Entire													
	Undulate													
	Lobate													
	Erose													
	Other													
Colony Consistency	Butyrous													
	Viscid													
	Membranous													
	Brittle													
	Other													
Colony Optical Character	Opaque													
	Translucent													
	Dull													
	Glistening													
	Other													
Colony Surface	Smooth													
	Rough													
	Other													
Colony Color Hemolysis														
	Type													
Other														

[a] MSA = Mannitol salt agar, SBA = Sheep blood agar.   [b] See Appendix 1 for description of colony terminology.

Exercise 1
Data Table 5: *Staphylococcus* Knowns and Isolate

		Culture Age	S. aureus	S. epidermidis	S. saprophyticus	Your Isolate Number: _____
Catalase test						
Gram stain	Reaction					
	Morphology					
	Arrangement					
Novobiocin 5 µg disks	Inhibition, mm					
Fermentations	Mannitol (MSA)					
	Trehalose, acid					
	gas					
Nitrate	Reduction					
Clumping Test Coagulase Test						
Other						

Other Laboratory Results and Notes

Beta lactamase Test: Appearance and Results.
    Culture ages: _____ Date: _____

β-lactamase positive *S. aureus*: Result: _____ Color: _____

Stock _____: Result: _____ Color: _____

EXERCISE 2
Streptococcus and *Enterococcus*

SECTION 1:
INTRODUCTION AND STANDARD IDENTIFICATION METHODS

Both *Streptococcus* and *Enterococcus* contain members that are frequently agents of infection. The most significant human pathogens among the former genus are *S. pyogenes, S. agalactiae,* and *S. pneumoniae* (33), while among the *Enterococcus* (formerly members of the genus *Streptococcus*), *E. faecalis* is the most frequent isolate from disease (26). Several others produce infection in humans, though they are more commonly associated with lower animals. Table 2-1 summarizes those species that have been isolated from human sources, their usual habitat, and some infections with which they are associated. However, it is important to recognize that both genera contain species that vary greatly in their potential to cause infection; indeed, many are quite innocuous as exemplified by the lactic acid streptococci (25), *Lactococcus* (or *Streptococcus*) *lactis.*

As previously noted, these Gram-positive, facultatively anaerobic cocci, found singly, in pairs, and short to long chains (see Photo 2-1) are members of the family *Streptococcaceae.* These organisms are devoid of a catalase system, and with few exceptions, have no cytochrome system (Table 1-1, page 2). Many changes in Bergey's Manual have taken place in what was previously a single genus of *Streptococcus* (16), and current usage of alternative schemes of classifying this group of organisms can lead to confusion. It is important to recognize each, and where each species belongs in the various schemes since all are in use. *Enterococcus,* for example, was recently formed from what were species of *Streptococcus* because of nucleic acid homology differences (36), as well as unique phenotypic characteristics (5, 14). It now encompasses 12 species, most of which have been isolated from human disease (14). Also, the lactic acid bacteria group has recently been placed into its own genus, the *Lactococcus* (37).

Further categorization is quite complicated because of the wide variation, distribution, and effects of these organisms. Sherman (38) in 1937, for example, separated the genus *Streptococcus*

according to physiological and growth characteristics, especially concerning temperature limitations on growth. The four general groups are (i) pyogenic, (ii) viridans, (iii) enterococcus, and (iv) lactics. Pyogenic bacteria are those that induce pus formation. The enterococcus and lactics, as the names suggest, would now be more appropriately grouped as *Enterococcus* and *Lactococcus,* respectively. Viridans, a term derived from *viridis* (L) meaning green, includes streptococci that produce α-hemolysis, which is frequently green-colored, and cannot be placed in other groups. This category has become of reduced significance as relationships between groups have been shown to overlap, but the characters for species separation remain important (39).

The *Streptococcus* also may be designated according to the type of hemolysis they produce. Thus, α-hemolytic (Photo 2-2), β-hemolytic (Photo 2-3), or ahemolytic (or γ-hemolytic) streptococci are commonly used designations (see Ex. 1, *Part 2* A-3, page 11 or description of these) (8).

Also, Lancefield (23) developed a serological classification based on the presence of C substance, an extractible carbohydrate found in the cell wall. Now, there are at least 20 groups (8), each of which is separable from the others by antibody directed against it. (A further discussion of antigen-antibody reactions can be found in Section 4, page 42.) Each is given a capital letter. A, B, C, D, and G, for example, are most commonly isolated from humans. One serologic group may or may not correspond to more than one species (e.g. Group A corresponds to *S. pyogenes,* but Group D includes *E. faecalis, E. faecium, E. avium, S. bovis, S. equinus,* and others (14)). Thus, based on the forgoing information, *E. faecalis* could be categorized by its formal name, as an α-hemolytic or ahemolytic enterococci (depending on its reaction), or as a Group D streptococci. These relationships are further delineated in Table 2-2.

Several characteristics of *Streptococcus* spp. and *Enterococcus* spp. important in humans are also seen in Table 2-2. Some general observations are useful. For example, hemolysis may not be a

Table 2-1
Habitat and Some Infections Caused By Selected Members of the
***Streptococcus* and *Enterococcus* (5, 14, 26, 33)**

Species	Usual Habitat In Humans	Infections and/or Non-suppurative Sequelae
S. pyogenes	Throat, respiratory tract	Pharyngitis, wounds, scarlet fever, impetigo, rheumatic fever, acute glomerulonephritis, and others.
S. agalactiae	Genital, urinary tract	Infant sepsis and meningitis
E. faecalis	Oral cavity, intestinal tract	Endocarditis, urinary tract, wounds, abscesses
E. faecium	Intestinal tract	Endocarditis
S. bovis	Intestinal tract	Endocarditis
S. salivarius	Oral cavity, intestinal tract	Endocarditis
S. pneumoniae	Respiratory tract	Pneumonia, meningitis, otitis media, septicemia, and others.
S. mutans	Oral cavity	Dental caries, endocarditis

uniform characteristic within a single species, although *S. pyogenes* is dependably beta hemolytic when properly assayed, and *S. pneumoniae* is consistently alpha hemolytic on sheep blood agar.

Of the assays shown, important characteristics in identification for *S. pyogenes* include that it is the only member of Group A, it is β-hemolytic, inhibited by bacitracin (Photo 2-4), positive in the PYR test, but generally non-reactive in other tests. *S. agalactiae*, conversely, can hydrolyze sodium hippurate to benzoic acid and glycine (24), and yields a positive CAMP reaction (discussed further in a *Part 3*A-10, page 34). It is also the only Group B member among the streptococci. *S. pneumoniae*, besides being α-hemolytic, is unique by being lysed by bile (Photo 2-6) and inhibited by 1:400 optochin (ethylhydrocupreine HCl)-impregnated differentiation disks (Photo 2-5). Finally, Group D, even in this Table of selected organisms, can be seen to include *Enterococcus* and non-enterococcal species. These can readily be distinguished because they all (including 10 species not shown in Table 2-2) are positive in the PYR test (see page 34 or more information on this assay), grow in the presence of 40% bile and in 6.5% NaCl broth, and hydrolyze

esculin to esculetin in the bile esculin test (24). This exercise will show these and other relationships concerning some of these bacteria.

Also included as integral parts of this exercise are an introduction to the use of computers in laboratory identification of microorganisms, quantitative disk method of antimicrobial sensitivity testing, and a discussion of antigen-antibody reactions and their applications to rapid assays. These will be covered in separate sections below.

MATERIALS
(Reminder: Appendices 2, 3, and 4 contain stain, reagent, and media formulation, and 5 gives suppliers of many reagents and media):

Section 1 - *Part 1*
A. Per pair of students:
    One culture of: *Streptococcus pyogenes, S. agalactiae, S. pneumoniae,* and *E. faecalis*
    3 Sheep blood agar "X" plates
    3 Sheep blood agar standard plates
    4 Bacitracin disks
    4 Optochin disks
    4 Tubes each of:
    Mannitol fermentation broth

Table 2-2
Characteristics of Some *Streptococcus* and *Enterococcus* Species Isolated From Humans (4, 13, 21, 39)

Characteristic	Description for:								
	S. pyogenes	*S. agalactiae*	*S. pneumoniae*	*E. faecalis*	*E. faecium*	*S. bovis*	*S. salivarius*	*S. mitis*	*S. mutans*
Grouping based on physiol. & growth	Pyogenic	Pyogenic	Pyogenic	Enterococcus	Enterococcus	Viridans	Viridans	Viridans	Viridans
Antigenic group	A	B	None	D	D	D	K	None	E
Hemolytic type	β	β,α,Ahemol.	α	α, Ahemol	α	α, Ahemol	Ahemol.	α	α, ahemol.
Growth at 10°C	–	V	–[a]	+	+	–	–	–	–
Growth at 45°C	–	–	–	+	+	V[a]	V	V	V
Growth in:									
0.1% m. blue milk (13)	–	–	–	+	+	–	–	–	–
6.5% NaCl broth	–	+	–	+	+	–	–	–	–
Bile esculin	–	–	–	+	+	+	–	–	–
Hippurate hydrolysis	–	+	–	V	V	–	–	–	–
CAMP reaction	–	+	–	–	–	–	–	–	–
Acid produced in:									
Arabinose	–	–	(+)[a]	–	+	–	–	–	–
Inulin	–	–	+	–	–	+	V	–	+
Mannitol	–	–	–	+	+	+	–	–	+
Raffinose	–	–	+	–	–	+	+	–	+
Sorbitol	–	–	–	+	–	–	–	–	+
Bile solubility & Optochin inhibition	–	–	+	–	–	–	–	–	–
Bacitracin inhibit.[b]	+	–	–	–	–	–	–	–	–
PYR hydrolysis[c]	+	–	–	+	+	–	–	–	–

[a] + = ≥90% positive; – = ≥90% negative; V = 11 - 89% positive; (+) = slow.
[b] Disk concentration of 2 units/ml
[c] L-pyrrolidonyl-β-naphthylamide hydrolysis by β-pyroglutamyl aminopeptidase.

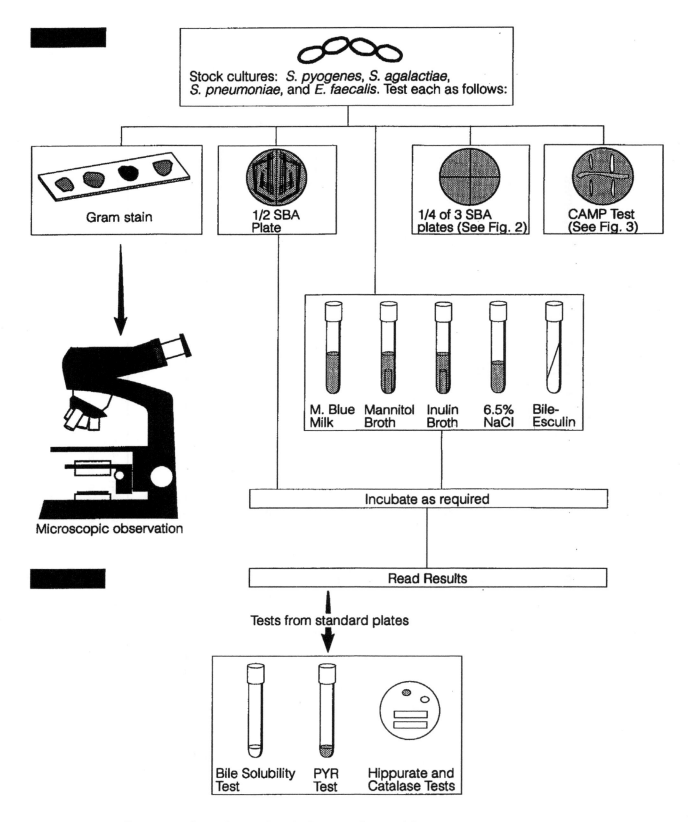

Figure 2-1: General procedure for known cultures of *Streptococcus* and *Enterococcus*.

Methylene blue milk
Inulin fermentation broth
6.5% NaCl broth
Bile esculin agar with 5% horse serum (HoS)

Per laboratory section:
2 cultures of β-lysin producing *Staphylococcus aureus*

Part 2
A. Per student:
1 tube containing 1 ml trypticase soy broth
1 tube with 15 ml melted blood agar base
1 tube with 1 ml sterile defibrinated sheep blood
1 sterile petri dish
1 sterile swab
1 tongue blade

Part 3
A. Per pair of students:
2-13 x 125 mm tubes containing 1.5 ml sterile physiological saline solution (PSS, 0.15 M NaCl)
2-12 X 75 mm tubes each of:
Sterile PSS, 0.5 ml/tube
Sterile 2% bile (Sodium deoxycholate) solution, 0.5 ml/tube
Sterile distilled water, 0.1 ml/disposable 12 x 75 mm tube
2 Hippurate test disks
3 PYR test swabs
2 Sterile swabs
5 12 X 75 mm disposable tubes

Per laboratory section:
3 Dropper bottles catalase reagent (3% H_2O_2 solution) stored in refrigerator
2 Dropper bottles ninhydrin reagent (store in refrigerator)
2 Dropper bottles PYR developing reagent (dimethylamino-cinnamaldehyde) stored in refrigerator.
2 Dropper bottles with sterile distilled water
2 sets McFarland Standards, No. 0.5 and 1.0, 1.5 ml each in 13 X 125 mm tubes
B. Per student:
2 Sheep blood agar plates
2 Bacitracin and optochin disks

Per bench:
1 Sheep blood agar plate
1 Culture β-lysin producing *S. aureus*
1 dropper bottle with oxidase reagent (store in refrigerator)

Part 4
Per bench:
1 bottle H_2O_2 (refrigerator)
1 bottle 10% bile solution
1 Culture of following on SBA (bile solubility control cultures):
S. pneumoniae
E. faecalis

Section 3 - *Part 1*
Per pair of students:
1 Sheep blood agar plate
1 Trypticase soy broth tube (4 ml)
1 Trypticase soy broth tube (5 ml)
1 Mueller-Hinton agar plate with 5% serum
2 Sterile cotton swabs (packaged separately)
1 Sterile Pasteur pipette
Antimicrobic disks
1 Pair forceps
95% Ethanol

Per laboratory section:
2 Mice previously inoculated with *S. pneumoniae*
3 0.5 McFarland barium sulfate turbidity standard
Vortex mixers

Section 1:
Standard Identification Methods

LABORATORY PROCEDURES

Part 1
(Reminder: Many organisms used here are *pathogens*. **BE CAREFUL. PLAN YOUR WORK BEFORE YOU START.**)
A. Each pair of students will be provided with stock cultures of *Streptococcus pyogenes, S. agalactiae, S. pneumoniae,* and *E. faecalis.* With each of these carry out the following steps (see Figure 2-1 for outline of this procedure):
1. To test for growth and hemolytic characteristics, streak for isolation on one-half sheep blood agar (SBA) plate.
2. Stab the agar plates at approximately a 45° angle with each organism using a needle or loop. Puncture the agar 2-3 times in an unused portion of the streaked plate with a single inoculum. This will allow for subsurface growth with reduced amounts of oxygen. Since one of the hemolysins, Streptolysin O, produced by *S. pyogenes* is

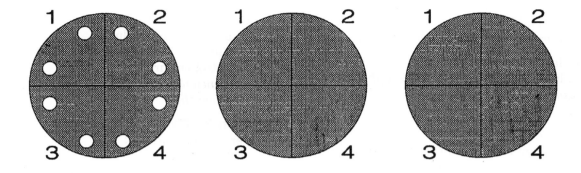

Figure 2-2: Arrangement of SBA "X" plates in *Part 1* A-3. Each plate is to contain one species in each quadrant. The left plate then has an optochin and a bacitracin disk located in each quadrant. This plate and one other are incubated at 35°C, the third plate at 45°C.

inactivated by oxygen, such growth gives better conditions for hemolysis by this organism (5, 14).

3. Inoculate each of the 4 species to:

a. Three sheep blood agar "X" plates to find the effects of growth temperature, and of optochin and bacitracin. Use a large inoculum of each species to obtain heavy growth of it over the surface of one quadrant of *each* of the 3 plates. Streaking in more than one direction will facilitate this. Each plate should contain all 4 species when completed.

Using one of the three "X" plates, aseptically place a bacitracin differentiation disk in one area of each quadrant. After this, aseptically place an optochin disk in each of the same quadrants, but in a location as far removed from the bacitracin disk as possible. Gently press each disk to make good contact with the agar. This and the other two plates will be incubated as described below. Figure 2-2 displays this set-up. (Note: Use sterile forceps as described in Ex. 1, *Part 1*A-2b, page 9).

b. 1 tube methylene blue milk to determine whether organisms can reduce methylene blue and clot milk.

c. 1 tube mannitol fermentation broth, and

d. 1 tube inulin fermentation broth to detect acid and gas production.

e. 1 tube 6.5% NaCl broth to assay for the capacity of the organisms to grow at this salt concentration.

f. 1 tube bile esculin agar with 5% HoS to find whether the organisms can grow in the presence of bile and, if so, also hydrolyze esculin.

4. Do the CAMP assay (10) as follows: Make a single heavy streak of β-lysin producing *Staphylococcus aureus* across the center of a blood agar plate. Next, streak each of the four streptococcal species in a single line perpendicular and up to the *S. aureus* streak, but not through it (Figure 2-3).

5. Incubate all cultures for 48 hours as follows:

a. All blood agar plates except the CAMP test plate at 35°C in a candle jar. This is a closed jar that has a lighted candle allowed to burn to extinction to increase atmospheric CO_2 concentration to about 3% (5). It *does not* produce anaerobic conditions. Incubate the CAMP test plate at this same temperature, but under normal atmospheric conditions outside the candle jar.

b. All tubes at 35°C under ambient atmospheric conditions.

c. Two "X" plates, including that containing bacitracin and optochin disks, at 35°C.

d. One "X" plate at 45°C. Do not use the plate containing disks for this.

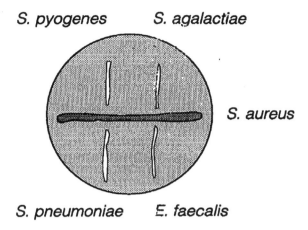

Figure 2-3: The CAMP test showing the arrangement of test organisms around *S. aureus.*

6. Prepare a Gram stain of each organism. Observe for differences in morphology, length of chains, etc. Also, compare these observations with those previously made on the staphylococci in Exercise 1. Results may be recorded on the forms provided at the end of this exercise.

Part 2

Many species of *Streptococcus* and *E. faecalis* are common representatives of the normal flora of the naso- and oropharyngeal cavity, and other areas of the host (see Table 2-1). Therefore, pathogenic streptococci must be isolated from among these. *Streptococcus pyogenes* isolation is aided by using blood agar pour plates to allow subsurface growth, giving improved conditions for this organism to give its typical β-hemolysis. *S. pneumoniae* does not require this condition to produce its characteristic α-hemolysis; indeed, it is an advantage to observe it on the surface so that colony morphology can be seen.

The following procedure is designed to bring out several facets. These include observations on the normal aerobic and facultatively anaerobic flora of the oropharyngeal cavity, and application of procedures for isolation and identification of *Streptococcus*. To accomplish this, each student is to attempt to isolate two species of *Streptococcus*, preferably *S. pyogenes* and *S. pneumoniae*, by the procedure given below and in Figure 2-4.

1. Moisten a sterile swab in a tube containing 1 ml of trypticase soy broth (TSB). Remove excess fluid from the swab by pressing against the wall of the tube while rotating it.

2. Ask your partner to swab your throat as previously described (Ex. 1, *Part 1*B, page 9).

3. Return the swab to the TSB tube and incubate for two hours in a 35-37°C water bath.

4. After incubation of the throat swab culture, place a sterile loop into the broth, drain it against the side of the tube, then inoculate this into a tube of melted blood agar base being held at 45-50°C. Warm the pre-measured sheep blood to an equal temperature (but be careful not to leave in the water bath for more than 5 minutes), and aseptically pour into the agar tube containing your inoculum.

5. Mix the contents by rolling the tube of SBA between your hands, then aseptically pour the tube contents into a sterile petri dish. Allow to solidify.

6. Inoculate the surface of the SBA plate by removing the throat swab from the broth, draining its excess liquid, then rubbing over a small portion of the agar surface. Streak for isolation with a loop.

7. Now use the swab to prepare a Gram-stained smear. Following this, the swab may be discarded. Microscopically examine the smear and describe as to kinds and relative numbers

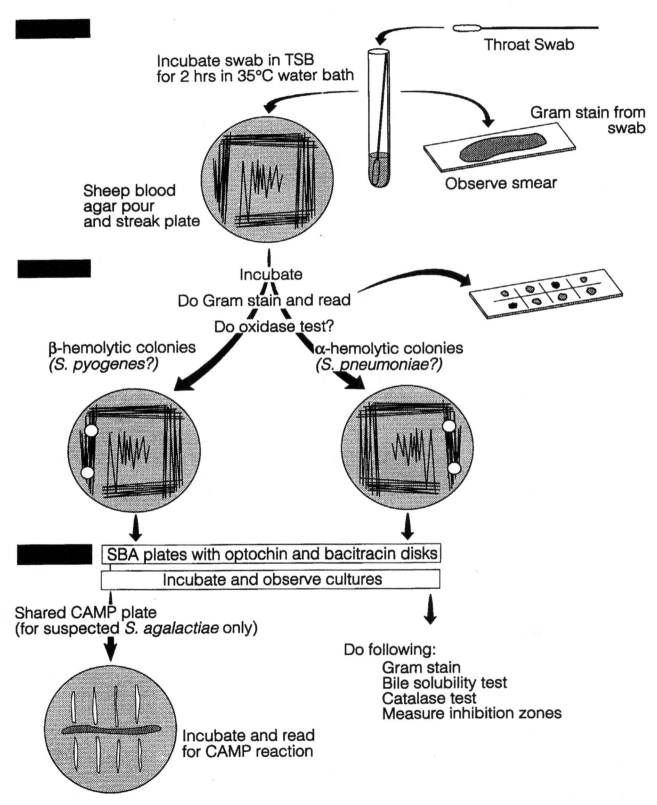

Throat Swab

Incubate swab in TSB
for 2 hrs in 35°C water bath

Gram stain from
swab

Sheep blood
agar pour
and streak plate

Observe smear

Incubate
Do Gram stain and read
Do oxidase test?

β-hemolytic colonies
(S. pyogenes?)

α-hemolytic colonies
(S. pneumoniae?)

SBA plates with optochin and bacitracin disks

Incubate and observe cultures

Shared CAMP plate
(for suspected *S. agalactiae* only)

Do following:
  Gram stain
  Bile solubility test
  Catalase test
  Measure inhibition zones

Incubate and read
for CAMP reaction

Figure 2-4: Steps for isolation of streptococci from throat swab.

of organisms. For example, there may be "rare" (i.e. <1/oil immersion field), "few" (2-5/oil immersion field), "moderate" (6-20/oil immersion field), or "many" (>20/oil immersion field) Gram-negative cocci, Gram-positive bacilli, yeasts, and other forms. Closely observe this to obtain early information on kinds of organisms in your throat, many of which should grow out on your sheep blood agar plate (but, not necessarily all types. Why?).

8. Incubate your SBA plate for up to 48 hours at 35°C in a candle jar (although it should be noted that anaerobic or CO_2-free atmospheres are preferred for isolation of *S. pyogenes* alone (19)). Examine at 18-24 hours if time permits. Following this, storage at 4°C is permissible, however the plate should first be observed, especially for types of hemolysis (circle several typical alpha and beta hemolytic types with a marking pen), before doing so. Such storage can lead to changes in the appearance of lysis.

Part 3

A. Observe cultures of known organisms as follows:

1. Blood agar plates: Observe for the presence of α- or β-hemolysis (Photo 2-2, 2-3), colony morphology, size, and other characteristics of the 4 streptococcal species employed. Also, note differences in surface and sub-surface hemolytic patterns. It is known that the kind of blood used in the medium can influence the type of reaction obtained. Sheep blood in a sugar-free medium appears to give most characteristic hemolysis with Group A streptococci. Furthermore, this medium is less likely to allow the growth of *Haemophilus haemolyticus*, which in human blood agar, for example, may culturally appear similar to, and give hemolytic reactions that can be confused with Group A streptococci.

2. Sheep blood agar "X" plates:
   a. Compare growth for cultures incubated at 35°C and 45°C.
   b. Using any of the plates that contain growth, test each species for catalase production using the filter paper strip technique (Ex. 1, *Part* 2A-7, page 11). Observe for gas evolution. (Use proper precautions.)

   c. Compare (by measurement) the inhibition of growth due to bacitracin and optochin (Photo 2-4, 2-5). Any inhibition by bacitracin is considered positive; the inhibition zone size due to optochin depends on the diameter of the disk. If the disk is 10 mm in diameter, an inhibition zone of 16 mm or more is considered positive; if it is 6 mm, a zone size of 14 mm or more is positive.

3. The bile solubility test (14): Remove several colonies of *S. pneumoniae* with a sterile swab from the surface of the standard blood agar plate incubated at 35°C. Use care not to remove bits of agar or red cells. Suspend the bacteria in 0.5 ml sterile physiological saline solution (PSS) by rubbing the swab against the side of tube under the surface of the liquid. The final turbidity should be between a No. 0.5 to 1 McFarland turbidity standard. (McFarland barium sulfate standards are prepared as described in Appendix 3. *Shake well* before using.) Deliver 0.5 ml of this suspension to two 12 X 75 mm tubes, one containing 0.5 ml PSS and the other with 0.5 ml bile solution. For controls, prepare similar suspensions of *E. faecalis* in PSS and 2% bile solution. Place all tubes in the 35-37°C water bath for up to two hours. Observe for turbidity. Does the culture turbidity disappear (Photo 2-6)? This is mainly a characteristic of pneumococci, though some are refractory (5). However, a positive test here is more indicative of *S. pneumoniae* than is inhibition by the optochin disk test. Therefore, if the latter shows a marginal degree of inhibition (i.e. 10-16 mm for a 10 mm disk; 6-14 mm for a 6 mm disk), the suspected organism should be retested by the bile solubility assay (14).

   A procedural variation of the bile solubility test is to carry it out directly on colonies growing on the surface of plates. This method is described in *Part 4*A-2 (page 35)

4. Milk cultures: Observe for growth and reactions in methylene blue milk (i.e. methylene blue reduction and clot formation). If no change is apparent (i.e. negative methylene blue reduction), microscopically examine a loopful of material

from the culture to assure that growth is present. To do this, it is usually helpful, after fixing the smear, to flood the slide with xylene to remove fats and lipids. After draining the xylene from the slide, allow the residual to evaporate, then stain as usual. (Note: Xylene should be used within a fume hood. Used liquid can be accumulated in a capped bottle for later disposal. Do not pour it into the sink.)

5. Sodium hippurate hydrolysis test: Emulsify 1-3 colonies of *S. pyogenes* and *S. agalactiae* in 0.1 ml sterile distilled water contained in 12 X 75 mm disposable test tubes. Aseptically place a hippurate disk into each tube. (Note: Disks described here obtained from Remel, Lenexa, KA; other commercial sources are given in Appendix 5. Always follow manufacturer's instructions for proper use.) Incubate in a 35-37°C water bath for 2 hours. Add two drops ninhydrin reagent, then reincubate for up to 30 minutes. Read. A blue to purple color appears in a positive test, a characteristic of Group B streptococci (Table 2-2); colorless to light grey shows a negative test. (What is the reaction taking place to allow the appearance of the purple color with ninhydrin?)

6. The PYR (pyroglutamyl aminopeptidase) test: Now, add one drop of sterile distilled water to a 12 X 75 mm disposable tube. Select three fully-grown colonies from the *S. pyogenes* culture growing on the standard SBA plate with the tip of the swab containing PYR, L-pyrrolidonyl-β-naphthylamide (Note: This chemical is a carcinogen, therefore do not allow it to make contact with your tissue.) (Swabs and reagents available from DPC, Los Angeles, CA). Place the swab into the tube. After incubating 10 minutes at room temperature, add 2 drops of PYR-developing reagent (dimethylaminocinnamaldehyde). Wait no longer than one minute and read. A positive test is indicated by the appearance of a red to pink color; a negative by a light yellow-green to colorless solution. Repeat these steps with *S. agalactiae* and *E. faecalis*. Record your results.

Both *E. faecalis* and *S. pyogenes* produce L-pyroglutamyl aminopeptidase (Table 2-2), and therefore cannot be dis-

tinguished based on the PYR test alone. However, use of it and other character differences easily separate them. (Name six characteristics where these species differ.)

7. Sugar fermentation tubes: Presence of acid and gas?

8. 6.5% NaCl broth: Presence of growth? Of color change? Either or both of these indicates a positive test.

9. Bile esculin agar: Presence of growth? Presence of a blackened medium? (What causes the black color?)

10. Observe the CAMP assay. As noted in Table 2-2, this test should be positive for *S. agalactiae*. It is seen as enhanced hemolysis due to "CAMP factor," usually in an "arrowhead" or "crescent-shaped" pattern at the junction of the streak of this organism with that of *S. aureus*. Some *S. pyogenes* also produce a positive test if incubated in a candle jar or anaerobically (14).

This test also can be done using commercially-available beta-lysin disks (Photo 2-7). These contain staphylococcal β-lysin that, when placed on the surface of a blood agar plate, diffuses into the medium. The presence of CAMP factor-producing bacteria leads to the typical crescent-shaped zone of enhanced hemolysis where it and β-lysin overlap.

11. Tabulate your results. Bring out distinguishing characteristics of each species. Are they comparable to *generally* obtained characteristics given in Table 2-2? You should be aware of which tests are most significant for identification of each species. Those used here are not always employed for all cases involving the Gram-positive streptococci; however, the proper combination will separate and identify Groups A, B, D, and *S. pneumoniae*. It also should be noted that *S. pneumoniae* is the only organism in this group that requires 5% CO_2 on primary isolation, and has the greatest nutritional need for complex media.

B. Throat isolates: Each student attempt to isolate *S. pneumoniae* and a β-hemolytic streptococci from their throat isolation plate by the following procedure (Figure 2-4):

1. Select several typical α- and β-hemolytic streptococcal colonies. *S. pyogenes*, if present, are best seen as subsurface colonies, while the α-hemolytic organisms, though at surface or subsurface locations, are best seen on the surface. *S. pneumoniae* form α-hemolytic, usually small, flattened (i. e. effuse to raised), transparent surface colonies with a moist surface. Mark the bottom of the plate as to the location of each colony you select to investigate. Make colony descriptions, then prepare a smear from each (several small smears can be made on a single slide). Gram stain and observe. When you have located a suspected *S. pneumoniae*, restreak it for isolation on a plate of sheep blood agar. Place an optochin disk and a bacitracin disk on the *heavily* inoculated portion of the plate. Incubate appropriately. Streak and stab your β-hemolytic streptococcal isolate on a second plate of SBA and apply optochin and bacitracin disks. Furthermore, carry out a CAMP test with this isolate on another SBA, sharing this plate with others at your bench. Be sure to include an *S. pyogenes* and an *S. agalactiae* control culture streak. Do not incubate this plate in a candle jar.

2. Note the wide variety of colonies present on the throat isolation plate. The normal throat may be the habitat for many bacterial species, including Gram-negative cocci as *Neisseria*, *Branhamella*, especially *B. catarrhalis*; Gram-negative rods of the genus *Haemophilus* and occasionally the coliforms; and Gram-positive diphtheroid bacilli. By microscopic examination, do these types of organisms appear on your plate?

   After you have completed the examination of your plate, and if you have microscopically observed colonies that contained Gram-negative cocci, test these with oxidase reagent (see Ex. 3, *Part 1* A-5, page 68). If the colony turns pink within 10 seconds, then to a dark purple within three minutes, this is a positive test, and these probably represent members of the *Neisseria* or *Moraxella*. These organisms are more thoroughly discussed in Exercise 3.

Part 4

A. *S. pneumoniae* (or other α-hemolytic) throat isolate:
   1. Examine SBA cultures inoculated with your throat isolate. Gram stain and observe the organism from an isolated colony.
   2. Measure the zone of optochin and bacitracin inhibition, and carry out the bile solubility test on an isolated colony directly on the plate. Do so by placing 1-2 drops of 2% bile solution on a colony. Allow the solution to remain on the colony for at least 5 minutes, then drain excess solution to the side of the plate. Observe for the presence of the colony by reflected light. Remember also to carry out this test with appropriate control cultures. Also do a catalase test by the filter paper method. Record your data.
   3. Is your isolate possibly *S. pneumoniae*? If you wished to identify it as such, what are the next steps you should carry out?

B. Beta-hemolytic throat isolate:
   1. Gram stain and record microscopic and colony characteristics. Have you obtained a pure culture? Is it inhibited by bacitracin or optochin?
   2. Do a catalase test. Be sure to use appropriate precautions. Is your isolate catalase positive?
   3. Read the results of the CAMP test given by your isolate and by the control cultures.
   4. What can you conclude concerning the species name of your isolate?

Part 5

Demonstrations

A. Serological identification of Group A streptococci by the precipitin reaction: The genus *Streptococcus* has been categorized into several antigenic groups (designated by capital alphabetical letters) based upon the presence of a "C substance" in its cell wall. Each group differs in antigenic specificity, thus enabling serological methods to be used in identification. Since "C substance" appears to be a subsurface antigen, cultures are subjected to treatment to release the antigen. Several procedures are available; however, that of Lancefield (23) will be demonstrated here. This involves extracting C antigen from

Tube No.	1	2	3	4	5
Streptococcal Group Antigen or Control	A	B	C	D	Saline
Streptococcal Group Antiserum	A	A	A	A	A

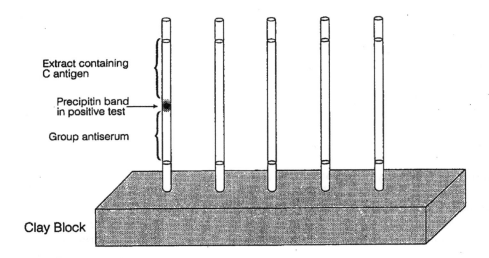

Extract containing C antigen

Precipitin band in positive test

Group antiserum

Clay Block

Figure 2-5: Capillary tube precipitin test for group identification of *Streptococcus* spp.

the organism by suspending in N/5 HCl, then placing in a boiling water bath for 10 minutes. After clarifying and neutralizing the solution, the antigen is ready for use.

The extract is tested with a battery of commercially available known antisera against the group antigens. Each antiserum is drawn into a capillary tube, carefully followed by the antigen extract. These are then incubated at room temperature until a finely-divided precipitate appears, or up to a maximum of 30 minutes. Figure 2-5 shows the appearance of such a test in which Group A, B, C, and D antigens, and a saline control are being assayed against streptococcal Group A antiserum.

Examine the demonstration of *Streptococcus* grouping. Record your results and discuss.

Several alternative rapid methods for serologic grouping of the *Streptococcus* are available and will be discussed below along with the basis for serologic reactions (Section 4, page 42).

B. The Quellung reaction (14):

There are many serotypes of *S. pneumoniae* distinguishable by the presence of a specific antigen located in the capsule (Photo 2-8). This should not be confused with the "C substance" of other streptococci since the latter is not a surface antigen.

The type of antigen contained in a particular *S. pneumoniae* can be determined by several methods of which the Quellung (means "swelling" in German) reaction is one. The phenomenon is characterized by a swollen-like appearance of the capsule in the presence of specific antibody. For example, if Type III pneumococcus is placed in the presence of anti-type III serum, a capsular "swelling" will be noted. If antibody for any other type is employed, this characteristic is not seen. Typing is particularly important in the study of the epidemiology of a particular species of bacterium. In the case of the Quellung reaction, it also shows another consequence of an antigen-antibody reaction.

SECTION 2: APPLICATION OF COMPUTERS IN MICROBIAL IDENTIFICATION

The use of the computer as an aid for identification will be introduced in this exercise. Not designed, nor intended to provide an in-depth expertise in this topic, it will hopefully give an appreciation of some strengths and weaknesses of this technology for use in microbial identification. As has been mentioned in the discussion on antimicrobial sensitivity testing of microorganisms, computers may be either an optional or integral part of these. In many of those cases, data is fed directly from an automated reader to the computer, which analyzes the data, then provides the probable identification. Probability numbers are given as to the likelihood of the identification by matching the input data with computer-resident database. The latter is derived by obtaining results using the particular test method on known species and/or strains. It is important to note that the reference database used must (i) contain the taxon of the organism to be identified, and (ii) it must have been generated using the same procedures employed to gain data for the unknown organisms to be identified. This is because, for example, variations in results can be obtained by changing container size (e.g. test tube vs. well of a 96-well plate), incubation periods, or other environmental parameters (12). Therefore, data tables in most standard microbiology references (including this manual) are not entirely appropriate for identification patterns unless the standard tube assay is used.

Basically computer identification methods are a form of numerical taxonomy, the organization of organisms into groups through statistical analysis. The principles of Adansonian taxonomy are generally applied. Such principles include the (i) equal weight of test data (i.e. no emphasis is placed on any single character); (ii) a maximum number of tests is studied for all strains (the larger the number, the more accurate the identification); and (iii) phenetic (i. e. observed character, not ancestry) analyses define similarities that establish the taxa (31). Furthermore, (iv) Bayes probability model of an identification based on previously established likelihood is used (7, 20). That is, characteristics of an unknown are compared to others in the data base to establish a statistical likelihood of an organism's deduced taxon.

Obviously the emphasis in each of the above is on data. The choices of equal emphasis for the data collected, that it is only to have a phenetic basis, and the concepts of prior likelihood are all established working constants. However, the number of tests is not. There is no hard and fast rule for the latter, although it may range from one characteristic to over 300 (7). Statistical logic is that a large sample of properties will yield a greater likelihood of showing the true character of each strain, therefore one should be able to more confidently separate, group, and/or identify them. However, there are limitations in that not all types of data can be obtained for all strains (as, for example, inability to grow all strains under the same conditions; and variations in the antimicrobial sensitivity results of a single strain due to lack or presence of resistance plasmids). Also, available assays may over or under emphasize certain properties (as the same catabolic pathway yielding separate products that are detected by different assays). In any case, the practical range has been suggested to be between 50 and 200 characters (31).

Once the data are available it must be entered into the computer. This can be done manually through a keyboard, or by optical or mechanical readers. Automated data acquisition where values can be accumulated directly by the computer is less subject to error and is faster. Many analytical instruments, like light and fluorescent detecting photometers, chromatographs, and other instruments can be interfaced with a computer to accommodate direct data acquisition. However, for that data to be handled properly appropriate software programs are required for the computer (hardware) to receive, process, and then present the information in a desired form (7). Such presentations may be nothing more than the data itself, or could include data analysis, statistical comparisons, and identification of the microorganism and/or its antimicrobial sensitivity. This data also may be incorporated into a larger report for maintaining a record, for example, of tests requested by a particular physician for his or her patient, the results of those tests, and other pertinent information that might relate to that patient. Furthermore, data may be retrieved for other analytical purposes such as epidemiological studies (9).

There is no doubt that the use of computers will increase in medical microbiology. Their advantages, when properly interfaced, programmed, and used make them invaluable. However, they have their limitations, perhaps not least of which is the tendency for one to believe that any computer-generated information is an absolute fact. Far from being the case, critical analysis, appraisal, and interpretation of data are essential in their proper application for identification of microorganisms (22). Furthermore, as indicated by Cartwright (9) computerization has a high start-up cost, can be inflexible in handling and presenting data; they can be unreliable, and "inherently out of date."

In this exercise, you will be introduced to the use of the personal or microcomputer to identify one or more of the *Streptococcus* sp. The software program "MICRIDX" will be used (this and a companion program, MICRID, both developed by S. T. Kellogg (18, 20) and available from the American Society for Microbiology, Washington, D. C.). Krichevsky (22) poses the question as to "should the microbiologist learn about computers or should the computer specialist learn about microbiology?" Although some basic knowledge of computer hardware and software is essential his conclusion is still valid: ". . . it is far faster for the microbiologist to learn the rudiments of computers than the converse." Although MICRID can be used with practically no computer background, it is the case, as with any level of use involving computer-assisted microbial identification, the better the background, the better the understanding of the output data, and the better the control of the results.

Part 1

A. Computer-assisted identification of microorganisms (CAIM) of a "paper unknown" *Streptococcus* species using MICRIDX (18, 20):

The objective of this part of the exercise is to attempt to identify a species of *Streptococcus* listed in Table 2-2, and in so doing become acquainted with the operation of computer hardware and MICRIDX software. This will be done by providing you with data that is then to be analyzed in two ways. The first is to make a species identification by comparison to published literature (referred to here as the standard analysis), as Table 2-2 or other sources. This is then to be verified by use of MICRIDX, a data base customized for use in Exercises 2, 8, and 9. Your instructor will provide you with basic instruction con-

cerning the operation of the particular computers you are to use, and how to load MICRIDX into it. You also should read the Users Manual that is part of the documentation accompanying the program. This practice exercise is to follow completion of the standard analysis, therefore represents a verification of it. The general steps for use of MICRIDX, assuming the program has been loaded and the program title has appeared (Figure 2-6) on the computer monitor, are as follows.

```
            MICRIDX
   ** COMPUTER IDENTIFICATION OF
       MICROORGANISMS **
          Experimental

*DO YOU WANT HARDCOPY FOR THIS SESSION*?
```

Figure 2-6: The opening screen for MICRIDX.

1. The question "Do you want a hardcopy for this session?" will now be seen. Answer appropriately: **Y** for yes, **N** for no. If **Y**, on-screen instructions will appear guiding you through the next steps; if **N**:

2. The next question "Instruction in the use of this system?" will appear. Answer **Y** or **N**. If **Y** brief instructions will be presented; if **N**, this is by-passed. In both cases, the main menu will now show (Figure 2-7). To use MICRIDX choose "(9) --> Your Own Data Base." This selects the customized data base of this program.

3. From this point on follow on-screen instructions. For identification of the streptococci, type the following in response to queries from the computer:

   a. Question: "What is your ORGANISM NAME file?" For answer, type: **STR-ORG**

   The computer will respond with "9 organism names Is this correct? Type **Y**

b. Next question: "What is your TEST NAME file?" Type: **STR-TEST**

Again the computer will respond, this time with "16 test names found Is this correct?" Type: **Y**

c. Next question: "What is the name of your PROBABILITY DATA file?" Type **STR-DATA**

Computer should respond with "Data are complete"

```
---------  ---------------
(1)-->     Enterobacteriaceae
(2)-->     Vibrio,Aeromonas,Neisseriaceae,Pseudomonas(enteric tests),
           Alcaligenes,Achromobacter,Flavobacterium,Chromobacterium
           Pasteurella,Brucella,Bordetella,Cardiobacterium,Eikenella
(3)-->     Pseudomonas(non-enteric tests)
(4)-->     Unknown gram-negative (Groups 1-3 simultaneously)
(5)-->     Gram positive facultatives & aerobes(Bacillus,
           Streptococcus,Lactobacillus,Leuconostoc)
(6)-->     Anaerobic Bacteria
(7)-->     Actinomycetales(Streptomyces,Mycobacterium,Corynebacterium
           Listeria,Rothia,Arachnia,Bacterionema,Erysipelothrix)
(8)-->     Yeasts(clinical & non-clinical)
(9)-->     Your Own Data Base
*YOUR GROUP NUMBER*--> ?
```

Figure 2-7: Main menu for MICRIDX. For identification of *Streptococcus* select "Group 9." Other groups may be accessed through the use of MICRID.

4. Three other questions will follow to which you may respond **Y** or **N**. However, two should in particular be answered **Y**. These are "*Would you like an evaluation of your missing data*?, and the other is "*Do you wish tests to be printed vertically*?

5. Enter your strain number at the prompt. If none has been assigned, press **Enter** or **Return** key.

6. Type the appropriate data under each test. Note that the test names are abbreviated and shown vertically. Full names of each test with their abbreviation are shown in Table 2-3. Only + (for positive), - (for negative), or 0 (zero, for variable (V) response or missing data) are acceptable data input.

7. On completion of data entry, striking the **Return** or **Enter** key will cause the computer to carry out the identification. This will appear with names of one or more bacteria, each with an accompanying "Identification Score" arranged in descending order. Scores in the range of, for example, 0.95-0.99 represent a high probability of identification. If an identification is made by the computer, it should correspond to that species you earlier identified by stand-

Table 2-3
Test Names and Their Abbreviated Forms Used in MICRIDX for
Streptococcal and Enterococcal Identification

Full Test Name	Abbreviated Name
Beta hemolysis	Beta
Growth at 10°C	10°C
Growth at 45°C	45°C
Growth in methylene blue milk	MBM
Growth in 6.5% NaCl	NaCl
Bile Esculin growth and reaction	BE
Hippurate hydrolysis	Hipp
CAMP Reaction	CAMP
Arabinose fermentation	Arab
Inulin fermentation	Inul
Mannitol fermentation	Mann
Raffinose fermentation	Raff
Sorbitol fermentation	Sorb
Bile solubility and optochin sensitivity	Opt
Bacitracin inhibition	Bac
PYR hydrolysis	PYR

ard analysis. If these do not correspond, review the data used for both methods. Rerun the computer analysis. If correlation is still not obtained, find and explain the reason for the discrepancy.

8. Having earlier chosen Y for an evaluation of missing tests, the computer will now list these, if any, along with other information.

9. Print the results of your computer analysis and enter it, along with your standard analysis, into your notebook. Discuss.

B. CAIM confirmation of a known *Streptococcus* sp.

Repeat *Part 1* A above using data acquired from testing of *S. pyogenes*, *S. agalactiae*, *S. pneumoniae*, or *E. faecalis*. You must enter data for the same series of tests listed in Table 2-3. Again, print your results and analysis of data and enter into your notebook. Does this computer-assisted identification give the correct species name? Are any data listed not compatible for the species named by the computer? If so, what should be done in such cases, if anything?

Discuss the strengths and weakness of MICRIDX. Suggest ways of improving its capacity to aid in microbial identification. Having now become acquainted with the general operation of MICRIDX, you may wish to try MICRID. This program can be used with several groups of bacteria and yeast found in this manual by appropriately selecting Groups 1-8 from the main menu (Figure 2-7). For particulars on its use read the MICRID Users Manual.

SECTION 3: ANTIMICROBIAL SENSITIVITY TESTING

Antimicrobial sensitivity testing is an important function of the diagnostic microbiology laboratory and of critical significance to the patient and physician. A brief introduction to this topic is presented here. More in-depth discussions are provided in Balows, et al. (4), and accepted procedural and performance standards available in a series of publications published by the National Committee for Clinical Laboratory Standards (NCCLS), Villanova, PA.

Antimicrobial testing must, of course, be initiated as early as possible, usually when the offending agent is isolated and known. (However, it should be noted that not all isolates require testing, such as those bacteria that respond predictably and constantly to certain antimicrobials (34). Several variations in testing are possible. Those most commonly used include dilution methods using either agar or broth, disk diffusion assays, and automated or semi-automated tests.

Both agar and tube dilution methods may be used quantitatively to provide the minimum inhibitory concentration (MIC) of each chemotherapeutic compound. Alternatively, it may be used qualitatively to categorize sensitivities into "susceptible," "intermediate," or "resistant" using interpretive standard charts provided by NCCLS (27). The agar method consists of preparing dilutions of each antimicrobial compound over a desired range in sterile Mueller-Hinton (M-H) agar (with supplements if required for the growth of the organism(s) being assayed). Each dilution is poured into a petri dish and allowed to solidify. A standardized concentration of inoculum of the isolate is prepared and spotted onto each plate containing separate antimicrobial concentrations, along with appropriate control organisms. After incubation at 35°C for 16-20 hours, plates are read for the presence of growth. The lowest drug concentration (or highest dilution) showing lack of visible growth is the endpoint or MIC.

In the broth dilution methods, standard tubes (macrodilution), 96-well plates (microdilution), or other containers are used. Again dilutions of the chemotherapeutic compounds are prepared, these usually being done in M-H broth. After addition of a standardized inoculum of organism to be tested to each tube or well, containers are incubated as described for agar plates. The tubes or wells are visually or photometrically read to find optical density or turbidity. The lowest concentration of drug that does not allow growth (i.e. turbidity is comparable to an uninoculated and incubated tube of broth) represents the MIC. Again, to be a valid test, appropriate controls must be run, including growth controls containing the test organisms without any antimicrobial compound (5, 27, 35). Plates that contain panels of antimicrobials are commercially available. It is apparent that there are similarities in the agar and broth dilution methods. The former, however, offers the advantage of allowing up to 36 different organisms, including controls, to be run on a single plate. In the broth dilution technique, each organism requires a separate tube or well, or series of these containing different compounds and their dilutions. Conversely, the broth dilutions method lends itself to automation, especially the microdilution technique. Commercially-available systems generally employ some variation of this procedure.

Commercially-available automated and semi-automated systems provide reduced labor and time to obtain results over manual systems. However, they also are generally more costly per test, and frequently less flexible. They are all instrument-based, including at least an optical detector or reader, and perhaps diluters, inoculators, incubator, and computer-assisted analysis. These, along with the antimicrobial compound-containing plates provided by the manufacturer, operate as a system. Several are available, as Aladin™, Autobac™ Series II, Sensititre® Microbiology Systems, autoSCAN®-W/A, The Esteem™ System, and the Vitek System. The latter was briefly described in Exercise 1 (page 6) for microbial identification. To use for susceptibility testing, the appropriate plastic card containing the desired antimicrobial panel is filled with medium containing inoculum, incubated for 3-13 hours, then analyzed by computer as to MIC and the organism's category of susceptibility (sensitive, intermediate, or resistant). The system lacks flexibility for streptococcal susceptibility testing as there is a limited number of cards (and therefore panels of drugs) and databases are available for only Group B and D organisms at this time. However, it can be used for many species of *Staphylococcus*. For Gram-negative bacteria, there are also not only many standard panels available (called "Standard Flexible Susceptibility Cards"), but also cards with broader spectra of compounds, "Superflex Susceptibility Cards," and the possibility of a card with a customized set of antimicrobial drugs.

It is instructive to compare such automated systems as Vitek, autoSCAN W/A, or Sensititre to the MSI/Micro Media Systems Esteem. The latter may be used manually with a plate viewer, or semi-automated by adding modules such as a work station to produce an MIC and category susceptibility report, and a data managing computer. Microplates with 96 wells containing frozen antimicrobial panels (Fox Extra™) are available from the manufacturer. Although the total plate is inoculated, only those drugs appropriate to the organisms being tested are reported. In this case, plates must be incubated 18-24 hours.

In the category of disk diffusion antimicrobial sensitivity tests results are relatively qualitative. The method involves streaking a standardized inoculum of isolate over the surface of M-H agar, which, again, may be supplemented if required for proper growth of the organisms. After the surface of the plate has dried, selected antimicrobial-containing disks of single concentrations are place on the surface of the agar and pressed into place with sterile forceps. Although disks should be adequately separated to allow space for inhibition zones to develop, several disks can be place on a single plate. Appropriate control organisms also must be included with the drugs being assayed. After incubation for 16-18 hours, the diameter of the inhibition zones is carefully measured for each disk, then these values interpreted as susceptible, intermediate, or resistant using NCCLS interpretive charts such as shown in Table 2-4 (28). MIC equivalent breakpoint values are also available in such charts. Generally the disk diffusion test, though qualitative and not amenable to automation, does have the advantage of simplicity and flexibility. The panel of antimicrobial compounds tested, for example, can be tailored to individual needs merely by selecting the needed disks. However, it is limited in application since it cannot be used for organisms that grow slowly, are capnophilic, or anaerobic (6).

Part 1

A. Diffusion testing of antimicrobial compounds:

Here, *S. pneumoniae*, freshly isolated from an *in vivo* source will (i) be stained allowing observation of this organism from tissue material, and (ii) used to accomplish an antimicrobial sensitivity test by the disk diffusion test.

Mouse heart blood smear: The instructor will dissect one or more mice that have succumbed to pneumococcal infection. Prepare a smear of heart blood from one animal. Gram stain and observe. Compare the organisms seen here with earlier observations made on stock cultures of pneumococcus. Usually these organisms, when held in culture, tend to lose their typical *in vivo* appearance. Those from such sources (whether mouse or human) typically are found in pairs (an earlier name of the genus was *Diplococcus*) rather than short chains, and "lancet-shaped" with slightly pointed ends rather than rounded characteristic of other streptococci (Photo 2-9). Are the typical pneumococcus forms present in the smears from mouse blood?

B. Antimicrobial sensitivity tests (6, 28).

1. Streak a sheep blood agar plate for isolation using heart blood of one of the mice dissected in *Part 1*A above. Aseptically place an optochin disk in a heavily inoculated portion of the plate. Incubate overnight at 35°C in a candle jar.

2. Examine the isolation plate and identify pneumococcal colonies. Emulsify 5-10 of these isolated colonies in 4 ml trypticase soy broth. Incubate at 35-37°C water bath until the culture turbidity is equal to, or slightly exceeds that of a No. 0.5 McFarland barium sulfate turbidity standard. Alternately, you may suspend enough organisms directly from the isolation plate to give the required density.

3. Dilute the concentration of organisms in the broth if necessary by adding sterile TSB until the turbidity is visually equal to the barium sulfate standard. This is best seen holding the tubes over a well-lighted white background with black lines, as a printed page. Be sure the McFarland standard is adequately mixed on a vortex mixer just before use.

4. Now wet a cotton swab with the broth culture and wring out excess liquid against the tube wall. Streak the *entire* surface of a Mueller-Hinton supplemented with 5% serum agar plate in one direction with the swab. Turn the plate 60° and rub the agar surface in a second direction with the swab, then turn another 60° and repeat. This should give an evenly distributed inoculum. Replace the lid of the dish and allow the plate to sit for 5, but no longer than 15 minutes, to allow absorption of surface moisture.

5. Note the kinds and concentrations of antimicrobial disks available. Place one of each on the agar surface with sterile forceps. Do not situate disks closer than 24 mm from the center of each other. Gently, but firmly, press each disk against the agar so that good contact is made. Immediately (within 15 minutes) incubate at 35°C for 16-18 hours *without* added CO_2.

Part 2

Measure the inhibition zone surrounding each disk, if any, to the closest millimeter. (Note that a uniform lawn of pneumococcus may be almost transparent and difficult to see with transmitted light. Look for differences around an antimicrobial for which it is usually sensitive, as one of the β-lactam family, using reflected light.) Include the disk in this measurement. Record your results and interpret them with the aid of a zone size interpretive chart, Table 2-4. Report your results as susceptible, intermediate, or resistant in the data table provided at the end of this exercise. What is the equivalent MIC for compounds to which pneumococcus is susceptible? Which of the antimicrobials tested is most effective in inhibiting *S. pneumoniae*?

Recently a variant of the disk diffusion test used here has been introduced, the E Test™ (Photo 2-10). In this assay, a single strip contains a gradient of known concentrations of an antimicrobial agent. The strip is applied in the same manner of the standard disk test, but allows for direct determination of MIC as well as sensitivity categories. According to Baker, et al (3) and Ngui-Yen, et al (30) results obtained are reproducible, reliable, and comparable to both disk diffusion and MIC determination methods when compared by sensitivity category results.

SECTION 4: ANTIGEN-ANTIBODY REACTIONS AND RAPID TESTS FOR IDENTIFICATION OF STREPTOCOCCI

A myriad of commercially-prepared rapid tests are available for identification of the streptococci. Some of these are physiologically-based assays and similar in principle and technical use as those described for staphylococcal identification (page 5). The API® 20S™ Streptococcus Test, for example, uses miniaturized physiological and chromogenic tests for identification of both streptococci and aerococci, as do Minitek® and RapID STR™.

Practically all other rapid tests for streptococcal identification are based on the use of specific antibodies. Before proceeding it would be

Table 2-4
Zone Diameter Interpretive Standards and Equivalent Minimum Inhibitory Concentration (MIC) Breakpoints for Organisms Other than *Haemophilus* and *Neisseria gonorrhoeae*

| Antimicrobial agent | Disk Content | Zone Diameter, nearest whole mm | | | Equivalent MIC Breakpoints[c] (µg/mL) | |
		Resistant	Intermediate[a]	Susceptible[b]	Resistant	Susceptible
β-LACTAMS						
Penicillins						
Ampicillin[d]						
when testing gram-negative enteric organisms	10µg	≤13	14-16	≥17	≥32	≤8
when testing staphylococci[e]	10µg	≤28	-	≥29	β-lactamase[e]	≤0.25
when testing enterococci[f]	10µg	≤16	-	≥17[f]	≥16	-
when testing streptococci (not enterococci)[f]	10µg	≤21	22-29	≥30	≥4	≤0.12
when testing *Listeria monocytogenes*	10µg	≤19	-	≥20	≥4	≤2
Azlocillin when testing Pseudomonas[e,g]	75µg	≤17	-	≥18	≥128	≤64
Carbenicillin[e]						
when testing *Pseudomonas*	100µg	≤13	14-16	≥17	≥512	≤128
when testing other gram-negative organisms	100µg	≤19	20-22	≥23	≥64	≤16
Methicillin when testing staphylococci[h]	5µg	≤9	10-13	≥14	≥16	≤8
Mezlocillin[e]						
when testing *Pseudomonas*[g]	75µg	≤15	-	≥16	≥128	≤64
when testing other gram-negative organisms	75µg	≤17	18-20	≥21	≥128	≤16
Nafcillin when testing staphylococci[h]	1µg	≤10	11-12	≥13	-	≤1
Oxacillin						
when testing staphylococci[h]	1µg	≤10	11-12	≥13	≥4	≤2
when testing pneumococci for penicillin G susceptibility	1µg	≤19	-	≥20	-	≤0.06
Penicillin G						
when testing staphylococci[e]	10 units	≤28	-	≥29	β-lactamase[e]	≤0.1
when testing enterococci[f]	10 units	≤14	-	≥15[f]	≥16	-
when testing streptococci (not enterococci)	10 units	≤19	20-27	≥28	≥4	≤0.12
when testing *L monocytogenes*	10 units	≤19	-	≥20	≥4	≤2
Piperacillin[e]						
when testing *Pseudomonas*[g]	100µg	≤17	-	≥18	≥128	≤64
when testing other gram-negative organisms	100µg	≤17	18-20	≥21	≥128	≤16
Ticarcillin[e]						
when testing *Pseudomonas*[g]	75µg	≤14	-	≥15	≥128	≤64
when testing other gram-negative organisms	75µg	≤14	15-19	≥20	≥128	≤16
β-LACTAM/β-LACTAMASE INHIBITOR COMBINATIONS						
Amoxicillin/Clavulanic acid[j]						
when testing staphylococci[k]	20/10µg	≤19	-	≥20	≥8/4	≤4/2
when testing other organisms[j]	20/10µg	≤13	14-17	≥18	≥16/8	≤8/4
Ampicillin/Sulbactam						
when testing gram-negative enterics and staphylococci[i,k]	10/10µg	≤11	12-14	≥15	≥32/16	≤8/4
Ticarcillin/Clavulanic acid						
when testing *Pseudomonas*[g]	75/10µg	≤14	-	≥15	≥128/2	≤64/2
when testing other gram-negative organisms	75/10µg	≤14	15-19	≥20	≥128/2	≤16/2

Table 2-4
Zone Diameter Interpretive Standards and Equivalent Minimum Inhibitory Concentration (MIC) Breakpoints for Organisms Other than *Haemophilus* and *Neisseria gonorrhoeae* (Continued)

| Antimicrobial agent | Disk Content | Zone Diameter, nearest whole mm | | | Equivalent MIC Breakpoints[c] (μg/mL) | |
		Resistant	Intermediate[a]	Susceptible[b]	Resistant	Susceptible
CEPHALOSPORINS AND OTHER CEPHEMS						
Cefaclor[k]	30μg	≤14	15-17	≥18	≥32	≤8
Cefamandole[k]	30μg	≤14	15-17	≥18	≥32	≤8
Cefazolin[k]	30μg	≤14	15-17	≥18	≥32	≤8
Cefetamet[k,l]	**10μg**	**≤14**	**15-17**	**≥18**	**≥16**	**≤4**
Cefixime[k]	5μg	≤15	16-18	≥19	≥4	≤1
Cefmetazole[k]	30μg	≤12	13-15	≥16	≥64	≤16
Cefonicid[k]	30μg	≤14	15-17	≥18	≥32	≤8
Cefoperazone[k]	75μg	≤15	16-20	≥21	≥64	≤16
Cefotaxime[k]	30μg	≤14	15-22	≥23	≥64	≤8
Cefotetan[k]	30μg	≤12	13-15	≥16	≥64	≤16
Cefoxitin[k]	30μg	≤14	15-17	≥18	≥32	≤8
Cefpodoxime[k,l]	**10μg**	**≤17**	**18-20**	**≥21**	**≥8**	**≤2**
Cefprozil[k]	**30μg**	**≤14**	**15-17**	**≥18**	**≥32**	**≤8**
Ceftazidime[g,k]	30μg	≤14	15-17	≥18	≥32	≤8
Ceftizoxime[k]	30μg	≤14	15-19	≥20	≥32	≤8
Ceftriaxone[k]	30μg	≤13	14-20	≥21	≥64	≤8
Cefuroxime Axetil (oral)[k]	30μg	≤14	15-22	≥23	≥32	≤4
Cefurozime Sodium (parenteral)[k]	30μg	≤14	15-17	≥18	≥32	≤8
Cephalothin[k,m]	30μg	≤14	15-17	≥18	≥32	≤8
Loracarbef[k,n]	30μg	≤14	15-17	≥18	**≥32**	**≤8**
Moxalactam[k]	30μg	≤14	15-22	≥23	≥64	≤8
CARBAPENEMS						
Imipenem[k]	10μg	≤13	14-15	≥16	≥16	≤4
MONOBACTAMS						
Aztreonam	30μg	≤15	16-21	≥22	≥32	≤8
GLYCOPEPTIDES						
Teicoplanin[l]	30μg	≤10	11-13	≥14	≥32	≤8
Vancomycin[l]						
when testing enterococci[o]	30μg	≤14	15-16	≥17	≥32	≤4
when testing other gram-positives	30μg	≤9	10-11	≥12	≥32	≤4
AMINOGLYCOSIDES						
Amikacin[p]	30μg	≤14	15-16	≥17	≥32	≤16
Gentamicin[p]	10μg	≤12	13-14	≥15	≥8	≤4
Kanamycin	30μg	≤13	14-17	≥18	≥25	≤6
Netilmicin[p]	30μg	≤12	13-14	≥15	≥32	≤12
Streptomycin	10μg	≤11	12-14	≥15		
Tobramycin[p]	10μg	≤12	13-14	≥15	≥8	≤4
MACROLIDES						
Azithromycin	**15μg**	**≤13**	**14-17**	**≥18**	**≥8**	**≤2**
Clarithromycin	**15μg**	**≤13**	**14-17**	**≥18**	**≥8**	**≤2**
Erythromycin	15μg	≤13	14-22	≥23	≥8	≤0.5
TETRACYCLINES						
Doxycycline[q]	30μg	≤12	13-15	≥16	≥16	≤4
Minocycline[q]	30μg	≤14	15-18	≥19	≥16	≤4
Tetracycline[q]	30μg	≤14	15-18	≥19	≥16	≤4

Table 2-4
Zone Diameter Interpretive Standards and Equivalent Minimum Inhibitory Concentration (MIC) Breakpoints for Organisms Other than *Haemophilus* and *Neisseria gonorrhoeae* (Continued)

Antimicrobial agent	Disk Content	Zone Diameter, nearest whole mm			Equivalent MIC Breakpoints[c] (μg/mL)	
		Resistant	Intermediate[a]	Susceptible[b]	Resistant	Susceptible
QUINOLONES						
Cinoxacin[r]	100μg	$\leq$14	15-18	$\geq$19	$\geq$64	$\leq$16
Ciprofloxacin	5μg	$\leq$15	16-20	$\geq$21	$\geq$4	$\leq$1
Enoxacin	10μg	$\leq$14	15-17	$\geq$18	$\geq$8	$\leq$2
Nalidixic acid[r]	30μg	$\leq$13	14-18	$\geq$19	$\geq$32	$\leq$8
Norfloxacin[r]	10μg	$\leq$12	13-16	$\geq$17	$\geq$16	$\leq$4
Ofloxacin	5μg	$\leq$12	13-15	$\geq$16	$\geq$8	$\leq$2
OTHERS						
Chloramphenicol	30μg	$\leq$12	13-17	$\geq$18	$\geq$32	$\leq$8
Clindamycin[s]	2μg	$\leq$14	15-20	$\geq$21	$\geq$4	$\leq$0.5
Nitrofurantoin[r]	300μg	$\leq$14	15-16	$\geq$17	$\geq$128	$\leq$32
Rifampin	5μg	$\leq$16	17-19	$\geq$20	$\geq$4	$\leq$1
Sulfonamides[r,t]	250 or 300μg	$\leq$12	13-16	$\geq$17	$\geq$350	$\leq$100
Trimethoprim[r,t]	5μg	$\leq$10	11-15	$\geq$16	$\geq$16	$\leq$4
Trimethoprim/Sulfmethoxazole[r]	1.25/23.75μg	$\leq$10	11-15	$\geq$16	$\geq$8/152	$\leq$2/38

Note: Information in boldface type is considered tentative for one year.

Footnotes:
(Note: Tables given in these footnotes refer to those in Reference 28 and 29 that should be consulted for full information.)

a. **The category "intermediate" should be reported. MICs for these isolates approach usually attainable blood and tissue levels and response rates may be lower than for susceptible isolates. The "intermediate" category implies clinical applicability in body sites where the drugs are physiologically concentrated (e.g., quinolones and β-lactams in urine), or when high dosage of drug can be used (e.g., β-lactams). The "intermediate" category also indicates a "buffer zone" which should prevent small uncontrolled technical factors from causing major discrepancies in interpretation, especially for drugs with narrow pharmacotoxicity margins.**

b. Policies regarding generation of cumulative antibiograms should be developed in concert with the infectious disease service, infection control, and the pharmacy and therapeutics committee.

c. These values represent MIC breakpoints used in determining approximate zone size interpretive criteria. They relate to MICs determined by M7 methodology. Occasional discrepancies may exist between M2 and M7 due to methodological limitations.

d. Class disk for ampicillin, amoxicillin, bacampicillin, cyclacillin, and hetacillin.

e. Resistant strains of S. aureus produce β-lactamase and the testing of the 10-unit *penicillin G disk is preferred*. Penicillin G should be used to test the susceptibility of all penicillinase-sensitive penicillins, such as ampicillin, amoxicillin, azlocillin, bacampicillin, hetacillin, carbenicillin, mezlocillin, piperacillin, and ticarcillin. Results may also be applied to phenoxymethyl penicillin or phenethicillin.

f. **The "susceptible" category for penicillin or ampicillin implies the need for high dose therapy for serious enterococcal infections. If possible, this should be denoted by a** footnote on the susceptibility report form. **Enterococcal endocarditis requires combined therapy with high dose penicillin or high dose ampicillin, or vancomycin, or teicoplanin plus gentamicin or streptomycin for bactericidal action.** Detection of ampicillin or penicillin resistance for enterococci due to β-lactamase procution is not possible using the inoculum concentration recommended for routine disk or dilution methods. For blood and CSF isolates, a β-lactamase test using an inoculum of $\geq$ 10[7] CFU/mL (or direct colony growth) and a nitrocefin-based substrate is recommended. Synergy between ampicillin or penicillin and an aminoglycoside is best predicted for enterococci by screening for susceptibility to 500 or 2000 μg of gentamicin, or 2000 μg of streptomycin per mL.

g. *Pseudomonas aeruginosa* infections in granulocytopenic patients and serious infections in other patients should be treated with maximum doses of the selected anti-pseudomonal penicillins (carboxypenicillin or acylaminocillins) **or ceftazidime** in combination with an aminoglycoside.

h. Of the antistaphylococcal, β-lactamase-resistant penicillins, either oxacillin, methicillin, or nafcillin could be tested, and results can be applied to the other penicillinase-resistant penicillins, cloxacillin and dicloxacillin. *Oxacillin is preferred* due to more resistance to degradation in storage and its application to pneumococcal testing and because it is more likely to detect heteroresistant staphylococcal strains. Do not use nafcillin on blood-containing media. Cloxacillin disks should not be used because they may not detect methicillin-resistant S. aureus. When intermediate results are obtained with staphylococci, the strains should be further investigated to determine if they are heteroresistant.

i. The interpretive criteria for ampicillin should also be used for interpretation of ampicillin/sulbactam and amoxicillin/clavulanic acid when testing enterococci, streptococci, and other gram-positives.

j. The use of 500/125 mg Q8-hour doses of amoxicillin/clavulanic acid are necessary for clinical responses for β-lactamase producing susceptible stains of *E. coli, Klebsiella* spp., and *Enterobacter* spp. strains in cutaneous infections. Amoxicillin at high doses (≥500 mg) will be required for coverage of susceptible (≤ 8 μg/mL) gram-negative bacilli.

k. Staphylococci exhibiting resistance to methicillin, oxacillin, or nafcillin should be reported as also resistant to other penicillins, cephalosporins, **carbacephems,** carbapenems, and β-lactamase inhibitor combinations despite apparent *in vitro* susceptibility of some strains to the latter agents. This is because infections with methicillin-resistant staphylococci have not responded favorably to therapy with β-lactam antibiotics.

l. **Not applicable for testing *Morganella.***

m. Cephalothin **can** be tested to represent cephalothin, cefaclor (except against *Haemophilus*), **cefuroxime (except against *Enterobacteriaceae* and *Haemophilus*),** cephapirin, cephradine, cephalexin, cefadroxil, cefazolin **(except against *Enterobacteriaceae*), cefprozil, (except against *Enterobacteriaceae* and *Haemophilus*)** and loracarbef **(except against *Enterobacteriaceae* and *Haemophilus*).** Cefazolin, **cefuroxime, or loracarbef (urinary tract isolates only)** can be tested additionally against *Enterobacteriaceae* because strains resistant to cephalothin or other first generation cephalosporins may be susceptible to **these agents.**

n. **Because certain stains of *Citrobacter, Providencia,* and *Enterobacter* have been reported to give false susceptible results with loracarbef disks, strains of these genera should not be tested and reported with this disk.**

o. When testing vancomycin against enterococci, plates should be held a full 24 hours and examined using transmitted light; the presence of a haze or any growth within the zone of inhibition indicates resistance. If vancomycin is being considered for treatment of serious enterococcal infection, those organisms with intermediate zones should be tested by an MIC method.

p. The zone sizes obtained with aminoglycosides, particularly when testing *P. aeruginosa,* are very medium dependent because of variations in divalent cation content. These interpretative standards are to be used only with Mueller-Hinton medium that has yielded zone diameters within the correct range shown in Table 3 when performance tests were done with *P. aeruginosa* ATCC® 27853. Organisms in the intermediate category may be either susceptible or resistant when tested by dilution methods and should therefore more properly be classified as "indeterminate" in their susceptibility.

q. Tetracycline is the class disk for all tetracyclines, and the results can be applied to chlortetracycline, demeclocycline, doxycycline, methacycline, minocycline, and oxytetracycline. However, certain organisms may be more susceptible to doxycycline and minocycline than to tetracycline. (See footnote p, Table 1.)

r. Susceptibility data for cinoxacin, nalidixic acid, nitrofurantoin, norfloxacin, sulfonamides, and trimethoprim apply only to organisms isolated from urinary tract infections.

s. The clindamycin disk is used for testing susceptibility to both clindamycin and lincomycin.

t. The sulfisoxazole disk can be used for any of the commercially available sulfonamides. Blood-containing media, except media containing lysed horse blood, are not satisfactory for testing sulfonamides. The Mueller-Hinton agar should be as thymidine-free as possible for sulfonamide and/or trimethoprim testing. (See NOTE for Table 3.)

Permission to use portions of M2-A4 (Performance Standards for Antimicrobial Disk Susceptibility Tests - Fourth Edition; Approved Standard) has been granted by NCCLS. The interpretive data are valid only if the methodology in M2-A4 is followed. NCCLS frequently updates the interpretive tables through new editions and supplements to the standard. Users should refer to the most recent edition. The current standard may be obtained from NCCLS, 771 E. Lancaster Avenue, Villanova, PA 19085.

profitable to examine briefly the principles and some types of antibody assays used for detection of *Streptococcus* and other organisms.

Antibodies are serum glycoproteins classified as immunoglobulins or Igs. They are directed toward, and highly specific for the antigen(s) used to induce them. They react with small sites on the antigen, the epitope. A preparation of antibodies may be directed against an epitope of a single chemical configuration, a characteristic of monoclonal antibodies, or epitopes of multiple chemical forms, polyclonal antibodies. To be of differential and diagnostic usefulness, the antibodies must not be reactive with epitopes on unwanted organisms. A simple example of this principle is that if it were wanted to identify Group A streptococci with an antibody-based assay, the Igs must not be reactive with epitopes of Group B, C, D, or any other serological group.

Several methods are available to show an antigen-antibody reaction. These are briefly described below. Further introductory information concerning these is readily available in most general textbooks on Immunology. However,

Stanfield's *Serology and Immunology. A Clinical Approach* (40), Turgeon's *Immunology and Serology in Laboratory Medicine* (42), or Balows, et al. 5th edition of *Manual of Clinical Microbiology* (4) are suggested.

A. Agglutination-type reactions: Agglutination results from an antibody reacting with an antigen that is *particulate* in nature, leading to a visible lattice of antigen-antibody complexes, the agglutinate. A particulate antigen can be considered, for convenience, to be one that is visible in the light microscope. Therefore, a bacterial cell is a particulate antigen, as are red cells, yeasts, or other particles of similar size. Agglutination tests can be of a direct or indirect type.

1. Direct agglutination tests: Direct agglutination refers to a reaction of antibody to epitopes that are an integral part of the reacting particle. Thus, an epitope that is a part of the cell wall of a microorganism will yield a direct agglutination test. These reactions necessarily must involve a surface epitope (Figure 2-8).

(a) Direct agglutination reaction

Particulate Antigen   Antibody   Agglutination

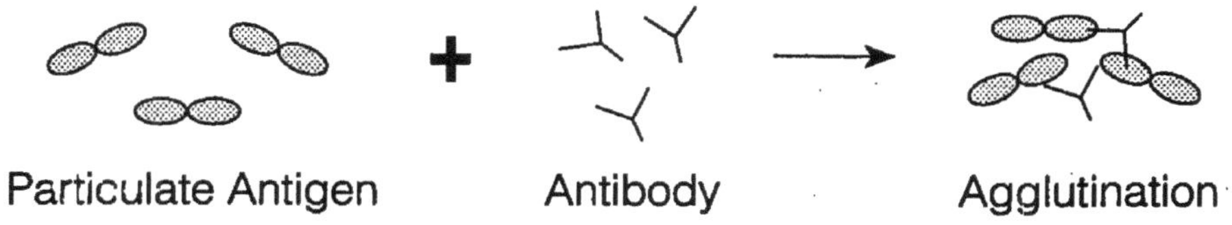

(b) Indirect or passive agglutination reaction

Soluble   Adsorbent   Antigen-coated   Antibody   Agglutination
Antigen   Particles   Particles

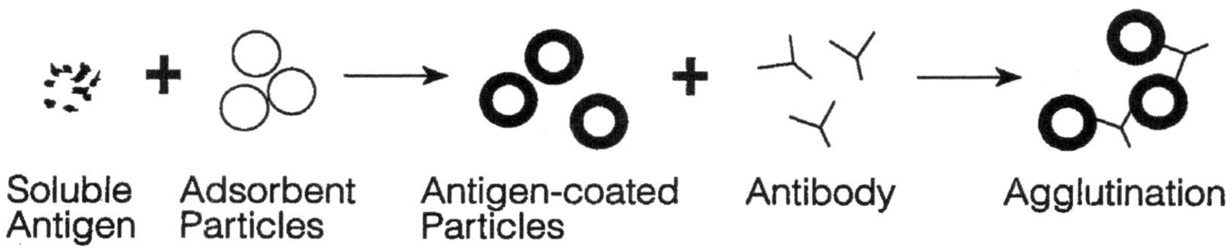

Figure 2-8: (a) Direct agglutination and (b) indirect agglutination. Note that antigen was not a part of original particle in indirect type.

2. Indirect agglutination tests and its variations (41): Indirect (or passive) agglutination tests refer to agglutination occurring when antibody reacts with epitopes adhering to a particle (or vise versa), but the component on the particle was not originally an integral part of it. Thus, the epitope (or antibody) is "passively" adherent to the surface of the particle. The particles themselves may be latex beads, red cells, or others with sticky or adsorbent qualities. Usually the antigens will be *soluble*, which in contrast to particulate are not visible in the light microscope. Thus, soluble antigens may be any solution of protein molecules as serum or egg albumin, or other complex antigens as, for example, most viruses, and extracted streptococcal grouping antigen.

Latex agglutination (Photo 2-11) and indirect hemagglutination are examples of indirect agglutination matrices (see Figure 2-8). In both soluble antigen or specific antibody is adsorbed to the particle. Reaction of this with antibody (in the case of antigen adsorption) or antigen (if antibody has been adsorbed) will produce an agglutinate indistinguishable in appearance from a direct test.

A more recently developed variation of indirect agglutination is the use of liposomes that are constructed to contain a color indicator. Antigen or antibody contained on the surface of the liposome reacts with its corresponding ligand, causing agglutination to occur. Beyond this, however, a secondary reaction is induced causing a color from the indicator to appear. Thus a positive test is seen by the appearance of a color.

Coagglutination is also an interesting variation of indirect agglutination. This reaction uses *S. aureus* as the matrix particle. This organism, because of its Protein A, can bind certain subclasses of Igs by their non-antigen binding F_c part of the molecule. Antibody thus bound is still free to react with antigen because antigen-binding F_{ab} sites remain available. An agglutinate forms in a positive reaction because of the lattice that is formed similar to that of any other indirect agglutination reaction.

B. Reactions involving the use of labeled reactants:

1. Enzyme-linked immunoassays (EIA) (43): Enzyme-linked immunoassays are commonly used in rapid diagnostic tests. Its major advantage is its high sensitivity. In this case, usually the antibody is labeled with an enzyme (thus becoming a "reporter" molecule), though in many cases antigen also can be labeled if wanted. Following reaction with antigen and steps to remove or negate the effect of the unreacted enzyme-linked component, substrate is added. The enzyme on the antibody (or antigen) hydrolyses its substrate in proportion to the concentration of the former, which in turn is proportional to amounts of reacted antibody (or antigen). The hydrolysis of substrate will release a colored end product that can be visually or optically read. Common enzyme label and substrate combinations include horse radish peroxidase acting on o-phenylamine diamine, and alkaline phosphatase on p-nitrophenylphosphate. There are many possible variations to EIA, but the most common is ELISA, the enzyme-linked immunosorbent assay, where either antigen or antibody is adsorbed to a solid surface, such as polystyrene beads or wells of a polystyrene 96-well plate. Subsequent reactants form a complex that remains attached to that surface. The advantage of this is that washing of complexes to remove unwanted and unreacted components (as unattached labeled ligand) is greatly simplified (Figure 2-9).

2. Radioimmunoassays: Radioimmunoassays (RIAs) are quite similar in principle and sensitivity to EIAs. The major difference is, of course, that radioisotopic labels are used rather than enzymes. In turn, this requires an isotope counter to determine extent of antigen-antibody reactions. Furthermore, these assays have the disadvantage of accumulating radioactive waste, high cost, and usually limited shelf life due to short half-life of the commonly used isotopes.

3. Other labels: Other kinds of labels also may be used. Colloidal gold, for example, linked to antibodies are commercially available. The colloidal gold, when concentrated, as in an antigen·antibody·gold complex, leads to a pink or red color due to the gold itself. This has been adapted for use in at least one commercial rapid test for streptococci (see below).

C. Fluorescent antibody (FA)-based assays (32): Fluorescent antibody-based assays all use a fluorescent tag, as fluorescein isothiocyanate, linked to the antibody molecule at a site that does not interfere with antibody binding to its specific epitope. If the fluorescent-labeled antibody is directed, for example, toward a cellular antigen, it attaches to it. The concentration of the label on the cell surface can be detected by use of the fluorescent microscope using a wavelength of light that activates the fluorescent compound causing it to fluoresce. (An example of this technique will be demonstrated in Exercise 9, **page 148**. Also see Photos 3-5 and 13-2, and Figure 9-2). Several variations also exist for use of FA as will be seen in other exercises.

D. Precipitin-type assays: The precipitin assay relates to the use of soluble antigens and to the formation of a lattice of a finely divided precipitate. The precipitin reaction is especially dependent on obtaining a ratio of antigen:antibody that will allow a precipitate to become visible. This is known as the equivalence zone or equivalence ratio. Excess antigen or antibody leads to invisible soluble complexes, a false negative test. The capillary tube precipitin tube grouping test (Section 1, *Part 5*A) was prepared so as to assure as much as possible that such a ratio would be achieved, this occurring where the precipitate finally formed. Although antigen and antibody excess are most critical in inhibiting a visible reaction in precipitin reactions, it is important to recognize that it can occur in many different types of antigen-antibody reactions. Generally speaking tests based on the precipitin reaction are not useful for titration of antibody (why?), but are very good for detection of antigen. The grouping test demonstration is an example of this procedure. However, it also may also be carried out in gels (single and double diffusion tests), applied in electrophoretic methods (as countercurrent immunoelectrophoresis, CIE), or in other variations to identify antigen.

Antibody based tests for detection and identification of *Streptococcus* may be found in all of the above categories. However, most of the rapid

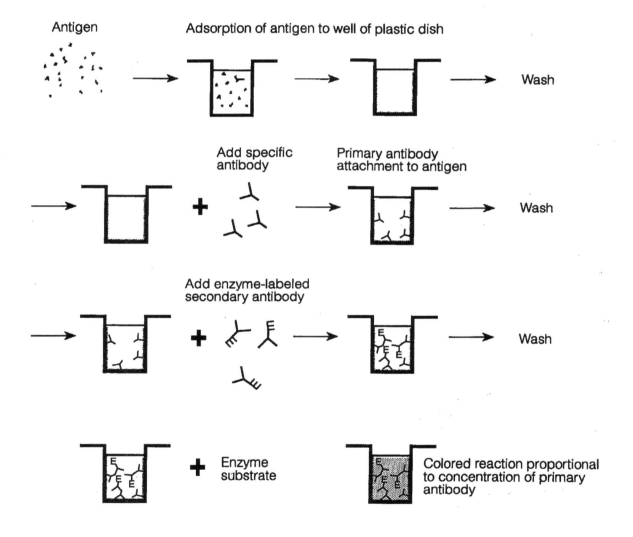

Figure 2-9: Outline of the enzyme immunosorbent assay (ELISA reaction. In this example antigen is adsorbed to the well, followed by specific antibody. This is then detected by the use of enzyme-linked (secondary) antibody. The intensity of color is related to the concentration of primary antibody.

assays fall into categories A (agglutination) and B (labeled reactants).

Somewhat rare at this time are assays that will reliably identify microorganisms directly from an original specimen. Perhaps more than in any others, this has been developed for streptococci where, for example, swabs from the throat and other sources may be used. Though highly specific, sensitivity varies from about 84-95% (e.g. 2, 17, and summarized in 5). Thus, care is required for optimal and reliable results. Even so, negative assays should be confirmed by culture tests. At this stage, they have not replaced more extensive and reliable methods of identification, but have promise for screening purposes.

A few examples of these types of rapid assays include Detect-A-Strep™, and Bactigen® Group A Streptococcus, which use patient throat swabs for latex agglutination tests to identify *S. pyogenes*. Additionally, Bactigen Group B Streptococcus-CS utilizes vaginal or cervical swabs and Wellcogen™, using CSF, urine and serum, identify *S. agalactiae* with latex agglutination (Photo 2-11). On the other hand, Directigen® 123™ Group A Strep Test employs lysosomal technology for rapid diagnosis from throat swabs. Enzyme-linked methods are used in Ventrascreen® Strep A, Cards® Strep A Test (Photo 2-12), and others. Finally, a simply and rapidly done test is the SMART™ (sensitive membrane antigen test) assay. Its reaction is based on the use of colloidal gold-labeled anti-Group A antibody (Anti-A·gold). Extracted antigen complexes with it to form "Group A antigen·Anti-A·gold." This is then immunologically bound to a membrane accumulating the colloidal gold resulting in a colored spot in a positive reaction (D. Trudil, New Horizons Diagnostic Corp., personal communication).

Several other tests for *Streptococcus* can be categorized as rapid tests, but require pure culture isolates, therefore overnight culture. Two examples of these include Phadebact® CoA System that detects Groups A, B, C, and G by, as the name suggests, coagglutination. PathoDx® Strep Grouping and Grouping kit DR 585 uses latex agglutination to identify Groups A, B, C, F, and G from cultured streptococci.

Pneumococcal typing using the Quellung reaction (Section 1, *Part* 5B) does not fall within any of the categories of antigen-antibody reactions listed above. Furthermore, its purpose is not strictly identification, but rather to type the

organisms following establishment of its species. However, there is a rapid identification test for this species. Bactigen *S. pneumoniae* has pooled rabbit antiserum against all the different types allowing detection of the presence of pneumococcus by latex agglutination. Phadabact CoA also detects at the species level using the coagglutination test. Both can identify the antigen in cerebrospinal fluid, serum, urine, or blood culture supernatant liquid. Since culturing is unneeded, in a disease such as meningitis the reduction in time for detection of the causative agent is a definite clinical advantage. However, these types of assays should be used only where clinically indicated and with the knowledge that some lack sensitivity and specificity (1, 15). Several products are also available for identification from culture as the BBL® Pneumoslide™ Test.

Finally, commercially available genetic probes are beginning to be applied for identification of the streptococci. Culture confirmation of *S. agalactiae* (n=100 cultures) and *Enterococcus* spp. (n=100) to a level of 100%, and for *H. influenzae* to 99.4% was achieved when compared to conventional methods with the Accuprobe™ DNA probe test (11). Accuprobe identification tests are also available for *S. pyogenes* and *S. pneumoniae*. Assays with as high a level of accuracy as this, which in this case can be completed in 40 minutes, could eventually replace what are now considered to be lengthy standard assays provided they can be shown to maintain a high degree of specificity and sensitivity. A more thorough discussion concerning this technology can be found in Exercise 3, **page 72**.

QUESTIONS

1. Prepare an identification flow-chart that will efficiently identify those organisms shown in Table 2-2, excluding the use of the grouping test.
2. Describe the anti-streptolysin O (ASO) test. Give its usefulness, and how it is carried out. Name two other antibodies whose detection is useful in the diagnosis of streptococcal disease, and the names of those diseases.
3. Other types of media not used in this exercise are available and useful for differentiation and identification of the streptococci. These include SF and other azide-containing media; and sufamethoxazole-trimethoprim (SXT)

blood agar. Describe the usefulness and application of these in streptococcal identification.

4. Give the factors that influence the diameter of an inhibition zone in the antimicrobial disk sensitivity test.

5. If more than one antimicrobial compound is effective in inhibition of a microorganism, what factors should be considered in choosing one for therapy?

6. Describe the methodology and applications of counterimmunoelectrophoresis (CIE). Of what advantage is it in the diagnosis of streptococcal (or other) infections over culture. For what streptococcal disease is it especially useful.

REFERENCES

1. Ajello, G. W., G. A. Bolan, P. S. Hayes, D. Lehmann, J. Montgomery, J. C. Feeley, C. A. Perlino, and C. V. Broome. 1987. Commercial latex agglutination tests for detection of *Haemophilus influenzae* type b and *Streptococcus pneumoniae* antigens in patients with bacteremic pneumonia. J. Clin. Microbiol. **25**:1388-1391.

2. Anhalt, J. P., B. J. Heiter, D. W. Naumovitz, and P. B. Bourbeau. 1992. Comparison of three methods for detection of Group A streptococci in throat swabs. J. Clin. Microbiol. **30**:2135-2138.

3. Baker, C. N., S. A. Stocker, D. H. Culver, and C. Thornsberry. 1991. Comparison of the E Test to agar dilution, broth microdilution, and agar diffusion susceptibility testing techniques by using a special challenge set of bacteria. J. Clin. Microbiol. **29**:533-538.

4. Balows, A., W. J. Hausler, Jr., K. L. Herrmann, H. D. Isenberg, and H. J. Shadomy (ed.). 1991. Manual of clinical microbiology, 5th ed. American Society for Microbiology, Washington, D. C., p. 59-136; 1059-1202.

5. Baron, E. J., L. R. Peterson, and S. M. Finegold. 1994. Bailey & Scott's diagnostic microbiology, 9th ed. Mosby-Year Book, Inc., St. Louis. p. 79-122; 168-188.

6. Barry, A. L., and C. Thornsberry. 1991. Susceptibility tests: diffusion test methods, p. 1117-1125. *In* A. Balows, W. J. Hausler, Jr., K. L. Herrmann, H. D. Isenberg, and H. J. Shadomy (ed.), Manual of clinical microbiology, 5th ed. American Society for Microbiology, Washington, D. C.

7. Bascomb, S. 1989. Computers in taxonomy and systematics, p. 65-102. *In* T. N. Bryant, and J. W. T. Wimpenny (ed.), Computers in microbiology. A practical approach. IRL Press, Oxford.

8. Bisno, A. L. 1990. Classification of streptococci, p. 1518-1519. *In* G. L. Mandell, R. G. Douglas, Jr., and J. E. Bennett (ed.), Principles and practices of infectious diseases, 3rd ed. Churchill Livingstone, New York.

9. Cartwright, K. A. V. 1989. Computers in clinical microbiology, p. 161-182. *In* T. N. Bryant, and J. W. T. Wimpenny (ed.), Computers in microbiology. A practical approach. IRL Press, Oxford.

10. Christie, R., N. E. Atkins, and E. Munch-Peterson. 1944. A note on a lytic phenomenon shown by Group-B streptococci. Aust. J. Exp. Biol. Med. **22**:197-200.

11. Daly, J. A., N. L. Clifton, K. C. Seskin, and W. M. Gooch III. 1991. Use of rapid, non-radioactive DNA probes in culture confirmation tests to detect *Streptococcus agalactiae*, *Haemophilus influenzae*, and *Enterococcus* spp. from pediatric patients with significant infections. J. Clin. Microbiol. **29**:80-82.

12. D'Amato, R. F., E. J. Bottone, and D. Amsterdam. 1991. Substrate profile systems for the identification of bacteria and yeasts by rapid and automated approaches, p. 128-136. *In* A. Balows, W. J. Hausler, Jr., K. L. Herrmann, H. D. Isenberg, and H. J. Shadomy (ed.), Manual of clinical microbiology, 5th ed. American Society for Microbiology, Washington, D. C.

13. Deibel, R. H., and H. W. Seeley, Jr. 1974. *Streptococcus* Rosenbach 1884, p. 490-509. *In* R. E. Buchanan, and N. E. Gibbons (ed.), Bergey's manual of determinative bacteriology, 8th ed. The Williams & Wilkins Co., Baltimore.

14. Facklam, R. R., and J. A. Washington II. 1991. *Streptococcus* and related catalase-negative Gram-positive cocci, p. 238-257. *In* A. Balows, W. J. Hausler, Jr., K. L. Herrmann, H. D. Isenberg, and H. J. Shadomy (ed.), Manual of clinical microbiology, 5th ed. American Society for Microbiology, Washington, D. C.

15. Forward, K. R. 1988. Prospective evaluation of bacterial antigen detection in cerebral spinal fluid in the diagnosis of bacterial meningitis in a predominantly adult hospital. Diagn. Microbiol. Infect. Dis. **11**:61-63.

16. Hardie, J. M. 1986. Genus *Streptococcus* Rosenbach 1884, p. 1043-1047. *In* P. H. A. Sneath, N. S. Mair, M. E. Sharpe, and J. G. Holt (ed.), Bergey's manual of systematic bacteriology, Vol. 2. Williams & Wilkins, Baltimore.

17. Hayden, G. F., J. C. Turner, D. Kiselica, M. Dunn, and J. O. Handley. 1992. Latex agglutination testing directly from throat swabs for rapid detection of beta-hemolytic streptococci from Lancefield serogroup C. J. Clin. Microbiol. **30**:716-718.

18. Kelley, R. W., and S. T. Kellogg. 1978. Computer-assisted identification of anaerobic bacteria. Appl. Environ. Microbiol. **35**:507-511.

19. Kellogg, J. A. 1990. Suitability of throat culture procedures for detection of Group A streptococci and as reference standards for evaluation of streptococcal antigen detection kits. J. Clin. Microbiol. **28**:165-169.

20. Kellogg, S. T. 1979. MICRID: a computer-assisted microbial identification system. Appl. Environ. Microbiol. **38**:559-563.

21. Koneman, E. W., S. D. Allen, W. M. Janda, P. C. Schreckenberger, and W. C. Winn, Jr. 1992. Color atlas and textbook of diagnostic microbiology, 4th ed. J. B. Lippincott Co., Philadelphia. p. 431-466.

22. Krichevsky, M. I. 1982. Coping with computers and computer evangelists. Ann. Rev. Microbiol. **36**:311-321.

23. Lancefield, R. C. 1933. A serological differentiation of human and other groups of hemolytic streptococci. J. Exp. Med. **57**:571-595.

24. MacFaddin, J. F. 1980. Biochemical tests for identification of medical bacteria, 2nd ed. Williams & Wilkins, Baltimore. p. 4-12, 141-162.

25. Mundt, J. O. 1986. Lactic acid streptococci, p. 1065-1066. *In* P. H. A. Sneath, N. S. Mair, M. E. Sharpe, and J. G. Holt (ed.), Bergey's manual of systematic bacteriology, Vol. 2. Williams & Wilkins, Baltimore.

26. Musher, D. M. 1990. Enterococcus species and group D streptococci, p. 1550-1554. *In* G. L. Mandell, R. G. Douglas, Jr., and J. E. Bennett (ed.), Principles and practices of infectious diseases, 3rd ed. Churchill Livingstone, New York.

27. National Committee for Clinical Laboratory Standards. 1990. Methods for dilution antimicrobial susceptibility tests for bacteria that grow aerobically-second edition. Approved standard. NCCLS document M7-2A. National Committee for Clinical Laboratory Standards, Villanova, PA. 32 p.

28. National Committee for Clinical Laboratory Standards. 1990. Performance Standards for antimicrobial disk susceptibility tests-fourth edition. Approved standard. NCCLS document M2-A4. National Committee for Clinical Laboratory Standards, Villanova, PA. 28 p.

29. National Committee for Clinical Laboratory Standards. 1992. Performance Standards for antimicrobial susceptibility testing; Fourth informational supplement. NCCLS document M100-S4. National Committee for Clinical Laboratory Standards, Villanova, PA. 28 p.

30. Ngui-Yen, J. H., E. A. Bryce, C. Porter, and J. A. Smith. 1992. Evaluation of the E test by using selected Gram-positive bacteria. J. Clin. Microbiol. **30**:2150-2152.

31. O'Brien, M., and R. Colwell. 1987. Characterization tests for numerical taxonomy studies. Meth. Microbiol. **19**:69-104.

32. Rosebrock, J. A. 1991. Labeled-antibody techniques: fluorescent, radioisotopic, immunochemical, p. 79-86. *In* A. Balows, W. J. Hausler, Jr., K. L. Herrmann, H. D. Isenberg, and H. J. Shadomy (ed.), Manual of clinical microbiology, 5th ed. American Society for Microbiology, Washington, D. C.

33. Ryan, K. J. 1990. Streptococci, p. 291-312. *In* J. C. Sherris (ed.), Medical microbiology. An introduction to infectious diseases, 2nd ed. Elsevier Science Publishing Co., Inc., New York.

34. Sahn, D. F., M. A, Neuman, C. Thornsberry, and J. E. McGowen, Jr. 1988. Cumitech 25: Current concepts and approaches to antimicrobial agent testing. Coordinating ed. J. E. McGowen, Jr. American Society for Microbiology, Washington, D. C. 17 p.

35. Sahn, D. F., and J. A. Washington II. 1991. Antibacterial susceptibility tests: dilution methods, p. 1105-1116. *In* A. Balows, W. J. Hausler, Jr., K. L. Herrmann, H. D. Isenberg, and H. J. Shadomy (ed.), Manual of clinical microbiology, 5th ed. American Society for Microbiology, Washington, D. C.

36. Schleifer, K. H., and R. Kilpper-Bälz. 1984. Transfer of *Streptococcus faecalis* and *Streptococcus faecium* to the genus *Enterococcus* nom. rev. as *Enterococcus faecalis* comb. nov. and *Enterococcus faecium* comb. nov. Int. J. Syst. Bacteriol. **34**:31-34.

37. Schleifer, K. H., J. Kraus, C. Dvorak, R. Kilpper-Bälz, M. D. Collins, and W. Fischer. 1985. Transfer of *Streptococcus lactis* and related streptococci to the genus *Lactococcus* gen. nov. System. Appl. Microbiol. **6**:183-195.

38. Sherman, J. M. 1937. The streptococci. Bacteriol. Rev. **1**:3-97.

39. Sneath, P. H. A., N. S. Mair, M. E. Sharpe, and J. G. Holt (ed.). 1986. Bergey's manual of systematic bacteriology, Vol. 2. Williams & Wilkins, Baltimore. p. 1043-1071.

40. Stanfield, E. D. 1981. Serology and immunology. A clinical approach. Macmillan Publishing Co., Inc., New York. 388 p.

41. Tinghitella, T. J., and S. C. Edberg. 1991. Agglutination tests and *Limulus* assay for the diagnosis of infectious diseases, p. 61-72. *In* A. Balows, W. J. Hausler, Jr., K. L. Herrmann, H. D. Isenberg, and H. J. Shadomy (ed.), Manual of clinical microbiology, 5th ed. American Society for Microbiology, Washington, D. C.

42. Turgeon, M. L. 1990. Immunology and serology in laboratory medicine. The C. V. Mosby Co., St. Louis. 415 p.

43. Voller, A., D. Bidwell, and A. Bartlett. 1980. Enzyme-linked immunosorbent assay, p. 359-371. *In* N. R. Rose, and H. Friedman (ed.), Manual of clinical microbiology, 2nd ed. American Society for Microbiology, Washington, D. C.

Exercise 2, Section 1
Data Table 1: *Streptococcus* and *Enterococcus* Known Culture Results

		Culture	S. pyogenes		S. agalactiae		S. pneumoniae		E. faecalis	
		Age	SBA	Other	SBA	Other	SBA	Other	SBA	Other
Colony size and Colony Form [a]	mm									
	Punctiform									
	Irregular									
	Circular									
	Rhizoid									
	Filamentous									
	Other									
Colony Surface	Flat									
	Raised									
	Convex									
	Pulvinate									
	Other									
Colony Margin	Entire									
	Undulate									
	Lobate									
	Erose									
	Other									
Colony Consistency	Butyrous									
	Viscid									
	Membranous									
	Brittle									
	Other									
Colony Optical Character	Opaque									
	Translucent									
	Dull									
	Glistening									
	Other									
Colony Surface	Smooth									
	Rough									
	Other									
Colony color Hemolysis										
	Surface									
	Subsurface									
Other										

[a] See Appendix 1 for description of colony terminology.

Exercise 2, Section 1
Data Table 2: *Streptococcus* and *Enterococcus* Known Culture Results

		Culture Age	S. pyogenes	S. agalactiae	S. pneumoniae	E. faecalis
Gram Stain Medium:	Morphology					
	Arrangement					
	Reaction					
Trypticase soy plates	Growth at 37°C					
	Growth at 45°C					
	Bacitracin inhib., mm					
	Optochin inhib., mm					
	Catalase production					
Methylene blue milk	Reduction					
	Clot formation					
	Growth					
Na Hippurate	Hydrolysis					
Mannitol	Fermentation					
Inulin	Fermentation					
Bile	Growth					
esculin	Blackening					
6.5% NaCl	Growth					
Bile solubility						
CAMP						
PYR						
Other						

Exercise 2, Section 1
Data Table 3: *Streptococcus* Throat Isolate Results

		Culture Age	Isolate No.							
			1	2	3	4	5	6	7	8
Colony size and Colony Form[a]	mm									
	Punctiform									
	Irregular									
	Circular									
	Rhizoid									
	Filamentous									
	Other									
Colony Surface	Flat									
	Raised									
	Convex									
	Pulvinate									
	Other									
Colony Margin	Entire									
	Undulate									
	Lobate									
	Erose									
	Other									
Colony Consistency	Butyrous									
	Viscid									
	Membranous									
	Brittle									
	Other									
Colony Optical Character	Opaque									
	Translucent									
	Dull									
	Glistening									
	Other									
Colony Surface	Smooth									
	Rough									
	Other									
Colony color Hemolysis										
	Surface									
	Subsurface									
Other	Oxidase									
	Catalase									

[a] See Appendix 1 for description of colony terminology.

Exercise 2, Section 1
Streptococcus and *Enterococcus* Results
Throat Isolates

Gram Stain Results from Throat Swab:

Cell Morphology and Arrangement	Relative Numbers in Smear[a]			
	Rare	Few	Moderate	Many

[a] Based on numbers/oil immersion field: Rare = <1; Few = 1 - 5; Moderate = 6 - 20; and Many = >20

Culture Observations

		Pneumococcus-like Isolate (No.)		Beta-hemolytic Isolate (No.)		Other Isolates Isolate (No.)		Isolate (No.)	
		Age		Age		Age		Age	
Gram	Reaction								
Stain	Morphology								
	Arrangement								
SBA	Bacitracin inhib., mm								
	Obtochin inhib., mm								
	Bile solubility								
CAMP									
	S. pyogenes								
	S. agalactiae								
Other									

Section 2: Notes on CAIM

Exercise 2
Streptococcus and *Enterococcus* Results
Section 3: Antimicrobial Sensitivity Testing

Part A: Mouse Heart Blood Smear

Observation:

Part B: *In vitro S. pneumoniae* Antimicrobial Sensitivity Test

Antimicrobial Compound[a]	Concentration	Culture Age, Hours	Inhibition Zone, mm	Interpretation[b]

[a] Name of antimicrobial compound and manufacturer. [b] From Table 2-4.

Exercise 2: *Streptococcus* and *Enterococcus*
LABORATORY NOTES

B. THE GRAM-NEGATIVE COCCI AND COCCOBACILLI, THE FAMILY *NEISSERIACEAE*

INTRODUCTION

The family *Neisseriaceae* includes aerobic, non-motile organisms that are Gram-negative cocci, commonly shaped as kidney beans in pairs or groups, and rods in pairs or short chains. Four genera are included in Bergey's Manual of Systematic Bacteriology, namely, *Neisseria, Moraxella* (with two subgenera, *Moraxella* and *Branhamella*), *Acinetobacter,* and *Kingella* (5). However, more recent RNA and DNA studies suggest the family be emended to exclude *Moraxella* and *Acinetobacter* spp. (34). These and other characteristics have prompted the proposal for two new families. The first, *Branhamaceae,* is to include the genera *Branhamella* and *Moraxella* (8). The second, *Moraxellaceae,* includes *Acinetobacter, Psychrobacter* (not discussed further here), and, again, *Moraxella* (35). While there is some species conflict with the latter appearing in both families, the point is made to remove these three genera (*Moraxella, Branhamella,* and *Acinetobacter*) from the *Neisseriaceae.* Simultaneously, it eliminates the need for subgenus categories of the former arrangement of *Moraxella.* In this manual we will follow these recommendations to designate *Branhamella* and *Moraxella* as separate genera in the family *Branhamaceae* fam. nov., and *Acinetobacter* in the family *Moraxellaceae* fam. nov.

Although all genera given above contain species that have been isolated from humans as parasites and as disease agents, *Neisseria* remains the most significant in the latter category (3, 23). The neisseriae, along with *Branhamella catarrhalis* is examined more thoroughly in Exercise 3, while *Moraxella* and *Acinetobacter* will be studied in Exercise 4. Major distinguishing characteristics of genera to be encompassed are shown in Table 3-1. From this it can be seen that rRNA/DNA hybridization studies have demonstrated groupings through G + C mole% that may not be strongly apparent through phenotypic characteristics (6).

It is useful to note that *Moraxella, Acinetobacter,* and *Kingella* also can be placed into the diagnostic category of "Non-fermenting Gram-negative Bacteria" (NFB). The characteristic common to this group (which includes *Pseudomonas aeruginosa,* the predominate species among NFB isolates from the many obtained from clinical sources) is that they are all obligate aerobes that use oxygen as their final electron acceptor. Thus, glucose fermentation, a common laboratory assay, is not used as such. Other clues that suggest NFB include a positive cytochrome oxidase reaction and a failure to grow on MacConkey agar (3, 20, 24). These non-fermenting bacteria are ubiquitous in the environment, as well as being mammalian parasites. Many produce infection in immunocompromised hosts, especially in nosocomial situations. We will discuss some of these further in future exercises.

Table 3-1
Features of Genera in the Family *Neisseriaceae* (5)

Genus	Morphology	Oxidase Reaction	Catalase	Acid produced from glucose	G + C Mole %
Neisseria	Coccus[a]	+[b]	+	+ and −	46.5 - 53.5
Moraxella	Short, plump rods	+	+	−	40 - 47.5
Branhamella	coccus	+	+	−	40 - 47.5
Acinetobacter	Rod	−	+	+ and −	38 - 47
Kingella	Rod	+	−	+	47 - 55

[a] Exception: *N. elongata* is a rod-shaped bacterium.
[b] + = usually positive; − = usually negative; + and − = both positive and negative strains within a genus.

EXERCISE 3
Neisseria and *Branhamella catarrhalis*

INTRODUCTION

Section 1: Identification by Standard Methods

Historically, the two species of major pathogenic importance in *Neisseria* are *N. meningitidis* (meningococcus), the causative agent of epidemic cerebrospinal meningitis, and *N. gonorrhoeae* (gonococcus), the inciter of gonorrhea. Although meningococcus can be isolated from the normal oral cavity, gonococcus is always a pathogen (23). These organisms are extremely fastidious and sensitive. Because of this certain precautions must be taken in isolating and culturing them, including the use of highly enriched media that has been warmed before inoculation, and incubation at an increased CO_2 tension in a humid atmosphere.

Parasitic, but usually non-pathogenic *Neisseria* are also found in the respiratory tract as normal inhabitants and include those given in Table 3-2, except for *N. gonorrhoeae* and *N. meningitidis*. *Branhamella catarrhalis* is also found in this location (3, 6, 29). Although this latter species is obviously not classified as a neisseriae, its morphology, habitat, and physiological characteristics make it more practical from a laboratory standpoint to include it with the study of the *Neisseria*. All of the usually non-pathogenic *Neisseria* species have been isolated as agents of disease, but are opportunistic in this role (29). *B. catarrhalis* is, however, being seen increasingly in the literature as causing diseases such as wound infection (14), respiratory tract infections, otitis media, bacteremia, etc., especially in immunocompromised patients (3, 16).

As noted in Table 3-1, characteristics common to each of the above species are that they are Gram-negative cocci, usually in pairs with flattened adjacent sides (see Photo 3-1). They produce cytochrome oxidase and catalase. *N. elongata*, however, is an exception since it is a rod and is catalase negative. Others characteristics that aid in separation and identification of species are shown in Table 3-2.

Clinically, an early suggestion of the presence of *N. gonorrhoeae* or *N. meningitidis* is the presence of Gram-negative intracellular, kidney bean-shaped diplococci within leukocytes of smears prepared from clinical materials of patients suspected of having disease due to these organisms (1, 19) (Photo 3-1). As seen in Table 3-2, both species will grow on modified Thayer-Martin medium. At this stage of the isolation procedure, the evolution of gas with the use of superoxol (30% H_2O_2), will strongly suggest gonococcus. Only this species and *N. gonorrhoeae* subsp. *kochii* (not shown in Table 3-2, but physiologically similar to gonococcus, and serologically like meningococcus) gives this reaction. However, recall that both coccus-shaped *Neisseria* and *Moraxella* are catalase-positive with the standard test with 3% H_2O_2. *N. meningitidis* and *N. polysaccharea* are also morphologically similar, but can be distinguished because the latter produces large amounts of polysaccharide on 1% sucrose agar.

Final speciation will require other assays shown in Table 3-2. Note that *N. gonorrhoeae* ferments only glucose, while *N. meningitidis* ferments both glucose and maltose. *N. lactamica* is the only member that attacks lactose while *B. catarrhalis* is the only one that produces deoxyribonuclease. *N. cinerea*, *N. flavescens*, and *B. catarrhalis* are assacharolytic, though the first of these may be weakly positive (29). Not seen in Table 3-2 is that *N. sicca* alone forms dry, adherent, wrinkled colonies. Furthermore, *Kingella denitrificans* can be confused with *N. gonorrhoeae* early in identification procedures. This is because both have similar morphology, grow on MTM agar but not on nutrient agar, and ferment only glucose. However, unlike gonococcus, *K. denitrificans* is negative in the standard and superoxol catalase assays, and positive in the nitrate test (23).

Many rapid assays are available for speciation of *N. gonorrhoeae* and *N. meningitidis* as well as serological identification of the latter. These will be discussed later after you have become acquainted with some of the standard speciation assays that follow.

Table 3-2

Distinguishing Characteristics of *Neisseria* and *Branhamella catarrhalis* (3,)[a]

| Organism | Growth @ 35°C on: | | Gas from Superoxol (30%H₂O₂) | Acid Produced From | | | | | Precipitate in 1% sucrose agar | DNase | Reduction of:[d] | | Colony Pigmentation |
	MTM agar	Nutrient agar		Gluc[c]	Fruc	Malt	Suc	Lac			NO₃	NO₂	
N. gonorrhoeae	+	−[b]	+	+	−	−	−	−	−	−	−	−	None
N. meningitidis	+	−	−	+	−	+	−	−	−	−	−	V	None
N. subflava	−	V	−	+	V	+	V	−	−	−	−	+	Yellow
N. cinerea	V	+	−	+	−	+	−	−	+	−	−	V	None
N. flavescens	+	+	−	−	−	−	−	−	+	−	−	−	Yellow
N. polysaccharea	+	+	−	+	−	+	−	−	+	−	−	V	None
N. sicca	−	+	−	+	+	+	+	−	+	−	−	+	White-Yellow
N. mucosa	−	+	−	+	+	+	+	−	+	−	+	+	None to sl. yellow
N. lactamica	+	+	−	+	−	+	−	+	−	−	−	+	None to sl. yellow
B. catarrhalis	V	+	−	−	−	−	−	−	−	+	+	+	None

[a] Listed here are 9 of 13 *Neisseria* spp., and 1 of 4 *Branhamella* spp.
[b] − = usually positive; − = usually negative; V = variable reaction.
[c] A medium such as cystine trypticase agar (CTA) (BBL Microbiology Systems, Cockeysville, MD and Remel, Lenexa, KA) or Cystine tryptic agar (Difco Laboratories, Detroit, MI) recommended for *Neisseria gonorrhoeae* and *N. meningitidis*. Gluc = glucose; fruc = fructose; malt = maltose; suc = sucrose; lac = lactose. The ONPG (o-nitrophenyl-β-D-galactopyanose) test can be used in place of the lactose fermentation test.
[d] Nitrate reduction determined in 0.2% enriched nitrate broth; nitrite reduction in 0.1% nitrite broth.

MATERIALS

Section 1

Part 1

A. Per pair of students:
 1 "Y" nutrient agar plate
 1 Modified Thayer-Martin "Y" plate
 3 tubes enriched nitrate broth with
  Durham tubes
 3 tubes enriched 0.01% nitrite broth with
  Durham tubes
 1 culture each of *N. gonorrhoeae, N.
  subflava,* and *B. catarrhalis*
 3 CTA glucose medium tubes
 3 CTA fructose medium tubes
 3 CTA maltose medium tubes
 3 CTA sucrose medium tubes
 Indophenol oxidase reagent
 Standard (3% H_2O_2) Catalase reagent
 Superoxol (30% H_2O_2) reagent
 Gram stain reagents
 Candle jar
B. Per pair of students:
 Clinical plates
 1 Modified Thayer-Martin plate
 1 Nutrient agar plate
 Gram stain reagents

Part 2

A. Per pair of students:
 Indophenol oxidase reagent
 Nitrate test reagents
B. Per pair of students:
 1 nitrate broth tube with Durham tube
 1 nitrite broth tube with Durham tube
 1 each CTA glucose, fructose, maltose, and
  sucrose medium
 Superoxol (30% H_2O_2) reagent
 Candle jar

Section 2

Per pair of students:
 1 culture of *N. gonorrhoeae, N. subflava,* or
  Branhamella catarrhalis
 1 Unknown culture
 4 Micropipetter tips to deliver 50 μl
  volumes
 2 Micropipetter tips to deliver 300 μl
  volumes
Per class:
 1 Gen-Probe AccuProbe™ *Neisseria
  gonorrhoeae* Culture Identification Kit
 3 Micropipetters for delivering 50 μl
  volumes

3 Micropipetters for delivering 300 μl
 volumes
1 60°C ($\pm$1°C) water bath or heating
 block
3 Vortex mixers
1 culture *N. meningitidis,* ATCC No. 13077

LABORATORY PROCEDURES
(Also see Procedural Flow Diagram, Fig. 3-1):

Part 1

A. Known cultures: Each pair of students will be given a culture of *N. gonorrhoeae* (gonococcus), *N. subflava,* and *Branhamella catarrhalis.* Carry out the following with each organism:
1. Prepare a Gram stain and observe. Note the tendency of these organisms to resist decolorization.
2. Streak for isolation on one sector of the following: (Note: Media to be used for the growth of gonococcus or meningococcus should be warmed to at least room temperature before inoculation.)
 a. "Y" nutrient agar plate (i.e. plate divided into 3 segments).
 b. "Y" plate of modified Thayer-Martin medium (MTM). This selective medium contains antimicrobial compounds which inhibit the growth of contaminants (41) (Photo 3-3). Several variations of the original medium are available. MTM containing vancomycin, sodium colistimethate, trimethoprim lactate, and nystatin, along with a defined supplement added to a chocolate agar base medium, has been reported to give superior recovery of *N. gonorrhoeae* from genital infections (4). The antimicrobial content is sufficient to inhibit some normal flora neisseriae and other bacteria, as well as some yeasts (41).
 c. Incubate plates at 35°C for 24 hours in a humidified candle jar (insertion of a dampened paper towel is satisfactory for providing a humid atmosphere).
3. Inoculate one tube of enriched nitrate and nitrite broths. Incubate as directed for the plates. Test for nitrate and/or nitrite reduction after 48 hours.
4. **Liberally** inoculate the following CTA carbohydrate-containing media immediately below the surface:

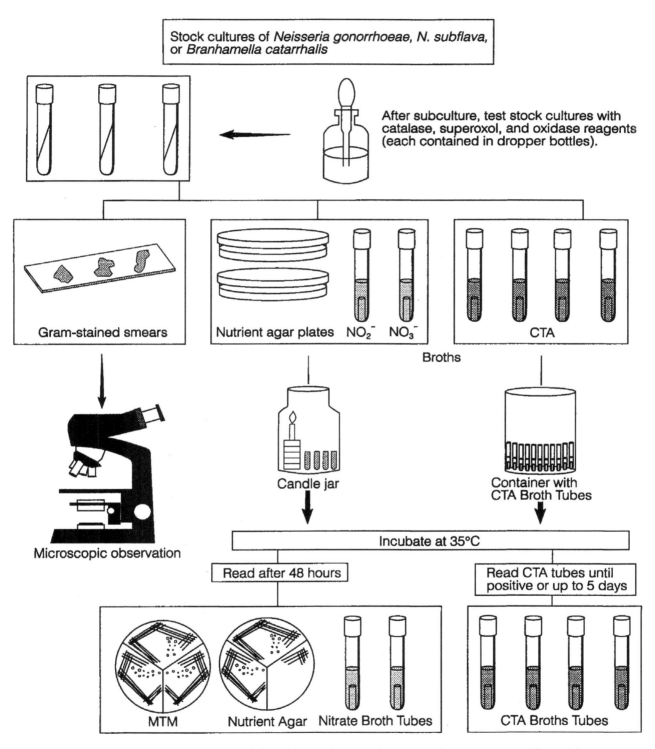

Test separate colonies for catalase reactivity with catalase and superoxol reagents, and for oxidase. Describe colony forms, test for nitrate and nitrite reduction, and read CTA carbohydrates for acid formation.

Figure 3-1: Procedural flow chart for examination of known cultures of *Neisseria gonorrhoeae, N. subflava,* and *Branhamella catarrhalis.*

a. Glucose
b. Maltose
c. Fructose
d. Sucrose

Tighten lids and incubate without increased CO_2. Examine daily up to 5 days or until acid production is seen by the appearance of a yellow color in the inoculated region.

If it is necessary to hold these cultures subsequent to incubation, do so at room temperature, not in the refrigerator; however, gonococcus usually does not survive beyond 4-5 days even under these conditions.

5. Apply 1-2 drops of oxidase reagent (Appendix 3; also see Appendix 5 for sources of prepared solution) to each stock culture and record results. A positive oxidase test is given by a darkening of the colony, eventually turning purple. This is due to enzymes contained by the organisms that oxidize the reagent to that color in the presence of cytochrome c and atmospheric oxygen (28). Reactions are positive for all *Branhamella, Moraxella,* most *Neisseria* and other organisms not included in this exercise such as *Alcaligenes,* pseudomonads, and certain other bacteria and yeasts sometimes found in the normal throat, cervix, urethra, and other body areas. Nevertheless, the test is very useful as an early indicator of a possible *Neisseria* sp. when coupled with isolation from the oral or genital tract.

It should be noted that application of the reagent to colonies will kill the organisms within 15 minutes. Therefore, if subcultures are to be made, they should be completed within this time. However, the test also can be done by rubbing some material from an isolated colony on to a filter paper strip wet with oxidase reagent, all contained within a petri dish. A sterile platinum loop or wooden tooth pick can be used to pick colony material. Nichrome loops should not be used since false-positive reactions may result. A pink to purple color will begin to develop within 10 seconds with the reagent in use here. Whichever method is used, be sure to include a known oxidase-positive (as *Pseudomonas fluorescens*) and -negative (such as *Escherichia coli*) control. In general, assays should not be done with organisms taken from selective and differential media, such as those used for isolation of enteric bacteria (see Exercises 8 and 9). Also, organisms taken from glucose-containing media should be avoided (why?). In order for an oxidizing reaction to take place, oxygen must make contact with the organisms. Therefore, excess fluid reagent must be drained from the colony (28).

Commercially prepared oxidase-containing strips, disks, sticks, or swabs are available from several sources. As always, to obtain reliable results, product manufacturer instructions should be followed.

6. Carry out the catalase test with each species using the standard 3% reagent using the filter paper strip method. Test using superoxol by removing a small amount of growth, place it on a slide contained within a petri dish, then apply the reagent. Place the cover on the dish and observe for bubbling. Is a positive test given in both cases for all species?

B. Isolate from clinical cases: If cultures from clinical cases of gonorrhea are available, each pair of students do the following (also see Fig. 3-2):

1. Examine the plate for typical gonococcus colonies, usually appearing as round, smooth, grayish-white, convex colonies with entire to crenated margins.
2. Prepare a Gram stain from each morphologic type of colony and observe.
3. If Gram-negative diplococci are found test the parent colony with oxidase reagent using the filter paper strip method.
4. Test the suspect colony with catalase and superoxol reagents as described above.
5. If positive tests occur in steps 3 and 4, streak the colony for isolation to:
   a. Modified Thayer-Martin medium
   b. Nutrient agar
   Care is always required to obtain a pure subculture for use in subsequent tests. Failure to do so appears to be a persisting reason, for example, of misidentification of gonococcus in public health laboratories (15).
6. Incubate at 35°C for up to 24 hours. Use the humidified candle jar as previously done.

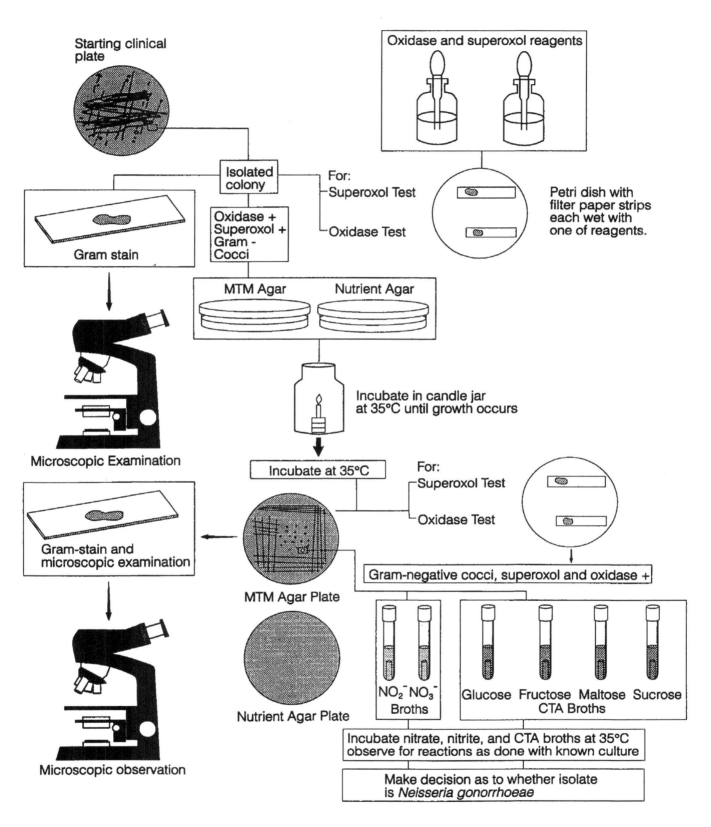

Figure 3-2: Procedural flow chart for attempted isolation of *Neisseria gonorrhoeae* from a clinical plate.

Part 2

A. Known cultures:
   1. Note the characteristics of typical isolated *N. gonorrhoeae*, *N. subflava*, and *B. catarrhalis* colonies on nutrient and modified Thayer-Martin agar. Describe.
   2. Test and observe the nitrate broth cultures for the reduction of nitrate and/or nitrite. (Reminder: Reagent formulation given in Appendix 3.) Is gas present in the Durham tubes? If so, what is the gas?
   3. Read the results of the sugar degradation tests. Are they comparable to data in Table 3-2?
   4. Tabulate results and discuss.
B. Isolates from clinical cases: Observe your isolation plates and describe. Select a typical gonococcus-like colony, prepare a Gram stain and observe. If Gram-negative cocci are seen, carry out the oxidase, catalase, and superoxol tests as described in *Part 1* B. If identifying reactions are given and if you have good reason for believing that you have *N. gonorrhoeae*, inoculate it to kinds of CTA sugar media and enriched nitrate and nitrite broths used in *Part 1*.

Part 3

Read and record reactions given by the clinical isolate in presence of carbohydrates and nitrate and nitrite broths. What is your conclusion concerning the identity of the organism isolated from clinical plates?

Further Notes on Identification Methods and Rapid Identification:

The use of modified Thayer-Martin medium for primary plating of specimens suspected of containing gonococcus has been very helpful in improving the number of successful isolations of this organism. Martin-Lewis medium, which substitutes the antifungal agent anisomycin for nystatin to improve shelf life, and New York City medium, which has translucent qualities, also may be used (3, 24). However, some strains of bacteria are sensitive to the antimicrobial compounds in these media, especially vancomycin (44). Furthermore, the fastidious nature of the organisms makes it much more demanding in terms of the quality of products used in preparation of the media and reagents. Both of these problems can be alleviated by (i) always including known control cultures on the media being used, and (ii) streak-

ing the clinical material on a second enriched medium that does not contain antimicrobial compounds, such as chocolate agar. Of course, if a specimen is from a source not usually containing normal flora bacteria, as blood, selective media need not be used at all.

The use of CTA base for carbohydrate degradation tests, though widely used, has certain deficiencies (20). These include failure by some fastidious stains to grow, slow growth by others causing delayed reactions, or false negative reactions through neutralization of small amounts of acid by alkaline end products (where could such end products come from?) or false positive reactions through non-specific acidification of the medium, as by exposure to excess CO_2.

Because of this and the importance of the pathogenic neisseriae, many rapid assays for the identification of *N. gonorrhoeae* and *N. meningitidis* have been developed (3, 20, 29). In gonorrhea, the Gram stain of smears made from clinical material alone can be considered a rapid test. Its sensitivity varies greatly, from 40-60% for a rectal swab smear to 95-100% for that from the male urethra. The specificity, whether urethra or endocervix is 95-100%, and for rectal smears, 90-95% (19).

Otherwise, the remainder can be categorized into three groups: (i) those that detect microbial enzyme activity; (ii) those that detect antigens derived from the microbe or antibodies from the patient; and (iii) DNA probes. All of the tests that detect microbial enzyme activity require pure colonies for testing and therefore are rapid only in the sense of identification, not in isolation and purification of cultures. Never the less, reduction of identification time of *Neisseria*, for example, from up to five days using the standard CTA carbohydrate tube tests to four hours in rapid assays is a significant savings of time. This is accomplished by using a heavy inoculum to provide large enzyme concentrations without the need for growth. In antigen- or antibody detection systems, the saving of time can be even more significant since most of these can be accomplished within 15 minutes, some within one minute.

Microbial enzyme assays include the non-commercial rapid carbohydrate or Brown method (7) and several commercially available assays as Minitek™, BACTEC®, and RIM™-M (Photo 3-4), Gonochek II™, Vitek Neisseria-Haemophilus identification card, and Biolog GN Microplates™. A brief discussion of some of these not previously covered follows to provide some idea of their features.

In the Brown method, one drop of a heavy suspension of a pure culture of a species of *Neisseria* harvested from the surface of a chocolate agar plate is mixed with one drop of a 20% concentration of the carbohydrate solutions to be assayed. After 4 hours of incubation at 37°C, the results are read. The Minitek system uses paper disks impregnated with high concentrations of carbohydrates to be assayed. These are placed in wells, and wet with a heavy suspension of bacteria, then read after incubation at 35-37°C. Although overnight incubation may be necessary, most reactions will occur within 4 hours. Finally, the RIM-N (*Rapid Identification Method for Neisseria*) assays the organism in 4 carbohydrates, glucose, lactose, maltose, and sucrose. Inoculation of these with a loopful of isolated bacteria will provide results in 30 minutes when incubated at room temperature because of the presence of enzyme catalysts.

A broader spectrum of substrates is included in the IDS RapID NH System. Ten different reagents are tested by adding a heavy suspension of culture to each. After 4 hours of incubation at 37°C, reagents supplied with the kit are added as required and results read. Besides glucose and sucrose degradation tests, this kit is also designed to detect nitrate and nitrite reduction, the enzymes β-galactosidase, phosphatase, urease, penicillinase, and several other component activities potentially produced by the organism. Biolog Microplates™ allow up to 95 carbon sources to be tested per isolate. After inoculation of wells with a uniform saline suspension of pure culture, plates are incubated at 33-35°C. A purple color develops in a positive test, usually within 4 hours, due to tetrazolium reduction. Identicult™ Neisseria detects *N. lactamica*, gonococcus, and meningococcus by use of a filter paper strip containing spots with β-galactosidase, γ-glutamylaminopeptidase, and prolylaminopeptidase chromogenic substrates. These correspond to enzymes produced by each of the respective species. Thus, *N. lactamica*, for example, causes development of a blue spot because of its β-galactosidase, etc.

Several of the nontraditional assays can be used in an automated or semi-automated mode by incorporating machine readers and computerized

identification methods. Vitek AMS^R and Biolog Microstation™, for example, both determine color changes in their microwells that are then numerically reported to a computer. The BACTEC method measures CO_2 release from substrates, after which data is computer-analyzed.

Many antigen and antibody-based systems are also available for rapid identification or culture confirmation of pathogenic neisseriae and other species. (See Exercise 2, Section 4, page 42 for information on antigen-antibody reactions and their use in rapid assays.) Detection systems for pathogenic neisseriae based on an agglutination-type reaction include the GonoGen™ test, Phadebact® Antibody Omni Monoclonal Coagglutination test, Directigen Latex Agglutination test, and Wellcogen™ Latex Agglutination test. The Wellcogen and Directigen tests also detect *Streptococcus pneumoniae*, Group B streptococci, *Haemophilus influenzae* Type b, as well as *N. meningitidis*, all agents of meningitis. Bartels Diagnostics and Syva Company also provides direct fluorescent antibody reagents for culture confirmation of *N. gonorrhoeae* (Photo 3-5).

Meningococcus especially among the pathogenic neisseriae exists in serogroups named A, B, C, D, E, H, I, K, L, W135, X, Y and Z (1), of which A-C, Y, and W135 are the most commonly isolated pathogens (29). However, rarely isolated types Y and Z may cause pulmonary and other types of infections in immunosuppression states, including HIV infection (30). As with pneumococcus detection of these depend on epitope variations of the capsule. Wellcogen™ *N. meningitidis* A, C, Y, W135 kit, Directigen *Neisseria meningitidis* Group A and Y, Group B, and Group C and W135 latex bead assays (Photo 3-6) are examples of typing reagents available. Direct slide agglutination typing antisera against many groups are also available from Difco Laboratories and E-Y Laboratories.

Assays for gonococcus using the enzyme-linked antibody assay are GonoGen™ II and the Gonozyme™ test. In the latter, the specimen, collected on a swab, is suspended in specimen dilution buffer, then tested directly by an enzyme-linked antibody assay. Culturing of the specimen is unnecessary.

Pure culture suspensions of gonococcus also can be speciated by making use of their property of being agglutinated by wheat germ and soy bean lectins. When these are used in combination with detection of gamma glutamyl aminopeptidase (10) and other enzymes (45), *N. gonorrhoeae* can be identified within 15 minutes.

A genetic approach to identification of microorganisms using DNA probes is commercially available. This will be the subject of Section 2 of this exercise, and will be discussed there.

Again, accuracy in laboratory testing is an obvious requirement in any situation. In the clinical microbiology laboratory this applies to traditional as well as non-traditional tests. Quality control is necessary in all aspects of testing. Furthermore, newly introduced assays require extensive validation of their accuracy, usually by comparing results with traditional assays. Extensive literature is available concerning these (e.g. 9, 13, 21).

Section 2: Identification of *Neisseria gonorrhoeae* with a Genetic Probe

All organisms exhibiting differences in detectable characteristics differ in their genetic constitution. Such differences in deoxyribonucleic acid (DNA) are detectable by hybridization methods providing a unique opportunity to identify such organisms based upon the code responsible for those phenotypic differences. Though still early in development, inroads are being made in turning research tools into commercially-available identification systems. The purpose of this section is to give some background concerning genetic methods and nomenclature as it relates to microbial identification. Also, a commercially-available system will be used to demonstrate one approach using DNA hybridization technology to identify *Neisseria gonorrhoeae*.

Recall that DNA is formed of two strands (except in some viruses) of repeating purine nucleotide bases, guanine (G), adenine (A); and pyrimidine bases, thymine (T), and cytosine (C). These pair with one another *between* strands such that A-T and G-C are bonded together through hydrogen bonds (Figure 3-3). The uniqueness between individuals is determined by the base sequence *along* the strand. Ribonucleic acid (RNA) similarly has four bases, but uracil (U) is used in place of thymidine. Also, it is single stranded, except, again, in some viruses.

During DNA replication the double stranded (ds) DNA briefly uncoils and separates to single stranded (ss) DNA allowing the duplication process to occur. Separation of these is also

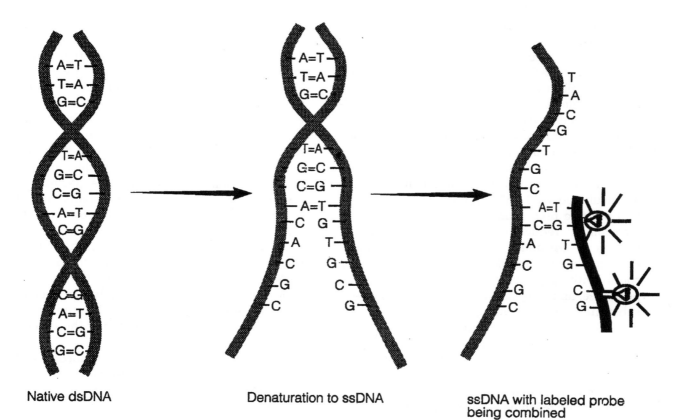

Native dsDNA   Denaturation to ssDNA   ssDNA with labeled probe being combined

Figure 3-3: Denaturation of dsDNA to ssDNA with hybridization of a labeled probe to a unique base sequence of the separated strand. (Adapted from Tenover (39).)

possible *in vitro* by denaturation, either through the use of heat or of chemicals (39). Indeed, the temperature at which half of the duplex chains become dissociated into single strands is called the temperature of melting or T_M (42). In turn, this is reflective of the mol% of G + C, thus it is a characteristic of DNA that has importance in microbial classification (e.g Table 3-1, **page 63**) (22).

Several general steps can be identified in the development and application of hybridizing methods to microbial identification. First, a unique base sequence, either DNA or RNA, must be determined or identified. (If RNA is chosen, it must be used to produce complementary DNA (cDNA) before proceeding.) This also requires what breadth of specificity is desired (that is, genus, species, or other level of identification). Second, a probe must be prepared that will detect the unique sequence. Third, a label to detect whether hybridization has occurred must be integrated into the probe. Finally, the probe must be tested to learn its usefulness. This is summarized in Figure 3-4.

Detecting unique base sequences within an organism requires the use of restriction endonucleases, a group of enzymes, each of which hydrolyzes ("cut") DNA between specific nucleotide sequences along the DNA strand. The nucleic acid may be from sources as chromosomal DNA from the whole cell, viral nucleic acid, sequence from a plasmid, or a portion of chromosomal DNA. The length of these cut pieces will vary depending on how frequently the specific sequences occur along the strand, and what endonucleases are employed. At this point, the location of the needed base sequence is unknown.

The next step is to splice enzymatically the entire preparation of cut DNA fragments (a "DNA library") into "cloning vectors," usually bacterial plasmids or to bacteriophage DNA. The cloning vector is then used to introduce the total sequence (integrated DNA fragments and DNA of the plasmid or phage) into their respective microbial hosts (*Escherichia coli* is commonly used). The host is plated and reproduces, amplifying the introduced sequence. Isolated phage or bacterial colonies are recovered, each containing an individually cloned sequence. The amplified DNA is recovered, purified, and again subjected to the appropriate restriction endonuclease. The desired sequence, by this process, is released from

plasmid or phage DNA, separated from contaminating nucleic acids by column chromatography and/or agarose gel electrophoresis, and recovered.

Alternatively, probes also may be prepared artificially. If the needed sequence is known, and it is an oligonucleotide of less than 100 nucleotides, it can be prepared in a nucleic acid synthesizer. This allows the preparation of a year's supply of probe in less than 24 hours (40). The purified sequences are now labeled so as to be able to test its usefulness. Probes are traditionally labeled with ^{32}P or other radioactive tracers to enable their detection. Other types will be discussed below. To screen the potential probes for a useful unique sequence, several methods can be used. One technique involves isolation of DNA or RNA from related strains or species of organisms, subject this to electrophoresis to obtain separation of fragments, then transfer these from the gel to a nitrocellulose (NC) membrane by Southern blotting (38), to which the nucleic acid avidly adheres (Figure 3-4). Alternatively, individual colonies of organisms to be tested may be blotted directly from growth plates to nitrocellulose, after which the nucleic acid is released from the cells, but held in place by the NC (17). In any case, application of a probe is now carried out. If a complementary sequence is present in the nucleic acid of the test organism, the probe will hybridize to it. After washing the nitrocellulose membrane with its adherent DNA and labeled probe to remove contaminants and non-bound probe, the location of the bound probe is determined by autoradiography. The probe can now be tested against DNA from other sources to find its specificity level.

It should be mentioned that specificity of reaction is not only a function of base sequence. It also can be influenced by (i) the length of the probe, and (ii) stringency conditions of hybridization. In the first case, generally the shorter the sequence in the probe, the higher the specificity, but the lower the sensitivity. Oligonucleotide probes (14-40 bp in length) may be capable of detecting a single nucleotide incompatibility on the target DNA by not hybridizing with it (43). However, this is also dependent on conditions under which hybridization is done that control stringency, the capacity of strands of DNA-DNA or DNA-RNA to maintain a stable double strand despite mismatched pairs (40). The conditions of stringency are dependent on temperature and/or

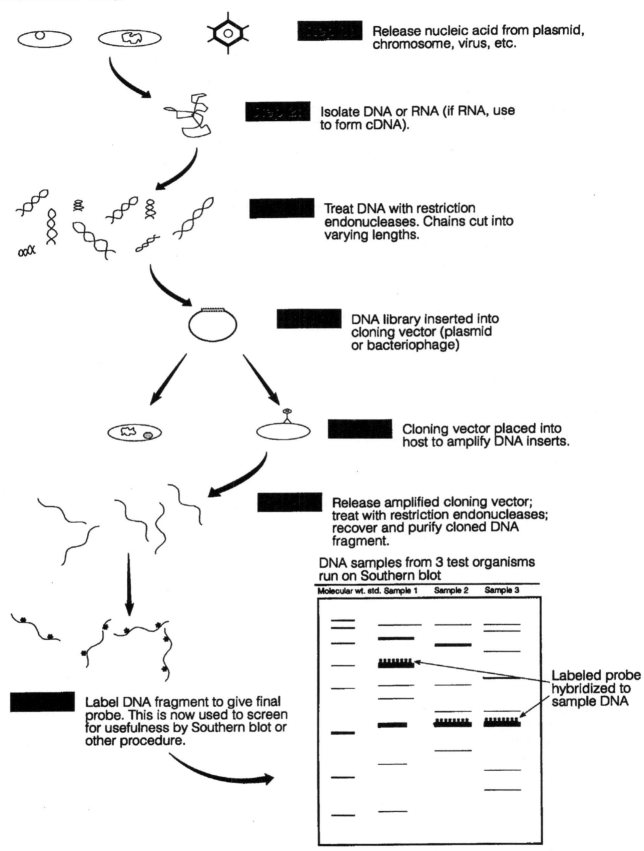

Release nucleic acid from plasmid, chromosome, virus, etc.

Isolate DNA or RNA (if RNA, use to form cDNA).

Treat DNA with restriction endonucleases. Chains cut into varying lengths.

DNA library inserted into cloning vector (plasmid or bacteriophage)

Cloning vector placed into host to amplify DNA inserts.

Release amplified cloning vector; treat with restriction endonucleases; recover and purify cloned DNA fragment.

DNA samples from 3 test organisms run on Southern blot

Molecular wt. std.   Sample 1   Sample 2   Sample 3

Labeled probe hybridized to sample DNA

Label DNA fragment to give final probe. This is now used to screen for usefulness by Southern blot or other procedure.

Figure 3-4: Outline of procedure for preparation and screening of genetic probe (adapted from Tenover (39).)

concentration of solutions used in hybridization. Probe stability between duplexes is reflected in T_M. For example, for hybrids of 20 bp or less, every mismatched pair causes about a 5°C decrease in T_M; for 150 bp, a mismatch of 1% of base pairs causes a T_M decrease of about 1°C. Hybridization should be done under the most stringent conditions.

Use of radioactively labeled probes, while sensitive, have obvious disadvantages. These include the radioactivity itself, which presents a health hazard and disposal problems, a short half-life for many of the most useful labels, as ^{32}P (half-life $= 14.3$ days), and cost. Furthermore, automation of the process to identify rapidly microorganisms with such probes is difficult. Fortunately these disadvantages can largely be overcome by using non-radioactive probes. Many possibilities exist, including the use of fluorochromes, a biotin-avidin system, antibodies, or enzymes (39). Of course, each of these must have a detectable component incorporated into the probe so hybridization can be detected. In the case of biotin-avidin, a nucleotide base is biotinylated and incorporated into the probe. After hybridization, this is detectable with an enzyme-labeled avidin, the latter having a high affinity for biotin. Addition of the enzyme substrate allows detection of the hybridization reaction. With antibodies, an antigenic fragment is incorporated into the probe, and the enzyme-labeled antibody used to detect the hybridization reaction. Finally, enzymes may be conjugated directly to the probes, then detected by applying their substrate. However, enzyme assays are slightly less sensitive than radiolabeled assays (11).

The sensitivity of DNA probes to detect their target is dependent on our capacity to detect the hybridization reaction. "Amplification" may be carried out by increasing the number of target molecules, as exemplified by the polymerase chain reaction (PCR) (12, 31). By this method a known nucleotide sequence (or target region), as a unique and identifying set of base pairs within a microorganism, can be increased in quantity *in vitro* to permit its identification. The process includes three general steps. First the dsDNA to be amplified is denatured to obtain ssDNA. Second, an oligonucleotide primer sequence (usually 15-30 nucleotides long) is hybridized to each ssDNA chain flanking the target region on the 5' and 3' sides, respectively. DNA polymerase, in the third

step, extends the primer sequence of each chain across the target region using free nucleotides in the medium, forming a complementary strand, and thus doubling the amount of the target region. By repeating this cycle, the newly formed dsDNA sequence can now serve as template resulting in another doubling of the target region (40). A calculation of $2n$, where $n=20$, demonstrates that an amplification of greater than one million times can occur in 20 cycles, assuming an efficiency of 100%. For various reasons, as polymerase denaturation and sample contamination, this is not achieved (36). However, its efficiency is sufficient that if a unique base sequence is being reproduced by PCR, potentially a single gene could lead to identification of a microorganism (or any other individual that produces DNA) (18, 37, 46). This technology is actively being pursued and nearing commercial application for diagnostic microbial identification.

Signal amplification also can be accomplished through non-radioactive labels attached to the probe. For example, horseradish peroxidase yields a higher substrate turnover using 2,2'-azino-di-(3-ethylbenzthiazoline sulphonate), ABTS, and higher sensitivity than alkaline phosphatase with p-nitrophenylphosphate substrate or β-galactosidase with o-nitrophenyl-β-D-galactopyranose substrate (33). Another example is the use of an acridinium-ester label on the probe. This compound is chemoluminescent in the presence of hydrogen peroxide with a high quantum yield, and equals the sensitivity of radioactive probes (2). The use of this probe has been developed into a commercially-available rapid test (Gen-Probe Inc.) for identification of several microorganisms or groups of microorganisms including *N. gonorrhoeae, Mycobacterium tuberculosis* complex, *Streptococcus agalactiae,* and *Coccidioides immitis.*

Another form of amplification is to use an enriched source of nucleic acid. Single stranded ribosomal RNA (rRNA), as an example, occurs at higher concentrations (approximately 10,000 copies of rRNA per cell (11) in the microbial cell than DNA, and therefore is more available for detection by a probe. Furthermore, rRNA, being single stranded, does not require denaturation and separation of complementary strands needed when dsDNA is used.

In the following procedure, the Gen-Probe AccuProbe system will be used. Although our assay will employ an isolated culture of *N. gonor-*

rhoeae (i.e. a culture confirmation test), the manufacturer also has available the PACE® system that is used directly on endocervical and urethral swabs. The culture confirmation test is 100% sensitive and specific (26); for endocervical swabs, it is 95% and 100%, respectively (27). The latter offers the added advantage of detecting gonococcus even after being in transport medium for an extended period (up to one month). Furthermore, the sample swab also can be used to test for *Chlamydia trachomatis*, agent of non-gonococcal urethritis. However, direct testing precludes the determination of β-lactamase sensitivity of gonococcus (32).

The Gen-Probe system, using a modification of the method of Lane, et al. (25) to develop sequencing information for appropriate genetic probes, involves hybridization of an acridinium-labeled DNA probe with rRNA. DNA•rRNA complexes protect the label from subsequent inactivation by added reagent, while unattached probe is inactivated. The hybridized acridinium ester is then activated to produce luminescence by addition of H_2O_2. The amount of luminescence, which is proportional to the amount of probe hybridized to rRNA, is determined in a luminometer (2).

The remainder of this exercise will be done according to the following protocol, with samples being done in pairs. Instructions provided by Gen-Probe must be followed. These are outlined below.

(Note: Another DNA probe system is available for use with the mycobacteria. See Exercise 21, Section 4 of the Introduction for further information.)

LABORATORY PROCEDURES

Each pair of students will be provided with a 24-48 hour culture of *Neisseria gonorrhoeae*, *N. subflava*, or *Branhamella catarrhalis*, **and** one other culture that will be an unknown, but may be *N. gonorrhoeae*. With these do the following.

A. Sample Preparation:
1. Remove two tubes containing lyophilized Probe Reagent from the foil pouch of the Gen-Probe AccuProbe kit. Label both with your Group No., the name of the known organism to one tube, and "unknown" to the second tube.

2. Remove the tube caps and, with a micropipetter, add 50 μl Specimen Diluent, *Reagent 1*, to each of the two tubes to dissolve the Probe Reagent. (Note: Reagents may be disposed of in sink, but must be flushed with large volumes of water to avoid accumulation of sodium azide.)
3. With an applicator stick, wire loop, or 1 μl disposable plastic loop, transfer the equivalent of a colony 1 mm in diameter (3-4 smaller colonies, or 1 μl loopful of cells) from your known culture to Tube 1, and an equivalent amount of your unknown to Tube 2. Use care not to include culture medium with your samples. Be sure your sample is well suspended by spinning the stick or loop.

B. Hybridization Steps:
1. To each sample tube, using a micropipetter with clean tips, add 50 μl Probe Diluent, *Reagent 2*. (If a precipitate has formed in this reagent, heat at 35-60°C and mix to dissolve.) Replace caps.
2. Mix the tube contents by shaking or using a vortex mixer.
3. Place your tubes in a 60°C (±1°C) water bath or heating block for no less than 15 minutes or longer than 20 minutes. It is critical that this temperature is maintained in this step and below in Step C-1. Also, be sure the reagent level in the tube is submersed in the water bath or below the top of the heating block.

C. Selection Steps.
1. Remove tubes from the 60°C incubator. Remove caps.
2. Add 300 μl Selection Reagent, *Reagent 3*, to each tube with a micropipetter.
3. Replace tube caps and *completely* mix reagents with a vortex mixer. (Lack of mixing can increase luminometer readings of negative control values above specified values.)
4. Again incubate tubes at 60°C (±1°C) in a water bath or heating block, this time for 5 minutes. Remove tubes and cool at room temperature for at least 5 minutes, but no longer than 30 minutes.

D. Detection Steps (Note: Your instructor will prepare the Gen-Probe PAL™ luminometer and explain its operation before this step):

1. Remove tube caps and discard. Wipe the outside of tubes with a damp paper towel or tissue to remove any surface residue.
2. Insert each tube into the luminometer as described by your instructor. Additions of Detection Reagents 1 and 2 are automatically made by the instrument. (Note: Detection Reagent 1 contains nitric acid; Detection Reagent 2 contains sodium hydroxide. Use appropriate precautions.)
3. Record the luminometer readings for your samples and that from other groups in the form provided at the end of this Exercise. After completion of readings, discard your tubes.
4. Compare luminometer readings obtained by you and others with cut-off values provided by Gen-Probe. These are as follows for the PAL Luminometer.

Luminometer Reading	Interpretation
≥1500 PLU[a]	Positive for *N. gonorrhoeae*
1200-1499 PLU	Inconclusive. Repeat sample run.
≤1200 PLU	Negative for *N. gonorrhoeae*

[a] PLU = PAL light units.

A recommended negative control for the Gen-Probe Accuprobe culture confirmation test is *N. meningitidis*, ATCC No. 13077; a positive control *N. gonorrhoeae*, ATCC 19424. These organisms should give values of <600 and >1500 PLU, respectively. Discuss your data and that for the class as a whole. Was your unknown *N. gonorrhoeae*? Do known non-gonococcal species including *N. meningitidis* ATCC No. 13077 give data comparable to that specified by Gen-Probe for a negative control?

QUESTIONS

1. From what kinds of specimens would one expect to isolate gonococcus? Meningococcus?
2. Outline precautions that should be taken in the transport of a clinical specimen suspected of containing gonococcus.

3. The oxidase test is very useful in the separation of Gram-negative facultatively anaerobic and aerobic rods. Give the chemical sequence of the oxidase reaction.
4. What is a lectin? How does it bring about the agglutination of gonococcus?
5. In the Gen-Probe *Neisseria gonorrhoeae* culture confirmation test, what is the purpose of:
   a. The lyophilized Probe Reagent contained in the tubes?
   b. Reagent 2, Probe Diluent?
   c. Reagent 3, Selection Reagent?
6. Many of the organisms used here and in other exercises are obtained from the American *Type Culture* Collection (ATCC). What is the function of this organization? Where is it located? What is its usefulness?

REFERENCES

1. Apicella, M. A. 1990. Neisseria meningitidis, p. 1600-1613. *In* G. L. Mandell, R. G. Douglas, Jr., and J. E. Bennett (ed.), Principles and practices of infectious diseases, 3rd ed. Churchill Livingston Inc. New York.
2. Arnold, L. J., Jr., P. W. Hammond, W. A. Wiese, and N. C. Nelson. 1989. Assay formats involving acridinium-ester-labeled DNA probes. Clin. Chem. **35**:1588-1594.
3. Baron, E. J., L. R. Peterson, and S. M. Finegold. 1994. Bailey & Scott's diagnostic microbiology, 9th ed. Mosby-Year Book, Inc., St. Louis. p. 123-167, 353-361, 386-405.
4. Bonin, P., T. T. Tamino, and H. H. Handsfield. 1984. Isolation of *Neisseria gonorrhoeae* on selective and nonselective media in a sexually transmitted disease clinic. J. Clin. Microbiol. **19**:218-220.
5. Bøvre, K. 1984. *Neisseriaceae*, Prévot 1933, p. 288-290. *In* N. R. Krieg, and J. G. Holt (ed.), Bergey's manual of systematic bacteriology, Vol. 1. Williams & Wilkins, Baltimore.
6. Bøvre, K. 1984. *Moraxella*, Lwoff 1939, p. 296-303. *In* N. R. Krieg, and J. G. Holt (ed.), Bergey's manual of systematic bacteriology, Vol. 1 Williams & Wilkins, Baltimore.
7. Brown, J. W. 1974. Modification of the rapid fermentation test for *Neisseria gonorrhoeae*. Appl. Microbiol. **27**:1027-1030.
8. Catlin, B. W. 1991. *Branhamaceae* fam. nov., a proposed family to accommodate the genera *Branhamella* and *Moraxella*. Int. J. Syst. Bacteriol. **41**:320-323.
9. Dillon, J. R., M. Carballo, and M. Pauze. 1988. Evaluation of eight methods for identification of pathogenic *Neisseria* species: Neisseria Kwik, RIM-N, Gonobio-test, Minitek, Gonochek II, GonoGen, Phadebact Monoclonal GC OMNI test, and Syva MicroTrak. J. Clin. Microbiol. **26**:493-497.
10. Doyle, R. J., F. Nedjat-Haiem, K. F. Keller, and C. E. Frasch. 1984. Diagnostic value of interaction between members of the family *Neisseriaceae* and lectins. J. Clin. Microbiol. **19**:383-387.
11. Enns, R. K. 1988. DNA probes: An overview and comparison with current methods. Lab. Med. **19**:295-300.
12. Erlich, H. A., D. Gelfand, and J. J. Sninsky. 1991. Recent advances in the polymerase chain reaction. Science **252**:1643-1651.
13. Gradus, M. S., C. M. Ng, and K. J. Silver. 1989. Comparison of the QuadFERM+ 2 hr identification system with conventional carbohydrate degradation tests for confirmatory identification of *Neisseria gonorrhoeae*. Sex. Transm. Dis. **16**:57-59.

14. Gray, L. D., R. E. Van Scoy, J. P. Anhalt, and P. K. W. Yu. 1989. Wound infection caused by *Branhamella catarrhalis*. J. Clin. Microb. **27**:818-820.

15. Griffin, C. W., III, M. A. Mehaffey, and E. C. Cook. 1983. Five years of experience with a national external quality control program for culture and identification of *Neisseria gonorrhoeae*. J. Clin. Microbiol. **18**:1150-1159.

16. Gröchel, D. H. M. 1990. Other Gram-negative cocci, p. 1632-1636. *In* G. L. Mandell, R. G. Douglas, Jr., and J. E. Bennett (ed.), Principles and practices of infectious diseases, 3rd ed. Churchill Livingston Inc. New York.

17. Grunstein, M., and D. S. Hogness. 1975. Colony hybridization: A method for isolation of cloned DNAs that contain a specific gene. Proc. Natl. Acad. Sci., U. S. A. **72**:3961-3965.

18. Guay, J.-M., D. Dubois, M.-J. Morency, S. Gagnon, J. Mercier, and R. C. Levesque. 1993. Detection of the pathogenic parasite *Toxoplasma gondii* by specific anplification of ribosomal sequences using comultiplex polymerase chain reaction. J. Clin. Microbiol. **31**:203-207.

19. Handsfield, H. H. 1990. Neisseria gonorrhoeae, p. 1613-1631. *In* G. L. Mandell, R. G. Douglas, Jr., and J. E. Bennett (ed.), Principles and practices of infectious diseases, 3rd ed. Churchill Livingston Inc. New York.

20. Howard, B. J., J. Klaas II, S. J. Rubin, A. S. Weissfeld, and R. C. Tilton. 1987. Clinical and pathogenic microbiology. The C. V. Mosby Co., St. Louis. p. 329-358.

21. Janda, W. M., and V. Sobieski. 1988. Evaluation of a ten-minute chromogenic substrate test for identification of pathogenic *Neisseria* species and *Branhamella catarrhalis*. Eur. J. Clin. Microbiol. Infect. Dis. **7**:25-29.

22. Johnson, J. L. 1984. Nucleic acids in bacterial classification, p. 8-11. *In* N. R. Krieg, and J. G. Holt (ed.), Bergey's manual of systematic bacteriology, Vol. 1 Williams and Wilkins, Baltimore.

23. Knapp, J. S. 1988. Historical perspectives and identification of *Neisseria* and related species. Clin. Microbiol. Rev. **1**:415-431.

24. Koneman, E. W., S. D. Allen, W. M. Janda, P. C. Schreckenberger, and W. C. Winn, Jr. 1992. Color atlas and textbook of diagnostic microbiology, 4th ed. J. B. Lippincott Co., Philadelphia. p. 185-242, 1075-1113.

25. Lane, D. J., B. Pace, G. J. Olsen, D. A. Stahl, M. L. Sogin, and N. R. Pace. 1985. Rapid determination of 16S ribosomal RNA sequences for phylogenetic analyses. Proc. Natl. Acad. Sci., U.S.A. **82**:6955-6959.

26. Lewis, J. S., D. Krainig-Brown, and D. A. Trainor. 1990. DNA probe confirmatory test for *Neisseria gonorrhoeae*. J. Clin. Microbiol. **28**:2349-2350.

27. Limberger, R. J., R. Biega, A. Evancoe, L. McCarthy, L. Slivienski, and M. Kirkwood. 1992. Evaluation of culture and the Gen-Probe PACE-2 assay for detection of *Neisseria gonorrhoeae* and *Chlamydia trachomatis* in endocervical specimens transported to a State health laboratory. J. Clin. Microbiol. **30**:1162-1166.

28. MacFaddin, J. F. 1980. Biochemical tests for identification of medical bacteria, 2nd ed. Williams & Wilkins, Baltimore. p. 249-260.

29. Morello, J. A., W. M. Janda, and G. V. Doern. 1991. *Neisseria* and *Branhamella*, p. 258-276. *In* A. Balows, W. J. Hausler, Jr., K. L. Herrmann, H. D. Isenberg, and H. J. Shadomy (ed.), Manual of clinical microbiology, 5th ed., American Society for Microbiology, Washington, D. C.

30. Morla, N., M. Guibourbenche, and J.-Y. Riou. 1992. *Neisseria* spp. and AIDS. J. Clin. Microbiol. **30**:2290-2294.

31. Mullis, K., F. Faloona, S. Scharf, R. Saiki, G. Horn, and H. Erlich. 1986. Specific enzymatic amplification of DNA in vitro: The polymerase chain reaction. Cold Spring Harbor Symp. Quant. Biol. **51**:263-273.

32. Panke, E. S., L. I. Yang, P. A. Leist, P. Magevney, R. J. Fry, and R. G. Lee. 1991. Comparison of Gen-Probe DNA Probe test and culture for the detection of *Neisseria gonorrhoeae* in endocervical specimens. J. Clin. Microbiol. **29**:883-888.

33. Porstmann, B., T. Porstmann, E. Nugel, and U. Evers. 1985. Which of the commonly used marker enzymes gives the best results in calorimetric and fluorimetric enzyme immunoassays: horseradish peroxidase, alkaline phosphatase or β-galactosidase? J. Immunol. Meth. **79**:27-37.

34. Rossau, R. G., G. Vandenbussche, S. Thielemans, P. Segers, H. Grosch, E. Göthe, M. Mannheim, and J. DeLay. 1989. Ribosomal ribonucleic acid cistron similarities and desoxyribonucleic acid homologies of *Neisseria, Kingella, Eikenella, Simonsiella, Alysiella*, and Centers for Disease Control groups EF-4 and M-5 in the emended family *Neisseriaceae*. Int. J. Syst. Bacteriol. **39**:185-198.

35. Rossau, R., A. Van Landschoot, M. Gillis, and J. De Lay. 1991. Taxonomy of *Moraxellaceae* fam. nov., a new bacterial family to accommodate the genera *Moraxella, Acinetobacter*, and *Psychrobacter* and related organisms. Int. J. Syst. Bacteriol. **41**:310-319.

36. Sardelli, A. D. 1993. Plateau effect - understanding PCR limitations. Amplifications: a forum for PCR users. Issue 9:1, 3-5.

37. Sauvaigo, S., V. Barlet, N. Guettari, P. Innocenti, F. Parmentier, C. Bastard, J. M. Seigneurin, J. C. Chermann, R. Teoule, and J. Marchand. 1993. Standardized nested polymerase chain reaction-based assay for detection of Human Immunodeficiency Virus Type 1 DNA in whole blood lysates. J. Clin. Microbiol. **31**:1066-1074.

38. Southern, E. M. 1975. Detection of specific sequences among DNA fragments separated by gel electrophoresis. J. Mol. Biol. **98**:503-517.

39. Tenover, F. C. 1988. Diagnostic deoxyribonucleic acid probes for infectious diseases. Clin. Microbiol. Rev. **1**:82-101.

40. Tenover, F. C. 1991. Molecular methods for the clinical microbiology laboratory, p. 119-127. *In* A. Balows, W. J. Hausler, Jr., K. L. Herrmann, H. D. Isenberg, and H. J. Shadomy (ed.), Manual of clinical microbiology, 5th ed., American Society for Microbiology, Washington, D. C.

41. Thayer, J. D., and J. E. Martin. 1966. Improved medium selective for cultivation of *Neisseria gonorrhoeae* and *Neisseria meningitidis*. Pub. Hlth. Rep. **81**:559-562.

42. Wahl, G. M., S. L. Berger, and A. R. Kimmel. 1987. Molecular hybridization in immobilized nucleic acids: Theoretical concepts and practical considerations. Meth. Enzymol. **152**:399-407.

43. Wallace, R. B., J. Shaffer, R. F. Murphy, J. Bonner, R. Hirose, and K. Itakura. 1979. Hybridization of synthetic oligodeoxyribonucleotides to ΦX174 DNA. The effect of a single base pair mismatch. Nucleic Acids Res. **6**:3543-3557.

44. Windall, J. J., M. M. Hall. J. A. Washington II, J. Douglass, and L. A. Weed. 1980. Inhibitory effects of vancomycin on *Neisseria gonorrhoeae* in Thayer-Martin medium. J. Infect. Dis. **142**:775.

45. Yajko, D. M., A. Chu, and W. K. Hadley. 1984. Rapid confirmatory identification of *Neisseria gonorrhoeae* with lectins and chromogenic substrates. J. Clin. Microbiol. **19**:380-382.

46. Yoon, K.-H., S.-N. Cho, M.-K. Lee, R. M. Abalos, R. V. Cellona, T. T. Fajardo, Jr., L. S. Guido, E. C. Dela Cruz, G. P. Walsh, and J.-D. Kim. 1993. Evaluation of polymerase chain reaction amplfication of *Mycobacterium leprae*-specific repetitive sequence in biopsy specimens from leprosy patients. J. Clin. Microbiol. **31**:895-899.

Exercise 3
Neisseria and *Branhamella catarrhalis*
Data Table 1: Known Cultures Results

		Age[a]	N. gonorrhoeae			N. subflava			B. catarrhalis		
			NA[b]	MTM[b]	Other	NA	MTM	Other	NA	MTM	Other
Colony size and Colony Form[c]	mm										
	Punctiform										
	Irregular										
	Circular										
	Rhizoid										
	Filamentous										
	Other										
Colony Surface	Flat										
	Raised										
	Convex										
	Pulvinate										
	Other										
Colony Margin	Entire										
	Undulate										
	Lobate										
	Erose										
	Other										
Colony Consistency	Butyrous										
	Viscid										
	Membranous										
	Brittle										
	Other										
Colony Optical Character	Opaque										
	Translucent										
	Dull										
	Glistening										
	Other										
Colony Surface	Smooth										
	Rough										
	Other										
Colony Color											
Other											

[a] Culture age. [b] NA = Nutrient agar; MTM = Modified Thayer Martin medium. [c] See Appendix 1 for description of colony terminology.

Exercise 3
Neisseria and Branhamella catarrhalis
Data Table 2: Known Culture Results

		Age[a]	N. gonorrhoeae			N. subflava			M. catarrhalis		
			NA[b]	MTM[b]	Other	NA	MTM	Other	NA	MTM	Other
Oxidase test											
Superoxol test											
Catalase test											
Acid Production	Glucose										
	Fructose										
	Maltose										
	Sucrose										
Nitrate test											
Nitrite test											
Gram stain (1000X)	Gram reaction										
	Morphology										
	Arrangement										
Other											

[a] Culture age. [b] NA = Nutrient agar; MTM = Modified Thayer Martin medium.

OTHER LABORATORY NOTES

Exercise 3
Neisseria* and *Branhamella catarrhalis
Data Table 3: Gonococcus Clinical Isolate Results

		Age[a]	NA[b]	MTM[b]	Other	Other	Other
Colony size and Colony Form[c]	mm						
	Punctiform						
	Irregular						
	Circular						
	Rhizoid						
	Filamentous						
	Other						
Colony Surface	Flat						
	Raised						
	Convex						
	Pulvinate						
	Other						
Colony Margin	Entire						
	Undulate						
	Lobate						
	Erose						
	Other						
Colony Consistency	Butyrous						
	Viscid						
	Membranous						
	Brittle						
	Other						
Colony Optical Character	Opaque						
	Translucent						
	Dull						
	Glistening						
	Other						
Colony Surface	Smooth						
	Rough						
	Other						
Colony Color							
Other							

[a] Culture age. [b] NA = Nutrient agar; MTM = Modified Thayer Martin medium. [c] See Appendix 1 for description of colony terminology.

Exercise 3
Neisseria and *Branhamella catarrhalis*
Data Table 4: Gonococcus Clinical Isolate Results

		Age[a]	NA[b]	MTM[b]	Other	Other	Other
Oxidase test							
Superoxol test							
Catalase test							
Acid Production	Glucose						
	Fructose						
	Maltose						
	Sucrose						
Nitrate test							
Nitrite test							
Gram stain (1000X)	Gram reaction						
	Morphology						
	Arrangement						
Other							

[a] Culture age. [b] NA = Nutrient agar; MTM = Modified Thayer Martin medium.

Identification of *Neisseria gonorrhoeae* with a Genetic Probe
Data Table 5: Gen-Probe AccuProbe Hybridization Test Results

Group No.	Name of Organism	Luminometer Units
Your Data:		

Class Data:

EXERCISE 4
Moraxella and *Acinetobacter*

Members of the genus *Moraxella* and *Acinetobacter* are considered to be of low virulence, and can produce infections usually only under opportunistic conditions. *M. nonliquifaciens,* one of the most frequent disease agents, has been isolated from ear, nose, throat, eye, urine, cerebrospinal fluid, and blood (5). *Acinetobacter* has been associated with bacteremia, pneumonia, peritonitis, wound and skin infections, etc., especially opportunistic in nature (1). However, both of these genera are usually of more importance in that they are common inhabitants of several areas of the body of humans and lower animals and therefore may be mistaken for more common pathogens. *Moraxella* is common on the mucous membranes, especially of the upper respiratory tract, although also found in the urogenital tract and skin (6). *Acinetobacter* inhabits many body locations including skin, vagina, sputum, urine and feces, and can be found extensively as a naturally-occurring free-living organisms in soil and water (1, 7).

Acinetobacter spp. are Gram-negative, oxidase negative, non-motile rods (7); *Moraxella* are oxidase-positive, non-motile rods and cocci (3). Both are strict aerobes, non-glucose fermenting, and catalase positive, and can morphologically be confused with pathogenic neisseriae (Photo 4-1). Many of the *Moraxella* spp., in contrast to the *Acinetobacter,* require complex media. Table 4-1 gives additional properties of selected species in these two genera (Note: *B. catarrhalis* characteristics are listed in Table 3-2). As noted in Table 4-1, one recommended classification of the genus *Acinetobacter* contains at least 6 species (2) instead of the single *A. calcoaceticus* used previously with or without Biotype names *anitratus, lwoffi, haemolyticus,* and/or *alcaligines* (3, 11).

There are several commercially available non-traditional assays for the identification of non-fermenting bacteria (NFB). Miniaturized assays that detect microbial enzyme production from heavy suspensions of purified isolates include API® Rapid* NFT, Biolog Microplates™, Sensititre®, BBL® Minitek™, and RapID™ NF Plus. The MIDI Microbial Identification System uses cellular fatty acid profiles by gas chromatography and subsequent MIS (Microbial Identification System) automated analysis. Identification here, as in other cases, can be accomplished by comparison of results with a database library.

MATERIALS

Part 1

Per pair of students
  Nutrient agar slant culture each of *Moraxella osloensis,* and *Acinetobacter calcoaceticus.*
  1 Nutrient agar (NA) plate
  1 MacConkey agar plate
  2 tubes triple sugar iron (TSI) agar slants
  4 tubes Oxidation-Fermentation medium containing glucose (O-F glucose)
  4 ml sterile petrolatum
  Oxidase and catalase reagents

LABORATORY PROCEDURES
(See Figure 4-1 for procedural diagram):

Part 1

Each pair of students will be provided with a nutrient agar slant culture of *M. osloensis* and *A. calcoaceticus.* Complete the following with each:
1. Prepare a Gram's stain and microscopically observe. Do the organisms appear as cocci or rods? Compare the typical colony morphology of each species and record on Data Table 2 at the end of this exercise.
2. Streak for isolation on one-half plate each of nutrient agar and of MacConkey agar. This latter medium is mildly selective for Gram-negative bacteria, and has compounds that help to differentiate glucose-fermenting bacteria from those that do not. More information concerning this and other selective and differential plating media is provided in the Introduction to Exercises 8 and 9, **page 126.**
3. Inoculate a triple sugar iron (TSI) agar slant by first stabbing it in the center of the tube with a straight bacteriological inoculating needle containing inoculum to the butt of the agar, then withdraw it and streak the slant in the same stroke. (See **page 127** for more information concerning the use of this medium.)

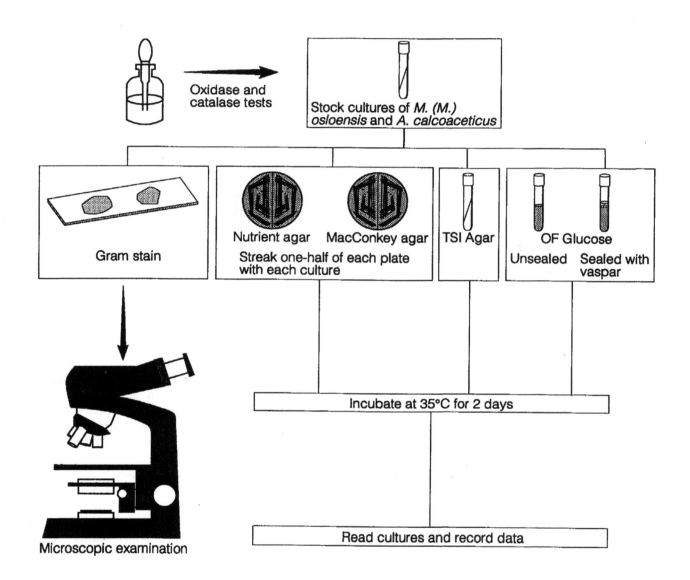

Figure 4-1: Procedural outline of Exercise 4. Similar steps are done for both *M. osloensis* and *A. calcoaceticus.*

Table 4-1
Selected Properties of Some *Moraxella* sp. and *Acinetobacter* sp. (2, 5, 8, 10)

Organism	Growth on MacConkey agar	Acid from glucose[b]	Nitrate reduction	Citrate Utilization	Gelatin liquifaction	L-Phenylalanine Utilization	41-42°C growth
Moraxella							
M. osloensis	V[c]	−	V⁻	−	−	V⁻	V
M. lacunata[d]	−	−	+	−	V⁺	V	−
M. phenylpyruvica	V	−	V	−	−	+	−
M. nonliquifaciens[d]	−	−	+	−	−	−	V
M. atlantae	+	−	−	−	−	−	−
Acinetobacter							
A. calcoaceticus	+	+	−	+	−	+	−
A. lwoffi	+	−	−	−	−	−	−
A. haemolyticus	+	V	−	+	+	−	−
A. baumannii	+	+	−	+	−	V⁺	+
A. johnsonii	+	−	−	+	−	−	−
A. junii	+	−	−	V⁺	−	−	+

[a] See Table 3-2 for information on *B. catarrhalis*. Five of six *Moraxella* spp. (4) and all presently accepted species of *Acinetobacter* shown here.
[b] Reaction in O - F medium.
[c] + = >90% positive; − = <10% positive; V⁺ = >70% positive; V⁻ = <30% positive; V = 11 - 89% positive.
[d] *M. lacunata* and *M. liquifaciens* can be separated by testing for Loeffler's slant digestion where only the former is positive for this test.

4. Inoculate a pair of O-F glucose tubes per species. Again, use a straight needle containing a heavy inoculum. Stab the medium several times to one-forth to one-half the depth of the medium. Overlay the medium of one of each pair of tubes with melted sterile petrolatum. (Why is this done?) If not liquid, melt the petrolatum by placing in a 60°C water bath.

5. Test cultures appropriately with oxidase and catalase reagents. Record your data.

6. Incubate your inoculated cultures at 35°C for 48 hours. Use of a candle jar is unnecessary.

Part 2

Observe your cultures of *A. calcoaceticus* and *M. osloensis* inoculated previously. Make at least the following observations:

1. Fully describe typical isolated colonies on nutrient agar plates for each species. (Also see Photo 4-2.) Record on Data Table 1 provided at the end of this exercise.

2. Note the relative amounts of growth on the MacConkey plates. This can be recorded as +1 (scant growth), +2 (marginal growth), +3 (moderate growth), or +4 (excellent growth) relating to whether growth occurs along the first, second, third, or fourth legs of the streak lines, respectively. Thus, growth only on the first streak is recorded as a +1, on the fourth streak as +4, and so on. Also note the color of the colonies, if any.

3. Record the following from your TSI agar slants:

    a. The slant reaction is "A" if it is yellow, showing the presence of acid from sucrose or lactose fermentation, or "K" if red indicating an alkaline reaction and no fermentation.

    b. If the butt is yellow indicating fermentation of sucrose, lactose, and/or glucose, record as acid ("A"), or alkaline ("K") if red showing no fermentation.

    c. H₂S is "+" or "-" depending on the presence of blackening in the agar due formation of hydrogen sulfide by the organism.

    d. Gas production is "+" or "-" indicating whether gas is produced as seen by fracturing of the agar.

4. Observe the O-F glucose tubes for the presence of oxidative (open tube) or fermentive (sealed tube) acid production from the substrate sugar. The weakly fermentive activity of bacteria can be more readily detected in this medium compared to standard phenol red broths. (Why?) (9).

5. Record and discuss your results.

OTHER NOTES

One should remember that both *Moraxella* and *Acinetobacter* may inhabit similar body locations as the pathogenic neisseriae studied in Exercise 3. It is worth repeating that it is easy to confuse them in such cases because of their similar morphological appearance on Gram's stain. Therefore, microscopic examination of clinical material should not be used as a definitive laboratory diagnosis in, for example, gonorrhea. Further confusion can arise because all of these organisms produce catalase, and *Moraxella* spp. are also oxidase positive. However, the genera can be distinguished from *N. meningitidis* and *N. gonorrhoeae* by further analysis. Examples of some of these differences should be evident by comparing your results herein with those of Exercise 3.

REFERENCES

1. Allen, D. M., and B. J. Hartman. 1990. Acinetobacter species, p. 1696-1700. In G. L. Mandell, R. G. Douglas, Jr., and J. E. Bennett (ed.), Principles and practices of infectious diseases, 3rd ed. Churchill Livingstone, New York.

2. Bouvet, P. J. M., and P. A. D. Grimont. 1986. Taxonomy of the genus *Acinetobacter* with the recognition of *Acinetobacter baumannii* sp. nov., *Acinetobacter haemolyticus* sp. nov., *Acinetobacter johnsonii* sp. nov., and *Acinetobacter junii* sp. nov. and emended descriptions of *Acinetobacter calcoaceticus* and *Acinetobacter lwoffi*. Int. J. Syst. Bacteriol. **36**:228-240.

3. Bøvre, K. 1984. *Moraxella* Lwoff 1939, p. 296-303. In N. R. Krieg, and J. G. Holt (ed.), Bergey's manual of systematic bacteriology, Vol. 1. Williams & Wilkins, Baltimore.

4. Catlin, B. W. 1991. *Branhamaceae* fam. nov., a proposed family to accommodate the genera *Branhamella* and *Moraxella*. Int. J. Syst. Bacteriol. **41**:320-323.

5. Graham, D. R., J. D. Band, C. Thornsberry, D. G. Hollis, and R. E. Weaver. 1990. Infection caused by *Moraxella, Moraxella urethralis, Moraxella*-like groups M-5 and M-6, and *Kingella kingae* in the United States, 1953-1980. Rev. Infect. Dis. **12**:423-431.

6. Gröschel, D. H. M. 1990. Other Gram-negative cocci, p. 1632-1636. In G. L. Mandell, R. G. Douglas, Jr., and J. E. Bennett (ed.), Principles and practices of infectious diseases, 3rd ed. Churchill Livingstone, New York.

7. Juni, E. 1984. *Acinetobacter* Brisou and Prévot 1954, p. 303-307. In N. R. Krieg, and J. G. Holt (ed.), Bergey's manual of systematic bacteriology, Vol. 1. Williams & Wilkins, Baltimore.

8. Koneman, E. W., S. D. Allen, W. M. Janda, P. C. Schreckenberger. and W. C. Winn, Jr. 1992. Color atlas and textbook of diagnostic microbiology, 4th ed. J. B. Lippincott Co., Philadelphia. p. 185-242.

9. MacFaddin, J. F. 1980. Biochemical tests for identification of medical bacteria, 2nd ed. Williams & Wilkins, Baltimore, p. 260-268.

10. Pickett, M. J., D. G. Hollis, and E. J. Bottone. 1991. Miscellaneous Gram-negative bacteria, p. 410-428. In A. Balows, W. J. Hausler, Jr., K. L. Herrmann, H. D. Isenberg, and H. J. Shadomy (ed.), Manual of clinical microbiology, 5th ed. American Society for Microbiology, Washington, D. C.

11. Rubin, S. J., P. A. Granato, and B. L. Wasilauskas. 1985. Glucose non-fermenting bacteria, p. 330-349. In E. H. Lennette, A. Balows, W. J. Hausler, Jr., and H. J. Shadomy (ed.), Manual of clinical microbiology, 3rd ed. American Society for Microbiology, Washington, D. C.

Exercise 4
Data Table 1: *Moraxella osloensis* and *Acinetobacter calcoaceticus* Results

		Culture Age[a]	M. osloensis		A. calcoaceticus	
			Nutrient agar	Other	Nutrient agar	Other
Colony size and Colony Form	mm					
	Punctiform					
	Irregular					
	Circular					
	Rhizoid					
	Filamentous					
	Other					
Colony Surface	Flat					
	Raised					
	Convex					
	Pulvinate					
	Other					
Colony Margin	Entire					
	Undulate					
	Lobate					
	Erose					
	Other					
Colony Consistency	Butyrous					
	Viscid					
	Membranous					
	Brittle					
	Other					
Colony Optical Character	Opaque					
	Translucent					
	Dull					
	Glistening					
	Other					
Colony Surface	Smooth					
	Rough					
	Other					
Colony Color						
Other						

[a] Culture age in hours.

Exercise 4
Data Table 2: *Moraxella osloensis* and *Acinebacter calcoaceticus* Results

		Culture Age[a]	M. osloensis		A. calcoaceticus	
			NA[b]	Other	NA	Other
Catalase test						
Oxidase test						
Gram stain	Reaction					
	Morphology					
	Arrangement					
MacConkey Agar	Amount of Growth					
Carbohydrate degradation assays	OF Glucose (Aerobic)					
	OF Glucose (Anaerobic)					
TSI[c]	Slant Reaction					
	Butt Reaction					
	H_2S					
	Gas					

[a] Culture age in hours. [b] NA = Nutrient agar; [c] Usual designations for TSI slant and butt reactions: K = alkaline; A = acid produced.

LABORATORY NOTES

INTRODUCTION TO THE GRAM-NEGATIVE AEROBIC AND FACULTATIVELY ANAEROBIC RODS

The Gram-negative aerobic and facultatively anaerobic rods comprise a heterogenous and complex group of organisms. Of those to be covered in this manual, the Gram-negative aerobic rods include members of the *Pseudomonadaceae* and several genera of doubtful affiliation such as *Brucella, Bordetella,* and *Francisella*. The Gram-negative facultative rods include the members of the families *Pasteurellaceae, Enterobacteriaceae* and *Vibrionaceae* (Table 5-1).

Unfortunately, the commonality of Gram reaction, morphology, and oxygen relationships give a massive group of organisms that vary in many other ways. This section is therefore approached based on a combination of other factors including

(i) those bacteria that have a need for complex nutritional requirements and inhabit the oropharyngeal cavity (*Haemophilus* and *Bordetella*); (ii) those most commonly associated with lower animals (*Brucella, Francisella, Pasteurella,* and *Yersinia*); (iii) those that are usually intestinal parasites (the *Enterobacteriaceae,* excluding *Yersinia*); and closely allied curving rods (*Vibrionaceae*). *Pseudomonas* and the *Legionellaceae* are linked to all of the above only by virtue of their being Gram-negative aerobic rods and their capability of being pathogens. Table 5-1 summarizes some of the pertinent properties of each of these groups as well as some of their more common associations.

Table 5-1
Differential Characteristics of Gram-Negative Aerobic and Facultatively Anaerobic Rods (16)

Family or genus	Oxygen Relationship	Size, μm	Oxidase Reaction	Catalase Reaction	Acid from Glucose	Flagellar Arrangement[c]	Strict Parasite	Common Associations
Pasteurellaceae	F[a]	0.2-0.3 x 0.3-2.0	+[b]	+	+	N	+	Vertebrates and birds
Bordetella	A	0.2-0.5 x 0.5-2.0	V[b]	V	−	N	+	Human respiratory tract; other vertebrates
Brucella	A	0.5-0.7 x 0.6-1.5	+	+	−	N	+	Intracellular parasite, usually of lower animals
Francisella	A	0.2-0.7 x 0.2-1.7	−	+	+	N	−	Lower animals
Enterobacteriaceae	F	0.3-1.0 x 1-6	−	+[b]	+	L, P, N	−	Plants, animals, and free-living
Vibrionaceae	F	0.3-1.0 x 1.0-3.5	+	+	+	P	−	Aquatic free-living and aquatic animals
Pseudomonadaceae	A	0.5-1.0 x 1.5-5.0	+	+	V	P	−	Environmental
Legionellaceae	A	0.3-0.9 x 2-20	− to ±	+	−	P, L	−	Environmental, especially in water

[a] F = facultatively anaerobic; A = Strictly aerobic. [b] + = usually positive; ± = weak reaction; − = usually negative; V = differs between genera or species. [c] N = no flagella; L = lateral flagella; P = polar flagella.

EXERCISE 5
Haemophilus and *Bordetella*

The species of *Haemophilus* and *Bordetella* found in humans frequently inhabit the same body locations and resemble each other in morphology, both being small, Gram-negative coccobacillary to rod-shaped bacteria (Photo 5-1, 5-2, and 5-3). Because of these practical similarities, they will be studied together. Taxonomically, however, the two groups are quite different. *Haemophilus* is a member of the family *Pasteurellaceae,* which also includes the *Pasteurella* and *Actinobacillus* (18). It is facultatively anaerobic and requires the blood components X (heme) and V (nicotinamide adenine dinucleotide, NAD, or NAD phosphate, NADP) factors for its growth.

Of 16 recognized species, the most important pathogenic species of *Haemophilus* are *H. para-influenzae,* the most common disease-causing member, and *H. influenzae,* potentially the most serious diseases-causing agent. Both generally cause infections in similar areas of the body as larynx, eyes, ear, brain, lungs, etc. (9). *H. influenzae,* especially type b, is the most frequent cause of meningitis in many countries, including the U. S., particularly in young children (1, 19), but is never the cause of influenza (what is the name of the agent that does?). Another pathogenic species is *H. aegyptius,* also called the Koch-Weeks bacillus and *H. influenzae* biotype aegyptius. It is responsible for contagious conjunctivitis and other conditions, including Brazilian Purpuric Fever, a fulminant pediatric disease that became recognized in the last decade (3). *H. aphrophilus* and *H. paraphrophilus* have also been isolated from infectious processes, as has *H. ducreyi,* the agent of soft chancre or chancroid, a venereal disease. However, all of the preceding except *H. ducreyi* and *H. aegyptius,* are more frequently isolated as normal flora bacteria. Also, *H. haemolyticus* (see Exercise 2, page 33), *H. parahaemolyticus* and *H. segnis* have been isolated as normal flora from the upper respiratory tract and oral cavity, and in *H. parainfluenzae,* from the urethra and vagina (9, 13).

Bordetella, unlike *Haemophilus,* is currently unaffiliated with any family. Furthermore, its member species are strict aerobes with a respiratory-type of metabolism, and do not have a strict requirement for X and V factors. The most important species in the *Bordetella* capable of causing human infection is *B. pertussis,* the etiologic agent of whooping cough. *B. parapertussis* and *B. bronchiseptica* also can be associated with whooping cough-like infections, although the latter is more commonly the cause of bronchopneumonia in lower animals (6, 20). Interestingly, these three species are genetically similar, differing primarily in their phenotypic ability to regulate toxin production (6). A commonly accepted fourth species, *B. avium,* (12) causes disease in turkeys, but its pathogenicity in other animals is unknown.

If *B. pertussis* is suspect, it is grown on Bordet-Gengou (B-G) agar where, as will be seen in the following exercise, it produces characteristic colonies. While Regan-Lowe and Jones-Kendrick agars, which give better recovery and have improved keeping qualities can be used (4), B-G yields the more typical colony forms expected from this organism. Antibiotics as cephalexin may be added to the medium of choice to inhibit normal flora of the nasopharyngeal cavity, especially *S. aureus,* which is antagonistic to the growth of *B. pertussis* (6). But, because some strains of *B. pertussis* are inhibited by this compound, culture should always include a medium free of antimicrobials (4). Furthermore, it should be noted that, *B. parapertussis* and *B. bronchiseptica,* unlike *B. pertussis,* will grow on standard sheep blood agar and less nutritionally complete media (6).

For primary isolation of haemophilae, highly enriched media is used. Chocolate agar containing 1% IsoVitalex, a chemically-defined supplement that provides V factor and other supporting growth factors (21), has been commonly used. Recently, GCYSB (GC base, yeast autolysate, sheep blood) agar has been reported to yield improved growth, while being easier to prepare and less expensive (22). If a heavily competing flora is expected to be present, addition of 300 mg/l bacitracin serves to provide selectivity for haemophilae (15).

Table 5-2 provides additional information and comparisons of selected properties of species of *Bordetella* and *Haemophilus.* The requirement of

Table 5-2
Some Differentiating Characteristics of *Haemophilus* and *Bordetella* (6, 13, 15, 20)[a]

Genus - species	β-lysis[b]	Catalase Reaction	Oxidase Reaction	ALA to Porphyrin	Requirement for		Nitrate Reduced	Urease	Acid produced from:			
					X factor	V factor			Glucose	Lactose	Sucrose	Mannose
H. influenzae[c]	−	+[d]	+[e]	−	+	+	+	V	+	−	−	−
H. aegyptius	−	+	+	−	+	+	+	+	+	−	−	−
H. parainfluenzae	−	V	+	+	−	+	+	V	+	−	+	+
H. ducreyi	−	−	+	−	+	−	+	−	−	−	−	−
H. haemolyticus	+	+	+	−	+	+	+	+	+	−	−	−
H. parahaemolyticus	+	+	+	+	−	+	+	+	+	−	+	−
H. paraphrohaemolyticus	+	+	+	+	−	+	+	+	+	−	+	−
H. segnis	−	V	−	+	−	+	+	−	+[W]	−	+[W]	−
H. aphrophilus	−	−	−	+[W]	−	−	+	−	+	+	+	+
H. paraphrophilus	−	−	+	+	−	+	+	−	+	+	+	+
B. pertussis	ND[d]	V	+	ND	−	−	−	−	NF	NF	NF	NF
B. parapertussis	ND	+	−	ND	−	−	−	+	NF	NF	NF	NF
B. bronchiseptica	ND	+	+	ND	−	−	+	+	NF	NF	NF	NF

[a] Hemolysis on rabbit or horse blood agar.
[b] Ten of sixteen species of *Haemophilus* and three of four species of *Brodetella* shown.
[c] *H. influenzae* consists of 6 Biovarieties and *H. parainfluenzae* includes 4 Biovarieties based upon biochemical patterns.
[d] + = 90% or greater positive; − = 10% or less positive; V = 11 - 89% positive; +[W] = weak reaction; NF = nonfermentive; ND = no data.
[e] Biovar. 4 gives variable reactions.

X or V factors by haemophilae is an important diagnostic characteristic. Species of *Bordetella* shown here can be distinguished from *Haemophilus* by the nitrate reduction and glucose fermentation tests. Also, the *Bordetella* do not have X and V factor requirements. Furthermore, this organism is relatively inert from a biochemical standpoint, which in itself can be helpful in laboratory identification. *B. parapertussis,* except for the oxidase reaction, is similar, at least for the set of reactions given in Table 5-2. This has led to the use of serological assays to distinguish *B. pertussis.*

There actually has been increasing reliance on serologic methods for identification of *B. pertussis.* The most acceptable is the direct fluorescent antibody (DFA) technique to identify the presence of the bacterial cell antigen. Unfortunately, the assay is subject to cross reactions and variability when done by different technical personnel.

Therefore it is recommended that this assay be used in conjunction with culture (4). Indeed, because of the lack of sensitivity and specificity of DFA assays, Halperin, Bortolussi, and Wort (8) recommend that culture and enzyme immunoassay be done in the pediatric population to detect antibodies against pertussis toxin (PT) and filamentous hemagglutination (FHA) antigens. Other approaches are also being taken, such as the use of monoclonal antibodies to detect antigens in the CIE assay (2), PT in nasal secretions in a dot blot immunoassay (5), FHA and lipopolysaccharide in a colony blot-dot test (7) and PCR assay(10). The blot dot assays involve the detection of the antigens adsorbed to nitrocellulose paper with the highly specific antibodies. The ELISA for identification of patient antibody in acute phase serum from pertussis patients also has potential as a means for laboratory confirmation of infection (17).

As noted in Table 5-2, *H. influenzae* can be categorized into 6 biovarieties (designated with Roman numbers) based on physiological properties. The reactions used for this are indole, urease, and ornithine decarboxylase production. However, serology is also important in identification of its serotype. These organisms may produce a capsular polysaccharide, enabling their separation into serotypes a-f. As stated earlier type b is almost exclusively associated with invasive disease, such as meningitis; indeed, over 95% of systemic disease of children due to this species is caused by this serotype (19). Most serotype b *H. influenzae* belong to biovar I (15).

The association of disease potential mostly to one of six serotypes makes identification of the correct type important in laboratory diagnosis. Furthermore, in an infection as meningitis, it is critical that the agent is identified rapidly. A stained smear (commonly a Gram stain) on the centrifuged sediment of suspected cerebrospinal fluid is always an important early step. If haemophilae are present, a variety of procedures can be used to serotype this organism. Agglutination, Quellung, immunofluorescence, and counterimmunoelectrophoresis (CIE) are available techniques. Also used are commercially available kits employing latex agglutination (as Directigen®; ImmunoScan™ for *Haemophilus influenzae* type b; Wellcogen™; and coagglutination (Phadebact® Haemophilus test)). The principles of these tests were described in earlier exercises. Several may be applied directly to the clinical sample without culture realizing a possible savings in time for diagnosis.

Haemophilus influenzae isolates also should be routinely tested for antimicrobial resistance. Resistant strains to both ampicillin and chloramphenicol, the antimicrobials most commonly used for meningitis, are encountered at 20% and up to 50% rates, respectively (19). This has led to the increased use of third generation cephalosporin compounds.

MATERIALS

Part 1

A. Per pair of students:
   1 culture of *H. influenzae*, *H. parainfluenzae*, and *B. pertussis*
   1 chocolate agar plate
   1 trypticase soy agar (TSA) "Y" plate

   1 strip each of X, V, and XV factors
   3 tubes δ-aminolevulinic acid (ALA)
   3 tubes trypticase soy broth (TSB)
   3 tubes enriched nitrate broth
   1 Bordet-Gengou (B-G) agar plate

Part 2
Catalase and oxidase reagents

LABORATORY PROCEDURE
(Also see Fig. 5-1 for diagram of procedures):

Part 1

A. Known cultures: Each pair of students will be given cultures of *H. influenzae*, *H. parainfluenzae*, and *B. pertussis*. With these, carry out the following:
   1. Streak each for isolation on the following plate media:
      a. One-third chocolate agar plate.
      b. One third B-G agar plate.
   2. Do the satellite test. Start by suspending several colonies of each organism in separate 1 ml tubes of TSB. This will dilute out contaminating X and V factors, if present. Following this, heavily streak each on separate areas of each of the 3 one-third segments of a "Y" TSA plate using a loop. Now, aseptically place a filter paper strip or disk containing X factor in one of the segments such that it covers the areas inoculated with all three organisms. Repeat with the V- and XV-containing strips or disks in each of the remaining segments. Be sure to press these down so as to make good contact with the medium. When finished your plate should appear similar to that shown in Figure 5-1, and when colonies appear, the satellite phenomenon will be apparent.

   It is also possible to carry out the satellite test using bacteria that provide X, V or X and V factors to the surrounding haemophilae. For this purpose, *Enterococcus faecalis* and *Staphylococcus aureus* are commonly used, being easily available in the microbiology laboratory. The procedure is similar to that described above using strips except that the bacteria are streaked in separate lines through the areas containing the originally inoculated haemophilae (and *Bordetella* in our case). As the

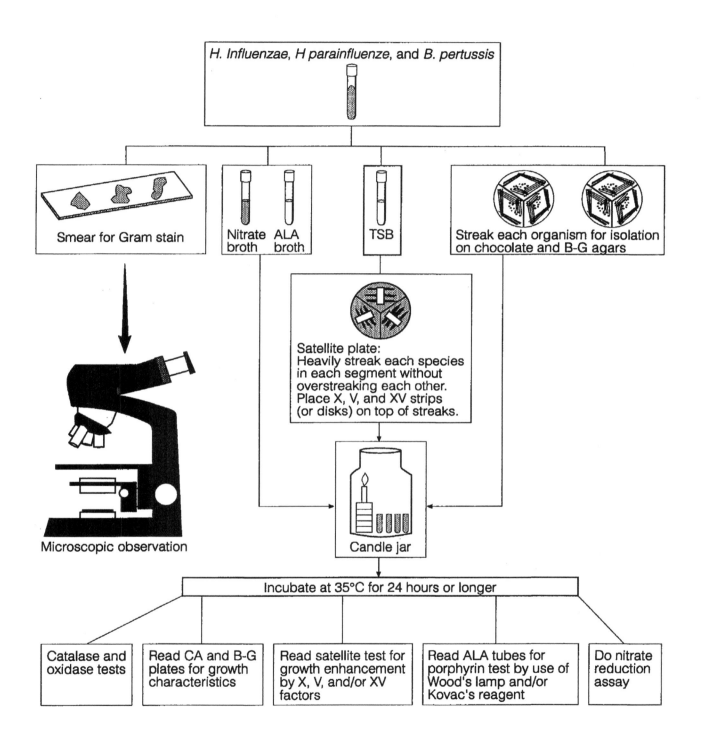

Figure 5-1: Procedural diagram for laboratory examination of *Haemophilus influenzae, H. parainfluenzae* and *Bordetella pertussis.* Steps for all species similar.

feeder streptococci and staphylococci grow, the X and V factors (or their equivalent) that they produce diffuse into the surrounding medium for haemophilae to use.

3. Do the porphyrin and nitrate tests by inoculating each stock organism into tubes of ALA and nitrate broth tubes, respectively. ALA tubes should receive a heavy inoculum. Incubate at 35°C for 24 hours (although generally ALA reactions can be read in 4 hours).

4. Gram stain each organism. Observe smears and describe your findings. Note any obvious differences in size of organisms in the two genera. Is there a tendency for *Haemophilus* spp. to be pleomorphic?

Incubate all plates for 24 hours at 35°C in a humidified candle extinction jar [(the growth of *Haemophilus* spp. are aided by the increased CO_2 and humidity, but is unnecessary for *Bordetella* (1), and in fact appears to be inhibitory for this organism (11)]. Examine for growth using a dissecting microscope if necessary. *B. pertussis* should be examined daily until growth appears, or up to 7 days.

Part 2
Known cultures:

1. Observe your chocolate and B-G agar plates for colony characteristics of *H. influenzae*, *H. parainfluenzae*, and *B. pertussis*. Are they similar? Does the latter produce minute colonies that appear as a "bisected pearl" or "droplets of mercury" on B-G agar? Is hemolysis produced by any of the bacteria on this medium? Tabulate your data and compare characteristics.

2. Determine whether the cultures have the capacity to reduce nitrate in nitrate broth.

3. Test each culture for oxidase and catalase production.

4. Observe your TSA plate for satellite growth. This should be seen, where X and/or V factor(s) are required, by enhanced growth of the bacteria around the strips or disks containing the growth-enhancing factor. Describe and explain your results.

5. Test for the synthesis of porphyrin from δ-aminolevulinic acid by exposure of the culture to a Wood's lamp within a darkened area. A red fluorescence will be seen in a positive test. (Note: Use caution so as not to expose your eyes or skin directly to the UV-emitting Wood's lamp.)

Testing also can be done with Kovac's reagent. Here, 10 drops of reagent are placed in the culture followed by vigorous shaking, then observing for the formation of a pink to red color due to the presence of porphobilinogen (15). A positive porphyrin test by either method shows that the organism does not require X factor.

The satellite test as done above has been a key assay for distinguishing *H. influenzae* from *H. parainfluenzae*, usually a non-pathogenic normal flora bacteria. Kilian (15), however, estimates that about 18% of results are erroneous in identification of the former due to the probable presence of small amounts of X factor in complex media that otherwise does not support the growth of *H. influenzae*. To avoid this problem, he devised the porphyrin test that measures the capacity of the organism to convert δ-aminolevulinic acid to porphobilinogen and porphyrins, intermediates in the synthesis of heme. This assay is now recommended over the use of the satellite test to assess X factor requirements of the haemophilae (1, 15).

Record and discuss your results. Do you note significant differences in the colony forms of *Bordetella pertussis* and the haemophilae? Does your data correlate with that of Table 5-2? If not, rationalize differences.

QUESTIONS

1. Explain the relationship of X factor and catalase.

2. Several types of blood agar (e.g. human, sheep, rabbit, horse, etc.) may be used for the culture of fastidious microorganisms. However, one type may be more useful than another for a particular organism. Indeed, some bacteria may not grow on certain types of blood agar. Therefore, what kind of blood medium would be most useful for the isolation of *S. pyogenes* from clinical material? Of *S. aureus*? Of *H. influenzae*? Why?

3. An important first step in the isolation of any organism in a clinical specimen is the method of specimen collection. This is particularly true of *B. pertussis*. Describe the proper methods of specimen collection for this bacteria, the media available for its transport from patient to the laboratory, and precautions that should be observed to assure that it is optimally handled.

4. X factor is heme. δ-aminolevulinic acid (ALA) is the substrate for the porphyrin test. By way of a flow diagram, show the intermediate major products of ALA change in the porphyrin test, and thereby show the relationships of ALA to porphyrin and to heme.

REFERENCES

1. Baron, E. J., L. R. Peterson, and S. M. Finegold. 1994. Bailey & Scott's diagnostic microbiology, 9th ed. Mosby-Year Book, Inc., St. Louis. p. 406-428.

2. Boreland, P. C., S. H. Gillespie, and L. A. E. Ashworth. 1988. Rapid diagnosis of whooping cough using monoclonal antibody. J. Clin. Pathol. **41**:573-575.

3. Brenner, D. J., L. W. Mayer, G. M. Carlone, L. H. Harrison, W. F. Bibb, M. C. C. Brandileone, F. O. Sottnek, K. Irino, M. W. Reeves, J. M. Swenson, K. A. Birkness, R. S. Weyant, S. F. Berkely, T. C. Woods, A. G. Steigerwalt, P. A. D. Grimont, R. M. McKinney, D. W. Fleming, L. L. Gheesling, R. C. Cooksey, R. J. Arko, C. V. Broome, and the Brazilian Purpuric Fever Study Group. 1988. Biochemical, genetic, and epidemiologic characterization of *Haemophilus influenzae* Biogroup Aegytius (*Haemophilus aegytius*) strains associated with Brazilian purpuric fever. J. Clin. Microbiol. **26**:1524-1534.

4. Friedman, R. L. 1988. Pertussis: The disease and new diagnostic methods. Clin. Microbiol. Rev. **1**:365-376.

5. Friedman, R. L., S. Paulaitis, and J. W. McMillan. 1989. Development of a rapid diagnostic test for pertussis: Direct detection of pertussis toxin in respiratory secretions. J. Clin. Microbiol. **27**:2466-2470.

6. Gilchrist, M. J. R. 1991. *Bordetella*, p. 471-477. *In* A. Balows, W. J. Hausler, Jr., K. L. Herrmann, H. D. Isenberg, and H. J. Shadomy, (ed.), Manual of clinical microbiology, 5th ed. American Society for Microbiology, Washington, D. C.

7. Gustafsson, B., and P. Askelöf. 1989. Rapid detection of *Bordetella pertussis* by a monoclonal antibody-based colony blot assay. J. Clin. Microbiol. **27**:628-631.

8. Haperin, S. A., R. Bortolussi, and A. J. Wort. 1989. Evaluation of culture, immunofluorescence, and serology for the diagnosis of pertussis. J. Clin. Microbiol. **27**:752-757.

9. Hand, W. L. 1990. Haemophilus species, p. 1729-1733. *In* G. L. Mandell, R. G. Douglas, Jr., and J. E. Bennett (ed.). Principles and practices of infectious diseases, 3rd. ed. Churchill Livingston, New York.

10. He, Q., J. Mertsola, H. Soini, M. Skurnik, O. Ruuskanen, and M. K. Viljanen. 1993. Comparison of polymerase chain reaction with culture and enzyme immunoassay for diagnosis of pertussis. J. Clin. Microbiol. **31**:642-645.

11. Hoppe, J. E., and M. Schlagenhauf. 1989. Comparison of three kinds of blood and two incubation atmospheres for cultivation of *Bordetella pertussis* on charcoal agar. J. Clin. Microbiol. **27**:2115-2117.

12. Kersters, K., K.-H. Hinz, A. Hertle, P. Segers, A. Lievens, O. Siegmann, and J. De Ley. 1984. *Bordetella avium* sp. nov., isolated from the respiratory tracts of turkeys and other birds. Int. J. Syst. Bacteriol. **34**:56-70.

13. Kilian, M., and E. L. Biberstein. 1984. *Haemophilus* Winslow, Broadhurst, Buchanan, Krumwiede, Rogers and Smith 1917, p. 558-569. *In* N. R. Krieg, and J. G. Holt (ed.), Bergey's manual of systematic bacteriology, Vol. 1. Williams & Wilkins, Baltimore.

14. Kilian, M. 1985. *Haemophilus*, p. 387-393. *In* E. H. Lennette, A. Balows, W. J. Hausler, Jr., and H. J. Shadomy (ed.), Manual of clinical microbiology, 3rd ed. American Society for Microbiology, Washington, D. C.

15. Kilian, M. 1991. *Haemophilus* p. 463-470. *In* A. Balows, W. J. Hausler, Jr., K. L. Herrmann, H. D. Isenberg, and H. J. Shadomy. (ed.), Manual of clinical microbiology, 5th ed. American Society for Microbiology, Washington, D. C.

16. Krieg, N. R., and J. G. Holt (ed.). 1984. Bergey's manual of systematic bacteriology, Vol. 1. Williams and Wilkins, Baltimore, pp. 140-600.

17. Lawrence, A. J., and J. C. Paton. 1987. Efficacy of enzyme-linked immunosorbent assay for rapid diagnosis of *Bordetella pertussis* infection. J. Clin. Microbiol. **25**:2102-2104.

18. Mannheim, W. 1984. *Pasteurellaceae* Pohl 1981a, p. 550-552. *In* N. R. Krieg, and J. G. Holt (ed.), Bergey's manual of systematic bacteriology, Vol. 1. Williams & Wilkins, Baltimore.

19. Moxon, E. R. 1990. Haemophilus influenzae, p. 1722-1729. *In* G. L. Mandell, R. G. Douglas, Jr., and J. E. Bennett (ed.), Principles and practices of infectious diseases. Churchill Livingston Inc. New York.

20. Pittman, M. 1984. Genus *Bordetella* Moreno-López 1952, p. 388-393. *In* N. R. Krieg, and J. G. Holt (ed.), Bergey's manual of systematic bacteriology, Vol. 1. Williams & Wilkins, Baltimore.

21. Power, D. A., and P. J. McCuen. 1988. Manual of BBL products and laboratory procedures, 6th ed. Becton Dickinson Microbiology Systems, Cockeysville, MD. p. 298-299.

22. Rennie, R., T. Gordon, Y. Yaschuk, P. Tomlin, P. Kibsey, and W. Albritton. 1992. Laboratory and clinical evaluations of media for the primary isolation of *Haemophilus* species. J. Clin. Microbiol. **30**:1917-1921.

Exercise 5
Data Table 1: *Haemophilus* and *Bordetella* Results

		Culture	H. influenzae			H. parainfluenzae			B. pertussis		
		Age	CA[a]	B-G[a]	Other	CA	B-G	Other	CA	B-G	Other
Colony size and Colony Form[b]	mm										
	Punctiform										
	Irregular										
	Circular										
	Rhizoid										
	Filamentous										
	Other										
Colony Surface	Flat										
	Raised										
	Convex										
	Pulvinate										
	Other										
Colony Margin	Entire										
	Undulate										
	Lobate										
	Erose										
	Other										
Colony Consistency	Butyrous										
	Viscid										
	Membranous										
	Brittle										
	Other										
Colony Optical Character	Opaque										
	Translucent										
	Dull										
	Glistening										
	Other										
Colony Surface	Smooth										
	Rough										
	Other										
Satellite Growth on TSA[a]	With X factor		■	■		■	■		■	■	
	With V factor		■	■		■	■		■	■	
	With XV		■	■		■	■		■	■	
Other											

[a] CA = chocolate agar; B-G = Bordet-Gengou agar; TSA = trypticase soy agar.

Exercise 5
Data Table 2: *Haemphilus* and *Bordetella* Results

		Culture	H. influenzae			H. parainfluenzae			B. pertussis		
		Age	CA[a]	B-G[a]	Other	CA	B-G	Other	CA	B-G	Other
Porphyrin test in ALA[a]	Wood's Lamp		███	███		███	███		███	███	
	Kovac's Reagent		███	███		███	███		███	███	
Nitrate Reduced			███	███		███	███		███	███	
			███	███		███	███		███	███	
Catalase test											
Oxidase test											
Gram stain (1000X)	Reaction										
	Morphology										
	Arrangement										
Other											

[a] CA = chocolate agar; B-G = Bordet-Gengou agar; ALA = δ-aminolevulinic acid.

Laboratory Notes

EXERCISE 6
Brucella and *Francisella*

Brucella and *Francisella* are both Gram-negative aerobic, small, coccoid to rod-shape bacteria unassociated with any family (6). They are primarily found as parasites of lower animals, causing zoonotic diseases. Human disease caused by *Brucella* (brucellosis, Malta fever, undulant fever, Bang's disease, etc.) is especially contracted through direct contact with cattle (*B. abortus*), swine (*B. suis*), and goats and camels (*B. melitensis*). Consumption of contaminated meat, milk, and milk products from these sources also lead to infection. The frequency of human brucellosis is low in the U. S. (200 or fewer cases per year 1980-89) (4), but it continues to be an occupational risk for microbiologists as exemplified by a 1988 outbreak in a clinical microbiology laboratory (15). In recent years a small number of cases has also been contracted from canines due to *B. canis*. Those found in sheep (*B. ovis*) and the desert wood rat (*B. neotomae*) have not yet been found to induce human infection (19).

F. tularensis, the agent of tularemia, in contrast to brucellae, is disseminated to humans by insect vectors, as deer flies and especially ticks, as well as by direct contact with infected animals. Over 100 species of wild animals have been identified as having been infected by this organism, but the important reservoirs for human disease in the U.S. include hares, rabbits, and muskrats, as well as ticks. Less commonly disease also occurs following animal bites and from contaminated water (1). Rarely *F. philomiragia*, a newly proposed species that has been isolated from water and muskrats, causes human infection in association with immunosuppression and near-drowning. Finally, *F. novicida* is now known also to cause symptoms similar to forms of tularemia. Because of its pathogenicity and genetic relatedness to *F. tularensis*, it has been recommended that this organism become a strain of it, namely *F. tularensis* biogroup Novicida (10).

Both brucellosis and tularemia are diseases with variable symptoms, and may be chronic in nature. However, in the former fever, chill, malaise, arthralgia, and weight loss are classic symptoms (19). In tularemia, the ulceroglandular form is most common (1).

Culturally, both *Brucella* and *Francisella* are fastidious in their nutritional requirements on primary isolation, though laboratory strains of *Brucella* can grow on simple media. In *Brucella*, plating media (as Brucella agar), has been formulated for its optimal growth although it will grow moderately well on, for example, sheep blood agar. CO_2 enhances the growth of some *B. abortus* Biovars (see Table 6-1). Due to their oxidative nature, except for *B. neotomae*, sugars are not fermented (6).

F. tularensis grows optimally on cysteine or cystine-containing medium, as cystine heart blood agar. The need for at least one of these amino acids is so strict, lack of growth on media without it is useful in differentiation of this species. Unlike many brucellae, increased CO_2 is unnecessary for *Francisella* (7).

Table 6-1 gives some additional characteristics for most species of *Brucella* and *Francisella*. As shown, there are several varieties of both genera. Also, it shows that most species can be distinguished based on physiological patterns (exception: *B. suis* Biovar 3 corresponds to *B. melitensis*). However, aside from initial isolation culture and either serological identification of organisms or patient antibody response, it is recommended that further analysis of laboratory culture is done by a reference laboratory. This is because both *Brucella* and *Francisella* are, as mentioned above, hazardous to handle. Data shows brucellosis and tularemia ranked in the top three diseases acquired in the laboratory (typhoid fever is the other) during the period 1930-1974 (5).

For *Brucella*, at least, the usual samples for primary isolation, namely blood cultures, can require incubation for up to 4 weeks with at least weekly subculture on plating media for isolation. Plates, in turn may need more than 3 weeks of incubation for growth to occur. For these reasons especially, serological methods have grown in importance to hasten diagnosis. However, some commercially-available culture systems have been useful in reducing detection times. BacT/Alert™ (Photo 6-1) may reduce detection time of *B. melitensis* in blood cultures, for example, to a few

Table 6-1
Characteristics of Some *Brucella* and *Francisella* spp. (7, 10, 13)[a]

Genus-species	No. of Biovars	Catalase reaction	Oxidase reaction	5% CO_2 required	H_2S produced[c]	Growth in Thionin[d]	Basic Fuchsin[d]	6% NaCl broth
B. abortus	7	+[b]	+	+[e]	+[f]	−[g]	+[h]	ND[i]
B. melitensis	3	+	+	−	−	+	+	ND
B. suis	5	+	+	−	−[f]	+[g]	−[h]	ND
B. canis	1	+	+	−	−	+	−	ND
F. tularensis	3	+[w]	−	−	−	ND	ND	−
F. philomiragia	1	− to +[w]	+	−	V	ND	ND	+

[a] Only *Brucella* and *Francisella* spp. most frequently causing infection in humans shown.
[b] + = mostly positive, +[w] = weakly positive, − = negative for most strains, V = variably positive, and ND = no data.
[c] Detected by use of lead acetate impregnated filter paper strips over tryptose agar slants for brucellae; TSI slants for *Francisella* spp.
[d] 40 μg/ml concentration thionin; 20 μg/ml basic fuchsin.
[e] Exceptions: *B. abortus* Biovars 5-7 are negative.
[f] Exceptions: *B. abortus* Biovar 5; *B. suis* Biovar 1.
[g] Exceptions: *B. abortus* Biovar 3; *B. suis* Biovar 2.
[h] Exceptions: *B. abortus* Biovar 2; *B. suis* Biovar 3.

days (14). This system, which can be applied to the detection of many types of bacterial and fungal organisms in blood culture (17), is based on the detection of CO_2 produced by these in culture.

Patient antibody response can be determined by several methods. In both brucellosis and tularemia, a four-fold increase in titer is diagnostic, although a single 1:160 titer is considered significant for the presence of disease (13). Agglutination techniques using killed brucellae or *F. tularensis* are most widely used (16) although anti-brucellae antibodies also cross react with *F. tularensis* and vice versa, and with *Vibrio cholerae* and *Yersinia enterocolitica* (12, 18). The use of other serological assays for anti-*Brucella* as latex agglutination (2), complement fixation (e.g 9, 18), enzyme immunoassay (e.g. 3, 11) and fluorometric assays (9) have been reported for testing both human and lower animal sera. For the identification of suspected *Brucella* culture isolates agglutination with monospecific serum is used (13).

With *Francisella*, agglutination is also used for microbial cell identification and culture confirmation (8). The direct fluorescent antibody test also can be employed to detect bacteria in histologic sections, exudate smears, or other patient samples (16).

Although this exercise will be demonstration, handle cultures with care. Do not open them. Keep them within the confines of a biohazard hood during all observations.

Part 1

A. Demonstrations of *Brucella abortus*, *B. suis*, and *B. melitensis*: Observe these cultures on days 2, 5, and 7 after inoculation, incubated at 35°C. in a candle jar.
   1. Observe differences in growth of these species in the presence of media containing 40 μg/ml thionin and 20 μg/ml basic fuchsin.
   2. Note any difference in rates of production of H_2S with time in the tryptose agar slants with lead acetate-containing strips. (Note: Lead acetate strips are replaced 24 hours before reading.)
   3. Are these species hemolytic? Show the relative growth rates of the 3 organisms that have been streaked for isolation on 5% sheep blood in Brucella agar plates.

B. Demonstration of *F. tularensis*:
   Observe colony forms on cystine heart blood agar plates, with and without cystine, incubated at 35°C. Describe colony characteristics and relative amounts of growth. Do *not* open these sealed containers. Do not remove from the biohazard hood.

C. Previously prepared Gram-stained preparations of *B. abortus*, *B. suis*, and *F. tularensis* will be made available for your microscopic examination.

Part 2

Record your observations from this demonstration. Does *F. tularensis* appear to have bipolar staining? *Francisella* has this property, as well as pleomorphism. Does it require cystine for its growth? Based on growth patterns, can *B. abortus*, *B. melitensis* and *B. suis* be distinguished?

QUESTIONS

1. *F. tularensis* and *B. abortus* are included in a group of antigens known as "febrile antigens." Name some other species that are included here. Why are they called "febrile antigens?"
2. Human brucellosis is accompanied by production of IgM and IgG antibodies. Indicate the temporal relationship of each of these during the course of infection (and thereby show the diagnostic significance of each). Furthermore, a type of IgM antibody may cause a false *negative* reading. What is this antibody called? How can its activity be eliminated?
3. Give the types of specimens that would be expected to contain the organisms studied in this exercise.

REFERENCES

1. Boyce, J. M. 1990. Francisella tularensis (tularemia), p. 1742-1746. *In* G. L. Mandell, R. G. Douglas, Jr., and J. E. Bennett (ed.), Principles and practices of infectious diseases, 3rd ed. Churchill Livingston, New York

2. Cambiaso, C. L., and J. N. Limet. 1989. Latex agglutination assay for human anti-*Brucella* IgM antibodies. J. Immunol. Meth. **122**:169-175.

3. Caravano, R., F. Chabaud, and J. Oberti. 1987. Applications of immunoenzymatic techniques for epidemiological surveys of brucellosis among human populations. Ann. Inst. Pasteur Microbiol. **138**:79-84.

4. Centers for Disease Control. 1989. Summary of notifiable disease, United States 1989. Morbid. Mort. Weekly Rep. **38**:53.

5. Collins, C. H. 1983. Laboratory-acquired infections: History, incidence, causes, and prevention. Butterworths, London. 227 p.

6. Corbel, M. J., and W. J. Brinley-Morgan. 1984. Genus *Brucella* Meyer and Shaw 1920, p. 377-388. *In* N. R. Krieg, and J. G. Holt (ed.), Bergey's manual of systematic bacteriology, Vol. 1. Williams & Wilkins, Baltimore.

7. Eigelsbach, H. T., and V. G. McGann. 1984. *Francisella* Dorofe'ev 1947, p. 394-399. *In* N. R. Krieg, and J. G. Holt (ed.), Bergey's manual of systematic bacteriology, Vol. 1. Williams & Wilkins, Baltimore.

8. Gelfand, M. 1987. Tularemia, p. 581-587. *In* B. B. Wentworth (ed.), Diagnostic procedures for bacterial infections, 7th ed. American Public Health Association, Inc., Washington, D. C.

9. Hall, S. M., and A. W. Confer. 1987. Comparison of TRACK XI fluorometric immunoassay system with other serologic tests for detection of serum antibody to *Brucella abortus* in cattle. J. Clin. Microbiol. **25**:350-354.

10. Hollis, D. G., R. E. Weaver, A. G. Steigerwalt, J. D. Wenger, C. W. Moss, and D. J. Brenner. 1989. *Francisella philomiragia* comb. nov. (formerly *Yersinia philomiragia*) and *Francisella tularensis* biogroup Novicida (formerly *Francisella novicida*) associated with human disease. J. Clin. Microbiol. **27**:1601-1608.

11. Larson, J. W. A., J. J. Webber, and L. D. Edwards. 1988. A field outbreak of bovine brucellosis—comparison of CFT, ELISA, and culture results. Austr. Vet. J. **65**:30-31.

12. Mikolich, D. J., and J. M. Boyce. 1990. Brucella species, p. 1735-1742. *In* G. L. Mandell, R. G. Douglas, Jr., and J. E. Bennett (ed.), Principles and practices of infectious diseases, 3rd ed. Churchill Livingstone, New York.

13. Moyer. N. P., L. A. Holcomb, and W. J. Hausler, Jr. 1991. *Brucella*, p. 457-462. *In* A. Balows, W. J. Hausler, Jr., K. L. Herrmann, H. D. Isenberg, and H. J. Shadomy (ed.), Manual of clinical microbiology, 5th ed. American Society for Microbiology, Washington, D. C.

14. Solomon, H. M., and D. Jackson. 1992. Rapid diagnosis of *Brucella melitensis* in blood: some operational characteristics of the BACT/ALERT. J. Clin. Microbiol. **30**:222-224.

15. Staszkiewicz, J., C. M. Lewis, J. Colville, M. Zervos, and J. Band. 1991. Outbreak of *Brucella melitensis* among microbiology laboratory workers in a community hospital. J. Clin. Microbiol. **29**:287-290.

16. Stewart, S. J. 1991. *Francisella*, p. 454-456. *In* A. Balows, W. J. Hausler, Jr., K. L. Herrmann, H. D. Isenberg, and H. J. Shadomy (ed.), Manual of clinical microbiology, 5th ed. American Society for Microbiology, Washington, D. C.

17. Thorpe, T. C., M. L. Wilson, J. E. Turner, J. L. DiGuiseppi, M. Willert, S. Mirrett, and L. B. Reller. 1990. BacT/Alert: an automated colorimetric microbial detection system. J. Clin. Microbiol. **28**:1608-1612.

18. Timoney, J. F., J. H. Gillespie, F. W. Scott, and J. E. Barlough. 1988. Hagan and Bruner's microbiology and infectious diseases of domestic animals, 8th ed. Comstock Publishing Associates, Ithica, NY. p. 132-152.

19. Wright, P. W. 1987. Brucellosis. Am. Family Phys. **35**:155-159.

Exercise 6
Data Table 1: *Brucella* spp. and *Francisella tularensis* Results

(Inoculation Date: _____)

		Culture	B. abortus			B. melitensis			B. suis			F. tularensis	
		Age	SBA[a]	Thionin	BF[a]	SBA	Thionin	BF	SBA	Thionin	BF	CHBA[b]	HBA[b]
Colony size and Colony Form	mm												
	Punctiform												
	Irregular												
	Circular												
	Rhizoid												
	Filamentous												
	Other												
Colony Surface	Flat												■
	Raised												■
	Convex												■
	Pulvinate												■
	Other												■
Colony Margin	Entire		■	■			■	■		■	■		■
	Undulate		■	■			■	■		■	■		
	Lobate		■	■			■	■		■	■		
	Erose		■	■			■	■		■	■		
	Other		■	■			■	■		■	■		
Colony Optical Character	Opaque		■	■			■	■		■	■		■
	Translucent		■	■			■	■		■	■		■
	Dull		■	■			■	■		■	■		■
	Glistening		■	■			■	■		■	■		■
	Other		■	■			■	■		■	■		■
Colony Surface and color	Smooth												
	Rough												
Hemolysis Growth rate	Type		■	■			■	■		■	■		■
			■	■			■	■		■	■		■
Rel. growth[c]													

[a] SBA = Sheep blood Brucella agar; BF = Basic fuchsin-containing agar.

[b] CHBA = cystine heart blood agar; HBA = heart blood agar.

[c] Record as +4 = maximum growth to +1 = minimum growth, and − = no growth.

Exercise 6
Data Table 2: *Brucella* spp. and *Francisella tularensis* Results

Inoculation Date: _____

		Brucella				F. tularensis	
		Age	abortus	melitensis	suis	Age	CHBA[a]
Gram stain (1000 X)	Reaction						
	Morphology						
	Arrangement						
H$_2$S production[b]	Day 2						
	Day 5						
	Day 7						
Other							

[a] CHBA = Cystine heart blood agar.

[b] Record relative amounts of H$_2$S produced as +4 to +1, or − (see footnote c, Data Table 1).

Other Notes:

EXERCISE 7
Pasteurella and *Actinobacillus*

Pasteurella and *Actinobacillus* of the family *Pasteurellaceae* are usually animal parasites. As noted in Table 5-1 members of this family are small coccoid to rod-shape, Gram-negative, non-motile, catalase-producing bacteria. The classification of members within the genera *Pasteurella* and *Actinobacillus* is undergoing modification, largely because of information based on genetic data (8, 9). Up to 18 species, some of which are unnamed, are accepted or proposed within the genus *Pasteurella* (compared to six in 1984 (3)), and seven in the genus *Actinobacillus* (contrasted to five in 1984 (7)), including *A. ureae*, which was reclassified from *P. ureae* (8). Table 7-1 gives some differentiating properties for some of those species in both genera that have been associated with human infection.

Overall the *Pasteurella* and *Actinobacillus* are most commonly commensal and pathogenic agents of lower animals (3, 7). Exceptions to this are the opportunistic agents of human disease, *A. actinomycetemcomitans* and *A. ureae*, which do not cause disease in lower animals (2, 7), but do so infrequently in humans. The former, a part of the normal oral flora, especially causes juvenile periodontitis, but is also associated with endocarditis and soft tissue infections (4, 6). *A. ureae*,

also found to be an occasional commensal of the mouth, uncommonly causing bronchial disease, pneumonia, meningitis and other conditions (3). In contrast, *P. multocida*, a more frequent cause of infection of humans, most frequently arises from cat and dog bites and scratches leading to soft tissue infections, osteomyelitis, or other complications. However, up to 15% may be upper respiratory or abdominal disease without evidence of animal contact, perhaps because this organism may be a part of the human normal flora (2). It can rarely cause meningitis as well (5). *P. haemolytica* and *P. pneumotropica* have also been associated with similar infections. The following laboratory work and demonstration will provide a brief exposure to these organisms.

MATERIAL

Per pair of students
1 plate culture each of *Pasteurella multocida, A. ureae,* and *A. actinomycetemcomitans.*
  Catalase reagent
  Oxidase-impregnated strips or disks
  Petri dish
  Gram and Giemsa stain reagents

Table 7-1
Some Differential Characteristics of *Pasteurella* and *Actinobacillus* spp.
Most Commonly Isolated from Humans (3, 8)

Genus-species	Catalase Reaction	Oxidase Reaction	Urease	Acid from Mannitol	Acid from Maltose	Acid from Sucrose	Indole	Ornithine Decarboxylase	Growth on MacConkey agar	Capnophilic
P. multocida	+[a]	+	−	V+	−	+	+	+	−	−[a]
P. haemolytica	V+	+	−	V	+	+	−	−	V+	−
P. pneumotropica	+	+	+	−	+	+	+	+	V	−
A. ureae	V	+	+	+	+	+	−	−	−	−
A. actinomycemcomitans	+	V−	−	V+	+	−	−	−	−	+

[a] + = 90-100% positive; V+ = 70-89% positive; V = 30-69% positive; V− = 11-29% positive; − = 0-10% positive.

LABORATORY PROCEDURES

Working in pairs, use the blood agar plate cultures of *P. multocida*, *A. ureae*, and *A. actinomycetemcomitans* (incubated in a candle extinction jar) provided to accomplish the following:

1. Observe and compare characteristics of isolated colonies. Note the odor of each culture. Does *P. multocida* have a "musty" odor? Its presence is useful in detecting this species.
2. Prepare two smears of each organism, noting the colony consistency of each at this time. Carry out the Gram stain procedure with one smear and a Giemsa stain (see Appendix 2 for procedure) with the second. Microscopically observe each bacteria stained by both methods, noting the small size, especially of *P. multocida* and *A. actinomycetemcomitans*. Also, bipolar staining, giving a "safety pin" appearance, is a feature of *Pasteurella*. Though visible by Gram stain, it is best seen by using Giemsa stain as follows (1):
   a. Fix smear in absolute methanol for 5 minutes, then dry slide.
   b. Stain in Giemsa stain (Appendix 2) for 30-60 minutes.
   c. Wash slide well with phosphate buffer, pH 6.4, blot dry, and examine.
   Is this characteristic visible in your preparation?
3. Using an empty petri dish to contain the following tests, determine for each culture:
   a. Catalase reaction.
   b. Oxidase reaction (following manufacturer's protocol for use of oxidase-impregnated strips or disks).

On completion of these assays, discard the petri dish containing the completed tests in the appropriate discard container.

DEMONSTRATION

Observe the following demonstration cultures of *P. multocida*, *A. ureae*, and *A. actinomycetemcomitans* that have been incubated at 35°C for 48 hours.

1. Christensen urea agar slant. Urease production is seen by the medium turning from a yellow to a deep pink color.
2. Mannitol, maltose, and sucrose fermentation tubes.
   Record all of your observations, and compare your results to those data given in Table 7-1. Discuss.

QUESTIONS

1. What is the literal meaning of "*multocida*" from the species name *P. multocida*? Of "*actinomycetemcomitans*" from "*A. actinomycetemcomitans?*"
2. Give the types of human clinical specimens where one would expect to find *P. multocida* and *A. actinomycetemcomitans*?
3. Give the reaction that describes the action urease on urea, and the production of the pink color in a positive test in Christiensen urea agar.

REFERENCES

1. Bell, R. H. 1987. Media, reagents and stains, p. 773-835. *In* B. B. Wentworth (ed.), Diagnostic procedures for bacterial infections, 7th ed. American Public Health Association, Inc., Washington, D. C.
2. Boyce, J. M. 1990. Pasteurella species, p. 1746-1748. *In* G. L. Mandell, R. G. Douglas, Jr., and J. E. Bennett (ed.), Principles and practices of infectious diseases, 3rd ed. Churchill Livingstone, New York.
3. Carter, G. R. 1984. *Pasteurella* Trevisan 1887, p. 552-557. *In* N. R. Krieg, and J. G. Holt (ed.), Bergey's manual of systematic bacteriology, Vol. 1. Williams & Wilkins, Baltimore.
4. Kaplan, A. H., D. J. Weber, E. Z. Oddone, and J. R. Perfect. 1989. Infection due to *Actinobacillus actinomycetemcomitans*: 15 cases and review. Rev. Infect. Dis. **11**:46-63.
5. Kumar, A., H. R. Devlin, and H. Vellend. 1990. *Pasteurella multocida* meningitis in an adult: case report and review. Rev. Infect. Dis. **12**:440-448.
6. McGowen, J. E., Jr., and C. Del Rio. 1990. Other Gram-negative bacilli, p. 1782-1793. *In* G. L. Mandell, R. G. Douglas, Jr., and J. E. Bennett (ed.), Principles and practices of infectious diseases, 3rd ed. Churchill Livingstone, New York.
7. Phillips, J. E. 1984. *Actinobacillus*, Brumpt 1910, p. 570-575. *In* N. R. Krieg, and J. G. Holt (ed.), Bergey's manual of systematic bacteriology, Vol. 1. Williams & Wilkins, Baltimore.
8. Pickett, M. J., D. G. Hollis, and E. J. Bottone. 1991. Miscellaneous Gram-negative bacteria, p. 410-428. *In* A. Balows, W. J. Hausler, Jr., K. L. Herrmann, H. D. Isenberg, and H. J. Shadomy. (ed.), Manual of clinical microbiology, 5th ed. American Society for Microbiology, Washington, D. C.
9. Sneath, P. H. A., and M. Stevens. 1990. *Actinobacillus rossii* sp. nov., *Actinobacillus seminis* sp. nov., nom. rev., *Pasteurella bettii* sp. nov., *Pasteurella lymphangitidis* sp. nov., *Pasteurella mairi* sp. nov., and *Pasteurella tehalosi* sp. nov. Int. J. System. Bacteriol. **40**:148-153.

Exercise 7
Data Table 1: *Pasteurella* and *Actinobacillus* Results

		Culture	P. multocida		A. ureae		A. actinomycetemcomitans	
		Age	SBA[a]	Other	SBA	Other	SBA	Other
Colony size and Colony Form	mm							
	Punctiform							
	Irregular							
	Circular							
	Rhizoid							
	Filamentous							
	Other							
Colony Surface	Flat							
	Raised							
	Convex							
	Pulvinate							
	Other							
Colony Margin	Entire							
	Undulate							
	Lobate							
	Erose							
	Other							
Colony Consistency	Butyrous							
	Viscid							
	Membranous							
	Brittle							
	Other							
Colony Optical Character	Opaque							
	Translucent							
	Dull							
	Glistening							
	Other							
Colony Surface and Color	Smooth							
	Rough							
	Other							
Hemolysis	Type			■		■		■
				■		■		■
				■		■		■
Other								

[a] Sheep blood agar

Exercise 7
Pasteurella and *Actinobacillus* Results

		Culture	P. multocida		A. ureae		A. actinomycetemcomitans	
		Age	SBA[a]	Other	SBA	Other	SBA	Other
Catalase test								
Oxidase test								
Gram stain	Reaction							
(1000X)	Morphology							
	Arrangement							
	Bipolar							
Giemsa stain	Bipolar							
Fermentation	Mannitol		■		■		■	
	Maltose		■		■		■	
	Sucrose		■		■		■	
Urease								

[a] Sheep blood agar

Laboratory Notes

C. THE *ENTEROBACTERIACEAE*

AN INTRODUCTION TO EXERCISES 8 AND 9

The family *Enterobacteriaceae* encompasses the most frequently encountered single group of bacteria in the clinical microbiology laboratory (1, 11). Its members, as the name suggests, inhabit the gastrointestinal tract of humans and lower animals (and therefore are frequently called the "enterics"). They are, however, ubiquitous, also being found in water, in the soil, and on plants (see Table 8-1).

From the view of human infection, many clinical conditions are caused by members of the *Enterobacteriaceae*. Typhoid fever due to *Salmonella typhi* and plague caused by *Yersinia pestis*, though uncommon in the U. S., represent the potentially most serious infections. Gastrointestinal infections due to other *Salmonella,* the *Shigella* spp., and urinary tract infections attributable to *Escherichia coli* are among the most frequent. There are, however, many types of disease caused by these organisms and others within the family. Pneumonia, urinary tract infections, abscesses, meningitis, bacteremia, and other diseases involving *Klebsiella pneumoniae, E. coli, Serratia* spp., *Enterobacter* spp., *Edwardsiella tarda, Proteus* spp., and additional species shown in Table 8-1 are not uncommon. In fact, they are a leading cause of nosocomial infections (8). In the following two exercises, space permits only a select group of enteric bacteria significant in clinical microbiology to be studied.

Because of nomenclatural confusion, combined with the frequency with which the members of the *Enterobacteriaceae* are isolated in the diagnostic laboratory, emphasis has been placed upon taxonomy by many workers in the field. The Division of Bacterial Diseases of the Centers for Disease Control (CDC) in Atlanta, Ga. has been especially influential, continuing development of a basic scheme developed by Edwards and Ewing (7). As with other groups of microorganisms, application of DNA hybridization studies to the enterics has helped to further delineate taxonomic relationships. This, as with other organisms we have studied, is partially reflected in the increased number of taxonomic groups. In 1985 there were 69 species and 29 biogroups in 22 genera included in this family (10). In 1991, this number has risen

to approximately 81 species and 22 biogroups or other recognized but unnamed groups in 28 genera (11). (This does not include serotypes or biotypes of *Salmonella.*) Furthermore, it has lead to a greater degree of agreement among workers in the field concerning currently existing taxa (e.g., 9, 11, 14). These are presented in Table 8-2. A significant difference in the listing seen in this table compared to that described by Ewing (9) is the exclusion of Tribes. He has continued to include these as a subdivision of the family. Many others (e. g. 11, 14), however, have excluded them based on the lack of scientific merit (14).

For study purposes, the *Enterobacteriaceae* is divided into two exercises. Exercise 8 will deal with the *Yersinia*; Exercise 9, the remainder of the family that are associated with humans. The reason for this division is that the general ecological distribution of yersiniae differs from the remainder of the animal-associated enterics. It resembles *Francisella* and *Pasteurella* in this respect. Furthermore, *Y. pestis,* as the agent of bubonic plague, is sufficiently different in its epidemiology, type of infection, and in its historical impact to warrant separate emphasis.

Description of the Family

The *Enterobacteriaceae* consist of species that are facultatively anaerobic, Gram-negative, oxidase negative, and straight rods (refer to Table 5-1) (Photo 8-1, 8-2, and 8-3). Their DNA G + C content falls in a range of 35-59%. Except *Xenorhabdus nematophilus* and *Shigella dysenteriae* Serovar 1, they all produce catalase. Also, excepting *Xenorhabdus* and some strains of *Yersinia,* they all reduce nitrate to nitrate. They all ferment glucose, and when motile, contain peritrichous flagella (11).

Approach Toward Identification of the Enterobacteria

In the isolation and identification of species within the *Enterobacteriaceae* a general pattern, such as shown in Figure 8-1 starting with a stool specimen, is followed. Such a scheme can vary depending in the specimen type and on the facility doing such analysis. Fecal specimens represent a major source where *Salmonella, Shigella,* diarrheal-producing *E. coli* and *Y. enterocolitica* are of prime interest. Also, urine, blood, sputum, throat

Table 8-1
Genera of the Family *Enterobacteriaceae* and Their Sources

Genus	No. species, bio- and/or subgroups(11)	Probable primary source(s)[a] (14)	Occurs in clinical samples (11)
Budvicia	1	Water	+[b]
Buttiauxella	1	Soil, water	−
Cedecea	5	Humans	Rare
Citrobacter	4	Environment	+ & −
Edwardsiella	4	Animals, environment	+ & −[c]
Enterobacter	13	Animals, environment	+ & −
Escherichia[d]	6	Humans, lower animals	+ & −
Ewingella	1	Humans, food	Rare
Hafnia	2	Humans, lower animals, diary products, water, soil	+ & −
Klebsiella	7	Humans, food, soil, sewage	+ & −
Kluyvera	2	Environment	+ & −
Leclercia	1	Humans, food	+ & −
Leminorella	2	Humans	+
Moellerella	1	Humans (11)	+
Morganella	2	Humans, lower animals	+
Obesumbacterium	1	Breweries	−
Pragia	1	Drinking water	−
Proteus	4	Humans, lower animals, environment (22)	+ & −
Providencia	5	Humans	+ & −
Rahnella	1	Water	Rare
Salmonella	7[e]	Human, lower animals (17)	+
Serratia	10	Environment	+ & −
Shigella[d,f]	4	Humans, primates (25)	+
Tatumella	1	Humans	Rare
Trabulsiella (18)	1	Humans, soil (18)	+
Yersinia	11	Animals, environment (3)	+ & −
Yokenella (15, 18)	1	Humans	+
Xenorhabdus	3	Nematodes	+ & −
Others[g]	7		+ & −

[a] Primary site of humans and lower animals is usually gastrointestinal that subsequently leads to contamination of food and water.
[b] + = found in clinical samples.
[c] − = not all species, biogroups, or subgroups isolated from clinical samples.
[d] *Escherichia* and *Shigella* very closely related and may represent a single genus.
[e] *Salmonella* placed into subgroups 1-6. Subgroup 1 contains *S. typhi, S. choleraesuis, S. paratyphi A, S. gallinarum, S. pullorum,* and other serotypes. Subgroup 3 includes *Arizona* strains.
[f] *Shigella* may be considered as consisting of *S. dysenteriae, S. flexneri, S. boydii,* and *S. sonnei,* or as *Shigella* O groups A, B, and C, respectively, and *S. sonnei.*
[g] Designated by numbers in the "Enteric Group."

swabs, spinal fluid, or wound samples may contain one or more species (9). If a urine specimen is being analyzed valuable information is obtained by assaying for the total number of bacteria present by quantitative plate counts. Generally 10^5 or more bacteria/ml is considered significant. Specimens other than stools or urine usually require culture on blood or other non-selective media to encourage the growth of fastidious and/or Gram-positive organisms. This is because they may be excluded by using selective and differential media used for enteric bacteria. Sometimes, however, one may want to isolate Gram-positive organisms to the exclusion of Gram-negative bacteria. This can be accomplished by using a medium as phenylethanol agar.

Usually, the sooner a specimen can be processed the better the chance for successful growth of desired pathogenic bacteria. For stool specimens, direct plating within one to two hours will

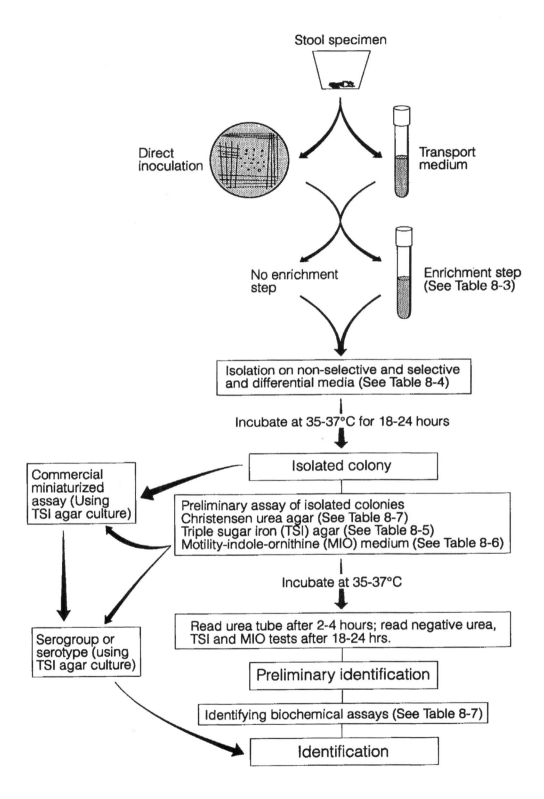

Figure 8-1: Basic schemes for isolation and identification of members of *Enterobacteriaceae* from stool samples using standard assays (9, 11)

Table 8-2
Comparison of Some Aspects of Commonly Used Classification Schemes for Enteric Bacteria Important in Clinical Microbiology

Edward's and Ewing's Identification of the *Enterobacteriaceae*, (9)	Bergey's Manual of Systematic Bacteriology, 1984 (4)	*Enterobacteriaceae* in Manual of Clinical Microbiology, 5th ed., 1991 (11)[a]
Tribe: *Escherichieae*		
Genus: *Escherichia* (5 species)	Genus: *Escherichia* (3 species)	Genus: *Escherichia*
Shigella (4 species)	*Shigella* (4 species)	*Shigella*
Tribe: *Edwardsielleae*		
Genus: *Edwardsiella* (3 species)	Genus: *Edwardsiella* (1 species)	Genus: *Edwardsiella*
Tribe: *Salmonelleae*		
Genus: *S. enterica* with 6 subspecies[b]	Genus: *Salmonella* Subgenus I-V[c]	Genus: *Salmonella*
Tribe: *Citrobactereae*		
Citrobacter (3 species)	Genus: *Citrobacter* (3 species)	Genus: *Citrobacter*
Tribe: *Klebsielleae*		
Genus: *Klebsiella* (7 species)	Genus: *Klebsiella*	Genus: *Klebsiella*
Enterobacter (10 species)	(2 species, 3 subspp.)	*Enterobacter*
Hafnia (3 species)	*Enterobacter* (6 species)	*Hafnia*
Serratia (9 species)	*Hafnia* (1 species)	*Serratia*
	Serratia (7 species)	
Tribe: *Proteeae*		
Genus: *Proteus* (4 species)	Genus: *Proteus* (3 species)	Genus: *Proteus*
Morganella (1 species)	*Morganella* (1 species)	*Morganella*
Providencia (4 species)	*Providencia* (3 species)	*Providencia*
Tribe: *Yersinieae*		
Genus: *Yersinia* (8 species)	Genus: *Yersinia* (6 species)	Genus: *Yersinia*
Tribe: *Erwinieae*		
Genus: *Erwinia* (no. species not given)	Genus: *Erwinia* (15 species)	Not provided.

[a] See Table 8-1 for complete listing of genera and number of species in each (from 11)
[b] All "biochemically typical" salmonellae and certain other bioserotypes included as *S. enterica* subspecies *enterica*, and therefore contains most strains.
[c] Serovars of *Salmonella* distributed among 5 subgenera based upon physiological characteristics (17).

give the greatest success in recovery of *Shigella* spp. These organisms are the most sensitive and fastidious of the clinically important *Enterobacteriaceae* (9, 11). If a longer period is required, a transport medium as Cary and Blair, Stuart's, or Amies may be used (11; also see Exercise 1, page 4 concerning these media).

If a pathogen is suspected in a stool specimen, especially if in low numbers as may happen with a carrier of *Salmonella typhi*, or if a food specimen suspected of containing *Y. enterocolitica*, enrichment should be considered. This will increase the relative numbers of desired organisms to better enable their isolation (Figure 8-1).

Enrichment Broths: Enrichment broths increase the possibility of isolating *Salmonella* and/or *Shigella* by *temporarily* inhibiting *Escherichia coli* and other normal inhabitants of stool speci-

mens. Table 8-3 shows those that are commonly used, their inhibitory components, and the usual application of each. It is important to use these media as directed by the manufacturer for best results.

Note that enteric enrichment broths are used to enhance the isolation of *Shigella* and/or *Salmonella*. If isolation of other genera are intended, excepting for certain *Yersinia*, an enrichment procedure should be avoided.

Yersinia also may be enriched, but not by the above methods. *Y. pestis* is, for example, increased in relative numbers by inoculation of guinea pigs, rats, or mice followed by isolation of the bacteria by plating methods (24). Other yersiniae, especially *Y. enterocolitica*, can be enriched using refrigeration temperatures. As might be expected, this may require an extended period of incubation to be successful (11).

Differential and Selective Plating Media
(Photos 8-4 through 8-21): Whether directly from patient or with an intermediate enrichment procedure, the next step, as shown in Figure 8-1, is to streak the sample or enrichment broth on to plates for isolation. If the sample is likely to contain one or two species, as in a blood specimen, only a single type of non-inhibitory medium is required. This is commonly sheep blood agar. However, if the specimen contains a mixture of microorganisms, as is the more common case, then both non-inhibitory and inhibitory selective and differential media are used. Selective media, as we have seen in some previous exercises, are helpful by allowing growth only of a desired group of organisms, while differential media allow one to distinguish organism(s) by their characteristic colonies on that medium. Table 8-4 gives properties of some types; the list is approximately grouped with least inhibitory media at the top and most inhibitory at the bottom.

Generally, except for *Y. enterocolitica*, at least two types of selective and differential media are used for stool specimens, along with a non-inhibitory medium. One of the former should be mildly inhibitory (and therefore less selective), but have good differential properties, such as MacConkey agar, eosin methylene blue (EMB) agar, or desoxycholate agar. The second should have moderate to strong inhibitory properties. This group includes desoxycholate citrate (DC), *Shigella-Salmonella* (SS), Hektoen enteric (HE), and xylose-lysine-sodium desoxycholate (XLD) agars. If *Salmonella typhi* is suspected, the strongly inhibitory bismuth sulfite (BiS) agar is included as a third type of medium. Brilliant green agar is also highly inhibitory, and useful for isolation of salmonellae other than *S. typhi* (1, 11).

For specimen sources of enteric bacteria other than the gastrointestinal tract two types of plating media are also used. In this instance, however, one is non-inhibitory and the other a mildly inhibitory and differential type, as MacConkey or EMB agar (1). *Yersinia enterocolitica* among the yersiniae especially can be isolated from stools of patients experiencing diarrhea. Although it will grow on MacConkey agar, cefsulodin-irgasan-novobiocin (CIN) agar is preferred. This is due to the strongly differential properties of this medium for yersiniae (Table 8-4). Other species of yersiniae are less commonly found in such specimens, but also will grow on CIN agar. Therefore, differential identification is required when characteristic colonies occur since the latter probably are not agents of gastrointestinal infection (11).

Important precautions should be noted concerning the use of all selective and differential media. First, non-growth of microorganisms, as normal flora bacteria, should be interpreted as *inhibition* of growth, not death. Thus, areas of an isolation plate that appear to have no growth can contain viable organisms. This also may be true of areas underlying growing colonies of wanted pathogens. This means that transfer of inhibited organisms to a non-inhibitory medium can lead to growth of these unwanted bacteria and therefore a mixed culture. Second, the "Groups Inhibited" and "Differential characteristics" shown in Table 8-4 are not absolute. For example, some Gram-positive bacteria will grow on mildly inhibitory media (e.g. enterococci on EMB agar). Furthermore, colony coloration giving differential characteristics is affected by culture age, kinds and density of adjoining colonies, and other factors.

Table 8-3
Enrichment Broths (9, 11)

Medium	Inhibitors or Selecting Condition	Application (For Isolation of:)
GN broth[a]	Sodium desoxycholate	*Shigella* and *Salmonella*
Selenite broth[a]	Sodium acid selenite	*Salmonella* spp. including *S. typhi*; some *Shigella* spp.
Tetrathionate broth of Mueller[a]	Sodium thiosulfate and iodine	*Salmonella* spp., including *S. typhi*; some *Shigella* spp.
Physiological saline, 2% peptone water, or sample itself	Refrigeration at 4-6°C for up to 3 weeks	*Yersinia enterocolitica*, *Y. pseudotuberculosis*

[a] These products available commercially (see Appendix 5).

Table 8-4
Properties of Enteric Bacteria Selective and Differential Plating Media (9, 11)

Medium[a]	Inhibitory Agents	Groups inhibited	Differential Characteristics
Mildly Inhibitory:			
Levine Eosin methylene blue (L-EMB) agar	Eosin Y; methylene blue	Gr (+)	*E. coli* form colonies with metallic green sheen; other lactose-fermenters pink, while non-lactose fermenters are colorless.[b]
MacConkey (Mac) agar	Bile salts, crystal violet	Gr (+)	Lactose fermenters form red colonies; non-lactose fermenters form colorless colonies.
Desoxycholate agar	Sodium desoxycholate	Gr (+)	Similar to MacConkey agar.
Moderately Inhibitory:			
Xylose-Lysine-Desoxycholate (XLD) agar	Sodium desoxycholate	Gr (+), some coliforms	Coliforms and some *Proteus* spp. form yellow colonies; some *Proteus* spp. form colorless colonies with black centers; most *Salmonella* spp. colonies red with black centers. *Shigella* form colorless colonies; *Citrobacter* are yellow with black centers.
Desoxycholate Citrate (DC) agar	Sodium desoxycholate	Gr (+), coliforms	Lactose fermenters form red to pink colonies; non lactose fermenters have colorless, translucent to opaque colonies; salmonellae may have brown centers.
Salmonella-Shigella (SS) agar	Bile salts, brilliant green	Gr (+), coliforms	Similar to MacConkey agar. Colonies with black centers due to H_2S formation.
Hektoen Enteric (HE) agar	Bile salts, acid fuchsin, bromthymol blue	Gr (+), coliforms and *Proteus*	Rapid lactose fermenters bright orange to salmon pink; *Salmonella* are blue to blue-green, usually with black (H_2S) centers; *Shigella* are more green then *Salmonella*; *P. mirabilis* gives greenish colonies with dark centers; H_2S-negative *Proteus* spp. similar to *Shigella,* but smaller colonies.
Strongly Inhibitory:			
Brilliant Green (BG) agar	Brilliant green	Gr (+), most Gr (−) except salmonellae (*S. typhi* inhibited)	*Salmonella* pink-white surrounded by red halo; others form yellow-green colonies with yellow-green halo.
Bismuth sulfite (BS) agar	Brilliant green, bismuth sulfite	Gr (+), most Gr (−).	*S. typhi, S. paratyphi B, S. enteritidis* form black colonies with metallic sheen; other salmonellae dark green colonies with or without black centers.
Other:			
Cefsulodin-irgasan-novobiocin (CIN) agar agar (26)	Cefsulodin, irgasan, and novobiocin	Gr (+), most Gr (−).	*Y. enterocolitica,* other *Yersinia* spp, and some *Citrobacter* form colonies with deep red centers and translucent periphery. Others that can grow form pink colonies without red centers.

[a] Media available form BBL Microbiology Systems; Difco Laboratories; and others.
[b] EMB agar also available with sucrose, as well as lactose. If both sugars present, additional species may present green sheen in colonies.

Testing of Isolates: Following growth of isolated colonies on streak plates, alternative routes of testing are available. The emphasis of this manual is on identification through standard biochemical testing. Figure 8-1 shows, however, that testing with commercially-available miniaturized, biochemically-based rapid assay kits can be used at this or later stages. (Many such kits are discussed in Exercises 1 and 2. Also, Photos 8-23 through 8-28 show several that can be used for enteric and other bacteria.) Indeed, this is a common step in many laboratories, using one or more of the many available. Some of these include, as examples, API® 20E, Rapid E*, and 20EC, Minitek®, Biolog GN Microplate™, The Fox Dual GNI Panel, Sensititre® Gram-Negative Autoidentification, the Vitek System using their GNI (Gram-negative identification) card, and others. As previously noted, these assays, besides saving space, have the advantage of also saving time. Thus, whereas biochemical identification may be accomplished within 4 to 24 hours after isolation of an organism using kits, standard tube methods usually require 48 hours or longer. However, as noted in Exercise 3, nontraditional assays require validation for accuracy. A particular laboratory facility should therefore thoroughly weigh these and other advantages against disadvantages of a preferred system before selecting it for use. References 2, 5, 12, 19, 20, 21, and 23 are selected examples of studies assessing non-traditional assays for identification of enteric bacteria.

Screening Tests: In the standard tube test, once having isolated colonies of a potential enteric pathogen on plates, the next task is to attempt to narrow it into a genus that could be responsible for the infection. The difficulty of this will in part depend, of course, on the concentration of contaminating flora on the plates. Especially confusing are bacteria that form colonies that resemble pathogenic groups, such as *Proteus* spp. Here a set of screening steps is useful. In our case, we will use triple sugar iron (TSI) agar, motility-indole-ornithine (MIO) medium, and Christensen urea agar (Figure 8-1).

TSI agar slants are inoculated by stabbing the agar deep with a straight inoculating needle. Without leaving the tube, the surface of the slant is then inoculated using a zig-zag streak pattern. Reactions are read after 18-24 hours incubation for the presence of sugar fermentation, gas

production, and H$_2$S production. Several possible reactions may be noted (Photo 8-22). These include a yellow butt and red slant due to the fermentation of glucose (phenol red indicator turns yellow due to the persisting acid formation in the butt; the slant remains red (alkaline) because of the limited glucose in the medium (0.1%) and therefore limited acid formation that does not persist); a yellow butt and slant due to the fermentation of lactose and/or sucrose (yellow slant and butt due to high concentrations (1%) of these sugars leading to excess acid formation in the entire medium); gas formation (noted by splitting of the agar); and H$_2$S formation (seen by blackening of the agar). If none of these reactions occur it means that none of the sugars were fermented (red butt and slant), and neither H$_2$S nor gas was produced. In such instances, *Acinetobacter, Pseudomonas,* or other non-fermenting bacteria should be suspected. (Remember, all members of the *Enterobacteriaceae* ferment glucose.) Table 8-5 gives usual TSI agar reactions expected from some more frequently encountered genera of the *Enterobacteriaceae*.

Extreme care must be employed when picking colonies from your selective and differential media to inoculate TSI slants or other types of media. As previously noted, many unwanted viable bacteria may be present on the surface of the plate. Therefore, it is poor technique to cool your needle by jabbing it into what may seem an uncontaminated portion. Always cool your needle in air, then touch only the very top of the needed colony for your inoculum.

Following inoculation of TSI agar, MIO medium can be stabbed to inoculate it. After streaking the TSI agar tube, and before removing the needle from the tube, touch its tip to the entry point of the stab. This will retrieve sufficient numbers of organisms to stab the MIO tube making it unnecessary to go back to the original colony (9). It is important that the needle is as straight as possible for this step. The stab is then made straight into the medium without forming a wide "groove" or broad cut in the agar. Following incubation, motility, indole production, and/or ornithine decarboxylation will be evident. Motility is visible by an increased turbidity in the tube distant from the stab line due to migration of organisms away from it. Ornithine decarboxylation causes the purple medium to become yellow in a negative test due to glucose fer-

Table 8-5
TSI Agar Reactions for Some Enteric Bacteria[a]

Genus-species	Occurrence of reaction	TSI Agar Reactions (Adapted from 13)[b]			
		Slant	Butt	H₂S	Gas
Citrobacter diversus		K[b]	A	−[b]	+
		A	A	−	+
C. freundii		K	A	+	+
		A	A	+	+
Enterobacter aerogenes		A	A	−	+
E. cloacae		K	A	−	+
Edwardsiella spp.		K	A	+[c]	+
Escherichia coli		K	A	−	+
		K	A	−	−
		A	A	−	+
		A	A	−	−
Klebsiella spp.	Usual	A	A	−	+
	Rare	K	A	−	−
	Rare	K	A	−	+
Morganella morganii	Usual	K	A	−	+
	Rare	K	A	−	−
Proteus vulgaris		K	A	+	+
		A	A	+	+
P. mirabilis	Usual	K	A	+	+
	Rare	A	A	+	+
Providencia spp.		K	A	−	+
		K	A	−	−
		A	A	−	−
Salmonella spp.	Usual	K	A	+	+
		K	A	+	−
	Rare	K	A	−	+
	Rare	A	A	+	+
S. paratyphi A		K	A	−	+
S. typhi	Usual	K	A	+	−
		K	A	−	−
Serratia spp.		A	A	−	+
		A	A	−	−
	Rare	K	A	−	−
	Rare	K	A	−	+
Shigella spp.		K	A	−	−
S. flexneri		K	A	−	+
Yersinia spp.		A	A	−	−
		K	A	−	−

[a] Readings based on a maximum of 48 hours incubation at 35-37°C.

[b] A = acid, K = alkaline. + = usually positive; − = usually negative.

[c] Of the *Edwardsiella*, only *E. tarda* produces H₂S on TSI agar. *E. tarda* biotype 1 and other *Edwardsiella* species do not produce this compound (11).

Table 8-6
Motility-Indole-Ornithine (MIO) Reactions of Enteric Bacteria (9, 11)[a]

Genus-species	Reactions on MIO		
	Motility	Indole	Ornithine Decarboxylation
Citrobacter diversus	+(−)	+	+
C. *freundii*	+(−)	−	+ or −
Enterobacter aerogenes	+	−	+
and E. *cloacae*	+	−	+
Edwardsiella tarda	+	+	+
Escherichia	+ or −	+	+ or −
Klebsiella spp.	−	−	−
Morganella morganii	+	+	+
Proteus vulgaris	+(−)	+(−)	−
P. *mirabilis*	+(−)	−(+)	+
Providencia spp.	+	+	−
Salmonella spp.	+ or −	−	+ or −
S. *paratyphi* A	+	−	+
S. *typhi*	+(−)	−	−
Serratia marcescens	+	−	+
Shigella spp.	−	+ or −	+[b] or −
Yersinia spp.	−	+ or −	+ or −
Y. *enterocolitica*	−ᵃ37°C	+ or −	+
	+25°C		

[a] + = usually positive; − = usually negative. (+) or (−) designate uncommon reactions.
[b] S. *sonnei* is positive; other species are negative.

mentation end products. If the medium again turns purple, the test is positive. (What is the biochemical reaction behind this?) Indole production is detected by addition of Kovacs' reagent. The formation of a pink to red color shows a positive test (6).

The test for urease using Christensen urea slants is also useful to consider. This is especially because *Salmonella* and *Shigella* are negative for this property, as shown in Table 8-7, while *Proteus, Morganella,* and some *Providencia* spp. are strongly positive. The importance of this in separation of genera is that all these, like the pathogenic *Salmonella* and *Shigella,* fail to ferment lactose. The earlier-developed selective and differential media as MacConkey, L-EMB, and desoxychlolate citrate agars contain this carbohydrate, and is a major basis for their differential property. Therefore, the lactose-negative genera cannot be distinguished on these media based on colony coloration, but most can be with the inclusion of the urease test. It is also helpful that those species positive for urease production are strongly so, and can induce a

positive test within 2-4 hours. Thus, if wanted, suspected colonies can be tested on the same day, but before inoculation of TSI and MIO media.

Following growth of TSI slants, other information also can be gathered that will be helpful in identification at the genus level. For, example, Gram stains, catalase, oxidase, and ONPG (o-nitrophenyl-β-D-galactopyanoside) tests can be readily and rapidly done. Therefore, using standard methods it is possible to isolate colonies, and find several key characteristics of the organism within 24-48 hours of receiving the sample. Colony characteristics, and TSI, MIO (Table 8-6), and urease reactions (Table 8-7) should show the possible genera present, including, most importantly, whether *Salmonella, Shigella,* or *Yersinia* is present. Subsequent steps are then designed to speciate and serotype your isolate.

Variations of this overall general procedure may be useful, and, at times, desirable. Early serological screening from non- or mildly-inhibitory plates may be possible, for example, and be helpful in detecting a *Salmonella, Shigella,* and pathogenic *E. coli* spp. Testing of an isolate on

Table 8-7
Biochemical Reactions of Enteric Bacteria (11)

Genus/species	Indole	MR[e]	VP[e]	Citrate[b]	Urease[c]	Arg	Lys	Orn	PA	Motility[d]	ONPG	Gas from glucose						Acid from[a]:											
													Adon	Arab	Dul	Inos	Lac	Malt	Mannit	Mucate	Raff	Rham	Salicin	Sorb	Suc	Trehal	Xylose
Citrobacter																											
diversus	+[a]	+	−	+	V+[e]	V	−	+	−	+	+	+	+	+	V	−	V	+	+	+	−	+	V−	+	V−	+	+
freundii	−	+	−	+	V+	V	−	V−	−	+	+	+	−	+	V	−	V	+	+	+	V−	+	−	+	V−	+	+
Edwardsiella																											
tarda[f]	+	+	−	−	−	−	+	+	−	+	−	+	−	−	−	−	−	+	−	−	−	−	−	−	−	−	−
Enterobacter																											
aerogenes	−	−	+	+	−	−	+	+	−	+	+	+	+	+	−	+	+	+	+	+	+	+	+	+	+	+	+
agglomerans	V−	V	V+	V	V−	−	−	−	V−	V+	+	V−	−	+	V−	V−	V	V+	+	V	V−	V+	V	V−	V+	+	+
cloacae	−	−	+	+	V	+	−	+	−	+	+	+	V−	+	V−	V−	+	+	+	V+	+	+	V+	+	+	+	+
Escherichia																											
coli[g]	+	+	−	−	−	V−	+	V	−	+	+	+	−	+	V	−	+	+	+	+	V	V+	V	+	V	+	+
Klebsiella																											
oxytoca	+	V−	+	+	+	−	+	−	−	−	+	+	+	+	V	+	+	+	+	+	+	+	+	+	+	+	+
pneumoniae	−	−	+	+	+	−	+	−	−	−	+	+	+	+	V−	+	+	+	+	+	+	+	+	+	+	+	+
rhinoscheromatis	−	+	−	−	−	−	−	−	−	−	−	−	+	+	−	+	−	+	+	−	+	+	+	+	V+	+	+
Morganella																											
morganii	+	+	−	−	+	−	−	+	+	+	−	+	−	−	−	−	−	−	−	−	−	−	−	−	−	−	−
Proteus																											
mirabilis	−	+	V	V	+	−	−	+	+	+	−	+	−	−	−	−	−	−	−	−	−	−	−	−	V−[e]	+	+
vulgaris	+	+	−	V−	+	−	−	−	+	+	−	V+	−	−	−	−	−	+	−	−	−	−	V	−	V−	V−	+
Providencia																											
alcalifaciens	+	+	−	+	−	−	−	−	+	+	−	V+	+	−	−	−	−	−	−	−	−	−	−	−	V−	−	−
rettgeri	+	+	−	+	V+	−	−	−	+	+	−	−	+	−	−	+	−	−	+	−	−	V+	V	−	V−	−	−
stuartii	+	+	−	+	V−	−	−	−	+	V+	−	−	−	−	−	+	−	−	−	−	−	−	−	−	V	+	−
Salmonella[h]																											
Subgroup 1	−	+	−	+	−	V+	+	+	−	+	−	+	−	+	+	V	−	+	+	+	−	+	−	+	−	+	+
choleraesuis (1)	−	+	−	V−	−	V[d]	+	+	−	+	−	+	−	−	+	−	−	+	+	−	−	+	−	+	−	−	+
paratyphi A (1)	−	+	−	−	−	V−	−	+	−	+	−	+	−	+	+	−	−	+	+	−	−	+	−	+	−	+	−
typhi (1)	−[d]	+	−	−	−	−	+	−	−	+	−	−	−	−	−	−	−	+	+	−	−	+	−	+	−	+	V+
arizonae (3a)[i]	−	+	−	+	−	V+	+	+	−	+	+	+	−	+	−	−	V−	+	+	+	−	+	−	+	−	+	+

	MR	VP	Arg	Lys	Orn	PA	ONPG	Adon	Arab	Dul	Inos	Lac	Malt	Mannit	Raff	rham	Sorb	suc	trehal	xylose
Serratia																				
liquifaciens	−	+	+	−	v−	−	v	v	−	−	−	v	+	+	−	v−	+	+	+	+
marcescens	−	v−	+	+	−	−	+	−	−	−	+	+	+	+	+	+	+	+	+	−
rubidaea	−	v−	+	+	−	−	+	v	−	+	+	v−	+	+	−	+	−	+	+	+
Shigella[j] (9)																				
dysenteriae (Gr.A)	v	+	−	−	−	−	−	−	−	−	−	−	v	v	−	v	−	−	v+	−
flexneri (Gr.B)	v	+	−	−	−	−	−	−	−	−	−	v	v	+	−	v	−	−	v+	−
boydii (Gr.C)	v−	+	−	v−	−	−	−	−	−	−	−	−	+	+	−	−	−	−	v+	v−
sonnei	−	+	−	+	−	−	+	v+	−	−	+	−	−	+	−	v+	−	−	+	−
Yersinia																				
enterocolitica	v	+	−	v+	−	−	+	−	v−	−	+	v−	+	+	−	−	−	+	+	v+
pestis	−	v+	−	−	−	−	v	−	−	−	+	−	v+	+	−	v+	v	+	+	+
pseudotuberculosis	−	+	−	+	−	−	v	v−	+	−	+	v−	−	+	+	v−	v+	−	+	+

[a] MR = methyl red reaction; VP = Voges-Proskauer reaction; Arg = Arginine dihydrolase; Lys = lysine decarboxylase; Orn = ornithine decarboxylase; PA = phenylalanine deaminase; ONPG = o-nitrophenyl-β-D-galactopyranoside. Abbreviations for carbohydrates: Adon = adonitol; Arab = L-arabinose; Dul = dulcitol; Inos = myo-inositol; Lac = lactose; Malt = maltose; Mannit = D-mannitol; Raff = raffinose; rham = L-rhamnose; Sorb = D-sorbitol; suc = sucrose; trehal = trehalose, and xylose = D-xylose.

[b] Citrate reaction determined on Simmon's citrate medium. [c] Determined using Christensen's urea medium. [d] Determined at 36°C.

[e] + = 90% or greater positive; V+ = 70-89% positive; V = 31-69% positive; V− = 11-30% positive; − = ≤ 10% positive. Results based upon a maximum incubation period of 48 hours at 35-37°C.

[f] *E. tarda* biogroup 1, unlike *E. tarda*, does not produce H_2S in TSI and uniformly produces acid in D-sorbitol.

[g] The strain "*E. coli* inactive" should be suspected if gas is not produced from glucose fermentation broth, and lactose is not fermented (V−). Other variations also occur.

[h] Farmer and Kelly (11) currently categorize *Salmonella* into Subgroups 1-6, with most serotypes belonging to Subgroup 1. *Arizona* strains fall into Subgroups 3a and 3b. Numbers shown in parenthesis designate subgroup.

[i] subgroup 3b (*Arizona*) biochemically differs from 3a in higher levels (V+) of lactose fermentation and lower levels (V−) of mucate fermentation.

[j] *Shigella* O groups A, B, and C are considered in Reference 11 to be a single biochemical group.

lysine iron agars (LIA) simultaneously as TSI helps to detect *Salmonella* spp. (11). Similarly, testing on phenylalanine deaminase (PA) agar will help to detect practically all *Proteus, Morganella,* and *Providencia.* Thus, although the general pattern above is one commonly used, flexibility in testing pattern should be included.

Identifying Steps: The identification of an enteric bacteria will necessarily involve a battery of biochemical tests. It also can include serological assays (Figure 8-1), procedures that will be discussed in Exercise 9.

Table 8-7 gives the expected results for many species in the *Enterobacteriaceae.* Though this can be used as a guide in identification, one should always be aware that many factors influence results of a particular test. Frequently, a method of "best fit" must be used, although additional tests will improve the certainty of identification. Also, more comprehensive references, many of which are listed at the end of this section, should be consulted.

Again, some additional precautions should be provided concerning these final steps. For example, despite your having done the MIO test, the ornithine decarboxylase test should be verified in the standard Moeller tube test (9). Also, confusing readings of motility should be verified in motility medium, although a wet mount and/or flagella stain may provide the needed information. The latter also has the advantage of providing information on the flagellar arrangement.

REFERENCES

1. Baron, E. J., L. R. Peterson, and S. M. Finegold. 1994. Bailey & Scott's diagnostic microbiology, 9th ed. Mosby-Year Book, Inc., St. Louis. p. 362-385.
2. Barr, J. G., G. M. Hogg, E. T. M. Smyth, and A. M. Emmerson. 1989. Comparison of identification of Enterobacteriaceae by API 20E and Sensititre Autoidentification System. J. Clin. Pathol. 42:649-652.
3. Bercovier, H., and H. H. Mollaret. 1984. *Yersinia* van Loghem 1944, p. 498-506. *In* N. R. Krieg, and J. G. Holt (ed.), Bergey's manual of systematic bacteriology, Vol. 1. Williams & Wilkins, Baltimore.
4. Brenner, D. J. 1984. *Enterobacteriaceae* Rahn 1937, p. 408-420. *In* N. R. Krieg, and J. G. Holt (ed.), Bergey's manual of systematic bacteriology, Vol. 1. Williams & Wilkins, Baltimore.
5. Cornaglia, G., B. Dainelli, F. Berlutti, and M. C. Thaller. 1988. Commercial identification systems often fail to identify *Providencia stuartii.* J. Clin. Microbiol. 26:323-327.
6. Difco Laboratories. 1984. Difco Manual, 10th ed. Difco Laboratories, Inc., Detroit, MI. p. 541-542.
7. Edwards, P. R., and W. H. Ewing. 1962. Identification of Enterobacteriaceae, 3rd ed. Burgess Publishing Co., Minneapolis, Minn. 258 p.
8. Eisenstein, B. I. 1990. Enterobacteriaceae, p. 1658-1673. *In* G. L. Mandell, R. G. Douglas, Jr., and J. E. Bennett (ed.), Principles and practices of infectious diseases, 3rd ed. Churchill Livingstone, New York.
9. Ewing, W. H. 1986. Edwards and Ewing's identification of Enterobacteriaceae, 4th ed. Elsevier Science Publishing Co., Inc. New York, p. 1-16, 27-45, 509-530.
10. Farmer, J. J. III, B. R. Davis, F. W. Hickman-Brenner, A. McWhorter, G. P. Huntley-Carter, M. A. Asbury, C. Riddle, H. G. Wathen-Grady, C. Elias, G. R. Fanning, A. G. Steigerwalt, C. M. O'Hara, G. K. Morris, P. B. Smith, and D. J. Brenner. 1985. Biochemical identification of new species and biogroups of *Enterobacteriaceae* isolated from clinical specimens. J. Clin. Microbiol. 21:46-76.
11. Farmer, J. J. III, and M. T. Kelly. 1991. *Enterobacteriaceae,* p. 360-383. *In* A. Balows, W. J. Hausler, Jr., K. L. Herrmann, H. D. Isenberg, and H. J. Shadomy (ed.), Manual of clinical microbiology, 5th ed. American Society for Microbiology, Washington, D. C.
12. Geers, T. A., and B. A. Backes. 1989. Evaluation of two rapid methods to screen pathogens from stool specimens. Am. J. Clin. Pathol. 91:327-330.
13. Howard, B. J., J. Klaas II, S. J. Rubin, A. S. Weissfeld, and R. C. Tilton. 1987. Clinical and pathogenic microbiology. The C. V. Mobsy Co., St. Louis. p. 289-328.
14. Jones, D. 1988. Composition and properties of the family Enterobacteriaceae. J. Appl. Bacteriol. Symp. Suppl. 65:1S-19S.
15. Kosako, Y., and R. Sakazaki. 1991. Priority of *Yokenella regensburgei* Kosako, Sakazaki, and Yoshizaki 1985 over *Koserella trabulsii* Hickman-Brenner, Huntley-Carter, Brenner, and Farmer 1985. Int. J. System. Bacteriol. 41:171.
16. Lelliott, R. A., and R. S. Dickey. 1984. *Ewinia* Winslow, Broadhurst, Buchanan, Krumwiede, Rogers and Smith, 1920, p. 469-476. *In* N. R. Krieg, and J. G. Holt (ed.), Bergey's manual of systematic bacteriology, Vol. 1. Williams & Wilkins, Baltimore.
17. Le Minor, L. 1984. *Salmonella* Lignières 1900, p. 427-458. *In* N. R. Krieg, and J. G. Holt (ed.), Bergey's manual of systematic bacteriology, Vol. 1. Williams & Wilkins, Baltimore.
18. McWhorter, A. C., R. L. Haddock, F. A. Nocon, A. G. Steigerwalt, D. J. Brenner, S. Aleksić, J. Bockenül, and J. J. Farmer III. 1991. *Trabulsiella guamensis,* a new genus and species of the family *Enterobacteriaceae* that resembles *Salmonella* subgroups 4 and 5. J. Clin. Microbiol. 29:1480-1485.
19. Miller, J. M., and D. L. Rhoden. 1991. Preliminary evaluation of Biolog, a carbon source utilization method for bacterial identification. J. Clin. Microbiol. 29:1143-1147.
20. O'Hara, C. M., and J. M. Miller. 1992. Evaluation of the autoSCAN-W/A system for rapid (2-hour) identification of members of the family *Enterobacteriaceae.* J. Clin. Microbiol. 30:1541-1543.
21. O'Hara, C. M., D. L. Rhoden, and J. M. Miller. 1992. Reevaluation of the API20E identification system versus conventional biochemicals for identification of members of the family *Enterobacteriaceae*: A new look at an old product. J. Clin. Microbiol. 30:123-125.
22. Penner, J. L. 1984. *Proteus* Hauser 1885, p. 491-494. *In* N. R. Krieg, and J. G. Holt (ed.), Bergey's manual of systematic bacteriology, Vol. 1. Williams & Wilkins, Baltimore.
23. Pfaller, M. A., D. Sahn, C. O. O'Hara, C. Ciaglia, M. Yu, N. Yamane, G. Scharnweber, and D. Rhoden. 1991. Comparison of the AutoSCAN-W/A rapid bacterial identification system and the Vitek AutoMicrobic System for identification of Gram-negative bacilli. J. Clin. Microbiol. 29:1422-1428.
24. Quan, T. J. 1987. Plague, p. 445-453. *In* B. B. Wentworth (ed.), Diagnostic procedures for bacterial infections, 7th ed. American Public Health Association, Inc., Washington, D. C.
25. Rowe, B., and R. J. Gross. 1984. *Shigella* Castellani and Chalmers 1919, p. 423-427. *In* N. R. Krieg, and J. G. Holt (ed.), Bergey's manual of systematic bacteriology, Vol. 1. Williams & Wilkins, Baltimore.
26. Schiemann, D. A. 1979. Synthesis of a selective agar medium for *Yersinia enterocolitica.* Can. J. Microbiol. 25:1298-1304.

EXERCISE 8
Yersinia

Of the eleven species of *Yersinia* (Table 8-2), three predominate in causing disease in both lower animals and in humans. Human plague due to *Y. pestis* is most notorious. Bubonic and pneumonic forms of this disease have been responsible for tremendous loss of life in human history. For example, probably one-third of the Western European population died between 1348 through 1350 because of this disease (7). It continues to occur today, fortunately, at a much lower rate of incidence. For 1990, the World Health Organization reported a world total of 1,250 cases with a 10.7% case fatality. The U. S. contributed only 2 cases to this total, with no deaths, however, over the previous 10 year period, a high of 40 cases was reported in 1983 resulting in 6 deaths (8).

Y. enterocolitica and *Y. pseudotuberculosis*, the other two species that cause human infection, have been isolated from a variety of conditions forming the disease entity "yersiniosis." In people this is usually acute mesenteric lymphadenitis and enterocolitis (2). Isolation of *Y. enterocolitica* from many extra-intestinal infections as pharyngitis, abscesses, cellulitis, etc. have also been reported (4).

As one could surmise from the distribution of diseases caused by *Y. pestis* compared to that of *Y. enterocolitica* and *Y. pseudotuberculosis*, the "lifestyles" of *Y. pestis* must differ from the others. It is, in fact, maintained *in vivo*, either in its flea vector or its rodent reservoir. In the U. S. these are mostly squirrels and prairie dogs; in other areas of the world they are rats (1, 2). Transmission to humans is usually from the bite of an infected flea, although aerosol transmission from a coughing infected individual also may occur (3).

Y. pseudotuberculosis and *Y. enterocolitica* also have lower animals as their primary reservoir. However, unlike the plague bacillus, except *Y. enterocolitica* serotypes 03 and 09, these organisms are spread into the environment through fecal excretions. Therefore, transmission to humans occurs through ingestion of contaminated food and water. Swine appears to be the reservoir for *Y. enterocolitica* serotypes 03 and 09. Because of this, this organism is not distributed widely in the environment (3). *Y. enterocolitica* infection occurs more frequently than those of either of the other species, though even it occurs infrequently in the U. S. compared to other diarrheal agents (2).

Morphological and physiological characteristics of *Y. pestis, Y. enterocolitica,* and *Y. pseudotuberculosis* are given in "Introduction to Exercises 8 and 9." However, some supplementary comments are provided here. Of course, all *Yersinia* have general characteristics typical of *Enterobacteriaceae*. Their temperature range for growth is comparatively broad for the medically important species, being 5°-45°C (1). This character has practical significance, as the use of refrigeration temperatures for enrichment of yersiniosis agents. *Y. enterocolitica* and *Y. pseudotuberculosis* are usually isolated from fecal samples, especially using CIN agar (Table 8-4), and incubated at 32°C for 24 hours (6). In identifying steps, *Yersinia* do not produce H_2S nor gas on TSI agar (Table 8-5), and both *Y. enterocolitica* and *Y. pseudotuberculosis* are motile at 20-25°C, but not at 35-37°C (*Y. pestis* is non-motile under both conditions) (6). These and other characteristics will become more evident in this exercise.

MATERIALS

A. per pair of students:
   1 slant culture *Y. enterocolitica*
   1 MacConkey agar plate
   1 Cefsulodin-irgasan-novobiocin (CIN) agar plate (Carr Scarborough Microbiologicals, Inc., Stone Mountain, GA; Remel, Lenexa, KA.)
   1 tube each of glucose and sucrose broths
   1 TSI agar slant
   2 tubes motility-indole-ornithine (MIO) medium
   Gram stain reagents
   Oxidase and catalase reagents
   Petri dish

LABORATORY PROCEDURES

Part 1

(Note: The proper use and reading of results of media used in this exercise are given in the introduction to exercises 8 and 9.)

A. Working in pairs, transfer the *Yersinia enterocolitica* stock culture to:
1. A MacConkey and a CIN agar plate, streaking for isolation.
2. Each of the following:
   a. TSI agar (stab and streak).
   b. Two tubes MIO medium (Stab with a *straight* needle).
   c. Christensen urea agar (streak)
   d. Glucose and sucrose broths.
   Incubate all cultures at 35°C for 48 hours, except one tube of MIO medium. This should be incubated at room temperature for 48 hours.
B. Prepare a Gram stain of *Y. enterocolitica* and examine microscopically.
C. Find the catalase and oxidase reactions for your stock culture. Do the catalase test on a filter paper strip in an empty petri dish, then do the oxidase test directly on a culture. Recall from Exercise 3 that the latter is to be done on colonies from non-selective and/or on a non-glucose containing medium. Otherwise, use the filter paper strip method for this also. After these steps, the stock culture can be discarded.

Part 2
A. Known culture:
1. Describe and compare colony characteristics of *Y. enterocolitica* grown on MacConkey and CIN agars. Can you decide whether the organism ferments lactose contained in MacConkey agar (See Table 8-4)?
2. Read the results of your tube inoculations. Compare reading of MIO medium incubated at 35°C with that kept at room temperature. Recall that motility is visible by turbidity extending away from the stab and ornithine decarboxylation by a purple color throughout the tube, while a bright yellow color is seen in a negative test. Indole production is tested by adding three to four drops of Kovacs' reagent to the culture. Development of a pink to red color is indicative of indole production, a yellow color is given in a negative test (5). Are glucose and sucrose fermented? What would you conclude if glucose were not? Was gas produced in the glucose tube? It should be noted that, although other fermentation broths may contain Durham

tubes, for enteric bacteria only gas production from glucose is significant. Therefore, it may be disregarded in other cases.
3. Tabulate and discuss your data. You should become aware of the key characteristics that not only differentiate species of *Yersinia*, but also separate this genus from others of the *Enterobacteriaceae*.
B. Demonstration of *Y. pestis*: (Note: Handle these cultures with extra care. Do *not* open plates or tubes, which have been taped shut for your protection. Keep cultures in a biohazard hood.)
1. Observe and record the colony characteristics of *Y. pestis* grown on blood agar at 35°C. Compare the amount of growth on this plate with that incubated at room temperature for an equal amount of time. What is the optimal temperature for this organism?
2. Record reactions obtained from TSI agar, urea slant, ornithine decarboxylase, motility medium, and glucose and sucrose broths. These were incubated at 35°C for 48 hours.
3. Compare these reactions with those of *Y. enterocolitica,* and those shown in Table 8-5 and 8-7. Based on these characteristics, which best differentiate it from *Y. pestis*? From *Y. pseudotuberculosis*?

QUESTIONS
1. *Y. pestis* was once classified as *Pasteurella pestis*. What characteristics better affiliate this organism (and other *Yersinia*) with the *Enterobacteriaceae* than the genus *Pasteurella*? Why is the genus *Pasteurella* not a part of the family *Enterobacteriaceae*?
2. The natural cycle of bubonic plague includes the rat and rat flea. How does this cycle differ from that of sylvatic plague?
3. Organisms such as *Y. enterocolitica* can be separated into "biotypes" and "serotypes." Give the basis of a biotype. How does it differ from a serotype? Of what importance is it to know an organisms' biotype and/or serotype?
4. With which genera in Tables 8-5, 8-6, and 8-7 of the family *Enterobacteriaceae* are *Y. enterocolitica* and *Y. pseudotuberculosis* most likely to be confused? Other than optimal growth temperature, give two other characteristics that will separate these *Yersinia* from each genus that you name.

REFERENCES

1. Brubaker, R. R. 1991. Factors promoting acute and chronic diseases caused by yersiniae. Clin. Microbiol. Rev. **4**:309-324.

2. Butler, T. 1990. Yersinia species (including plague), p. 1748-1756. *In* G. L. Mandell, R. G. Douglas, Jr., and J. E. Bennett (ed.). Principles and practices of infectious diseases, 3rd. ed. Churchill Livingston, New York.

3. Carniel, E., and H. H. Mollaret. 1990. Yersiniosis. Comp. Immu. Microbiol. Infect. Dis. **13**:51-58.

4. Cover, T. L., and R. C. Aber. 1989. *Yersinia enterocolitica*. N. Eng. J. Med. **321**:16-21.

5. Ederer, G. M., and M. Clark. 1970. Motility-indole-ornithine medium. Appl. Microbiol. **20**:849-850.

6. Farmer, J. J. III, and M. T. Kelly. 1991. *Enterobacteriaceae.*, p. 360-383. *In* A. Balows, W. J. Hausler, Jr., K. L. Herrmann, H. D. Isenberg, and H. J. Shadomy. (ed.), Manual of clinical microbiology, 5th ed. American Society for Microbiology, Washington, D. C.

7. Slack, P. 1989. The black death past and present. 2. Some historical problems. Trans. Royal Soc. Trop. Med. Hyg. **83**:461-463.

8. World Health Organization. 1991. Human plague in 1990. Weekly Epidemiol. Rec. **66**:321-324.

Exercise 8
Data Table 1: *Yersinia* Results

		Culture	*Y. enterocolitica*			*Y. pestis*	
		Age	MacConkey agar	CIN agar[a]	Other	Blood agar	
						35°C	RT
Colony size and Colony Form	mm						
	Punctiform						
	Irregular						
	Circular						
	Rhizoid						
	Filamentous						
	Other						
Colony Surface	Flat						
	Raised						
	Convex						
	Pulvinate						
	Other						
Colony Margin	Entire						
	Undulate						
	Lobate						
	Erose						
	Other						
Colony Consistency	Butyrous						
	Viscid						
	Membranous						
	Brittle						
	Other						
Colony Optical Character	Opaque						
	Translucent						
	Dull						
	Glistening						
	Other						
Colony Surface	Smooth						
	Rough						
	Other						
Colony	Color						
Hemolysis	Type						

[a] Cefsulodin-irgasan-novobiocin agar.

Exercise 8
Data Table 2: *Yersinia* Results

		Culture Age	*Y. enterocolitica*	*Y. pestis*
Catalase				
Culture Source				
Oxidase test				
Culture Source				
Gram stain	Reaction			
	Morphology			
	Arrangement			
TSI Agar	Slant[a]			
	Butt			
	H$_2$S			
	Gas			
MIO, 35°C	Motility			
	Indole			
	Ornithine			
MIO, RT[b]	Motility			
	Indole			
	Ornithine			
Urea				
Ornithine				
Motility	35°C			
Fermentation	Glucose, acid			
Broths	Gas			
	Sucrose			
Other				

[a] Usual designations for TSI agar reactions: A = Acid; K = Alkaline

[b] RT = Room Temperature.

Exercise 8
***Yersinia* Results**

Laboratory Notes

EXERCISE 9
The *Enterobacteriaceae*
(Excluding *Yersinia*)

This exercise emphasizes the isolation and identification of members of the family *Enterobacteriaceae* other than *Yersinia*. Earlier it was said that *Salmonella*, *Shigella*, and pathogenic *Escherichia coli* are of particular interest because of their disease-producing potential. Obviously, to recognize these organisms, it is necessary to be able also to identify what are usually normal flora organisms. It will be the objective of this exercise to expose you to both groups of bacteria. This will be done primarily through a physiological study of known stock cultures, followed by isolation and identification of enteric bacteria from a stool specimen. However, some added background concerning these organisms will prove useful.

Salmonella spp. are all considered to have disease-producing potential. They cause salmonellosis of two general types. The majority induce gastroenteritis, while a few cause enteric fever. The latter includes *S. typhi,* an organism whose host is restricted to humans, and *S. paratyphi* A, C, and some B (8). Other species occasionally also may cause enteric fever. All forms of this clinical entity are named paratyphoid fever, except that due to *S. typhi* that is responsible for typhoid fever. A common feature of all forms of enteric fever is bacteremia, therefore, blood samples, besides stools, may be useful in the isolation of the offending agents. However, agents of gastroenteritis, the second general type of infection associated with salmonellae, can cause bacteremia, as exemplified by *S. choleraesuis,* which is isolated less frequently from stools than from blood. Nonetheless, the most commonly isolated serotypes are derived from stools (5, 8). Other types of infections are also produced by salmonellae, including abscesses, respiratory tract infections, meningitis, and arteritis. Furthermore, human and animal carriers of *Salmonella* represent an important reservoir of disease, especially the human typhoid carrier.

Shigella spp. are all also considered to be pathogenic, though species markedly vary in their virulence. These and pathogenic *E. coli* are responsible for human gastrointestinal disease. That due to *Shigella* have been classically called bacillary dysentery or shigellosis. Pathogenic *E. coli* have been categorized by the four clinical entities they can cause. The first is enteropathogenic *E. coli* (EPEC), associated with watery diarrhea outbreaks in nurseries; enteroinvasive *E. coli* (EIEC) produce shigellosis-like symptoms; enterotoxic *E. coli* (ETEC) induce diarrhea due to production of heat labile and heat stable enterotoxins, and is an important cause of travelers' diarrhea; and, finally, enterohemorrhagic *E. coli* (EHEC) cause hemorrhagic colitis accompanied by bloody diarrhea, but without fever or gastrointestinal mucosal inflammation (3). Lower animals are also afflicted with pathogenic *E. coli*. For example, ETEC are an important cause of diarrheal disease in neonatal calves, lambs, and pigs. Also, EHEC cause diarrhea in calves (7).

Identification of *Salmonella* and *Shigella* to the genus level, and *E. coli* can be accomplished using morphological and physiological methods discussed earlier. Beyond this, special problems are encountered. *Salmonella*, for instance, consists of over 2200 serovars (or serotypes) (12), although only 10% of these accounts for over 70% of human isolates (8). It is quite possible the name of your home town or State is among the species since the location where the first isolate was obtained is frequently used for this. *Shigella* consist of four species (or alternately, *S. sonnei* and O-groups A, B, and C), and about 40 serotypes (1). *E. coli,* though a single species, unlike salmonellae and shigellae, can be non-pathogenic normal flora bacteria. However, it is known that pathogenic *E. coli* contain certain identifying antigens, and therefore can be selected by serotyping.

From this brief summary it should be apparent that antigenic typing may be important in either identification of the organisms, or deciding the epidemiology of the pathogenic salmonellae, shigellae, or *E. coli*. Serology is also used for similar purposes for *Serratia*, *Klebsiella*, and others (4).

Fortunately, the principles in serotyping all these organisms are similar. Basically, the epitopes of heat stable somatic antigen (or lipopolysaccharide, LPS), heat labile H antigen (or flagellar antigen), and/or K or V_i capsular or envelope antigens are determined for each isolate. Although typically all isolates contain LPS, the presence of others will vary. *Shigella*, for example, are non-motile, therefore obviously lack H antigens.

In no group is the number of serotypes (or serovars) more extensive than in the *Salmonella*. This genus will later be used in this exercise to demonstrate the principles of serotyping by slide agglutination. The classification of the *Salmonella* into serovars is based upon the Kauffmann-White Schema (9). Of the over 2,200 serovars, each is different from the other by the presence of one or more specific O antigens, which are given numbers; one or more "Phase 1" (relatively serovar-specific), indicated by lower case letters, or letters with subscript numbers) and "Phase 2" (relatively serovar nonspecific, shown by numbers, letters, or letters with subscript numbers) flagellar antigens; and V_i antigen. The latter occurs only on 3 serovars of salmonellae, *S. typhi*, *S. dublin*, and *S. paratyphi C*. If this antigen is present, it will mask O epitopes because of its surface location. This effect can be overcome by boiling the V_i-containing organisms suspended in physiological saline solution for 10-20 minutes (4).

Two examples of the application of the Kauffmann-White Schema are *S. typhi* and *S. typhimurium*. Both organisms belong to Group 1 (Table 8-7) of the *Salmonella*. *S. typhi* is serologically typed as 9, 12 [V_i]: d: -. Thus, its O antigens are 9 and 12; it contains a V_i envelope; and a Phase 1 "d" flagellar antigen. It does not have any Phase 2 H antigen. It is noted that the bracket around V_i antigen or any other term means that the antigen may not be present. For the second example, *Salmonella typhimurium* is serovar *1*, 4, [5,] 12 : i: 1, 2. Based on the above convention, it contains O antigens 1, 4, 12, and perhaps 5. Its Phase 1 flagellar antigen is "i"; its Phase 2 antigens are 1 and 2. In addition, the italicized O antigen 1 designates that it is present due to a lysogenic bacteriophage (4, 11).

The serovars of salmonellae are all categorized into groups based upon certain common O antigens. For example, serogroup $O_2(A)$ has three serotype members, all of which contain somatic antigen O_2. Group O9, 12 (D_1) contain all serotypes with O9 and O12 (including *Salmonella typhi*). Group O9, 46(D_2) differs by having common O antigen O46 instead of O12. As can be seen here, each group also has a capital letter desig-

nation, at least through "Y." Several of these are subdivided, as D_1 and D_2 shown above. Beyond this, they are designated by the common O antigen of that group (11).

The practical significance of placing salmonellae into groups based on common O antigens is that "grouping" antisera can readily be used to screen isolates to their serogroup using anti-Group A, anti-group B, etc. Many diagnostic laboratories may not proceed past this step in serological analysis of the salmonellae. Instead, the culture is forwarded to a reference laboratory that has the complete battery of typing antisera available for complete analysis of the isolate.

A similar convention of serotype designation is used for other *Enterobacteriaceae*, including *Shigella* and *E. coli*. *Shigella* are serologically grouped as A, B, C, and D. This fortunately corresponds to species designations of *S. dysenteriae*, *S. flexneri*, *S. boydii*, and *S. sonnei*, respectively (Table 8-7). Grouping antisera are available, and may be required to identify shigellae at the species level. Beyond this, the organisms may be typed into one of the 37 different serotypes using specific antiserum. Here, only O antigen content is used for serotyping (5), these being designated by numbers, or numbers with subscript letters (which designate subfactors). Thus, shigellae can be classified as Group B (i.e. *S. flexneri*), 1a, or Group A (i.e. *S. dysenteriae*), 12, etc. (4). While group determinations are useful as an aid for identification, serotyping is primarily used for epidemiological purposes.

Those serotypes of *E. coli* responsible for gastrointestinal disease have been identified. There are 26 serotypes that are ETEC, 21 EPEC, etc. These are based upon somatic and flagellar antigens, if any. Thus, common serotypes associated with diarrhea of the newborn due to an EPEC are O55:H6 and O55:NM (non-motile), and hemorrhagic colitis (due to EHEC) is O157:H7 (5). As should be apparent, serotyping of enteropathogenic *E. coli* is important for associating it with a particular infection, and ruling out several hundred of other serotypes that are normal flora.

As will be shown in this exercise, serotyping is primarily done employing the slide agglutination method using a saline suspension of the isolate and a desired grouping or typing antiserum. (See Exercise 2, page 46 for more information concerning the agglutination and other serological tests.) Several antisera are commercially available for this, as are latex agglutination tests designed to detect *E. coli* O157:H7 from isolation plates, and *Salmonella-Shigella* from GN broth.

Several other assays are available to aid in diagnostic testing. Titration of patient's serum for antibody levels has been useful, especially in typhoid fever, where the assay is called the Widal test. The detection of V_i antibodies has also been helpful in diagnosing typhoid carriers. *Shigella* and infectious *E. coli* have toxic and invasive properties. These characteristics can be detected by specialized assays, but are usually not done in the general diagnostic laboratory. DNA probes, ELISA, and bacterial toxicity and invasion of cells *in vivo* and in cells in culture are a few approaches being applied (5, 15). Two assays for *E. coli* heat-labile enterotoxin are commercially available. The Vet-RPLA is based on reverse passive agglutination; the Phadebact ETEC-LT uses a coagglutination test.

It also should be mentioned that O-1 phage can be useful in salmonellae detection because most strains are susceptible to it (11). The number of phage-resistant strains, a frequent problem with this procedure can be alleviated by use of two screening media, a double sugar tyrosine and an ONPG-urease-indole medium (16). Phage typing also can be applied to epidemiologic studies for some species as *S. typhi*, *S. typhimurium*, and *S. enteritidis*, having the advantage of being able to divide the species beyond the level of serovars. A recent study of the latter species, for example, differentiated 27 phage types, although the epidemiologic significance of this remains to be determined (6).

MATERIALS

Part 1

Per pair of students:
1 culture each of *Escherichia coli, Klebsiella pneumoniae, Salmonella typhi, Shigella dysenteriae,* and *Proteus vulgaris.*
(Note: Cultures may be given code letters or numbers in place of names.)
3 agar plates of each of the following:
Levine Eosin Methylene Blue (L-EMB)
Shigella-Salmonella (SS)
MacConkey (Mac)
Bismuth Sulfite (BS)
Hektoen Enteric (HE)

5 tubes of each of the following:
TSI agar slant
Christensen urea agar
Motility-indole-ornithine (MIO) semisolid agar
MR-VP broth, 0.5 ml per 13 x 100 mm tube
MR-VP broth, 2.5 ml per 16 x 100 mm tube
Simmons citrate agar
Arginine dihydrolase broth
Lysine decarboxylase broth
Phenylalanine agar
Glucose broth with Durham tube
Arabinose broth
Dulcitol broth
Lactose broth
Maltose broth
Mannitol broth
Mucate broth
Rhamnose broth
Sucrose broth
Trehalose broth
Xylose broth

Part 2

A. Reagents for:
Indole test (Kovac's Reagent)
Catalase test
MR-VP tests
Oxidase test
Phenylpyruvic acid (10% ferric chloride)
ONPG test (o-nitrophenyl-β-D-galactopyranoside disks and five 10 x 75 mm tubes, each containing 0.2 ml physiological saline
B. Per student:
Fecal specimen containing unknown enteric organism(s)
1 tube GN broth
2 standard plates of MacConkey or L-EMB agar
2 standard plates of SS or Hektoen agar

Part 3

Per student:
4 TSIA slants
4 Christensen urea slants
4 tubes MIO
4 tubes Simmons citrate agar
4 tubes MR-VP broth, 0.5 ml/tube
4 tubes MR-VP broth, 2.5 ml/tube
2 tubes of each of remaining biochemical media used in *Part 1* and:
Ornithine decarboxylase
Motility medium
Adonitol broth

Inositol broth
Raffinose broth
Salicin broth
Sorbitol broth
1 Miniaturized, commercially manufactured identification kit.

Part 4
Per pair of students:
1 tube with 0.25 ml anti-*S. typhimurium* serum
1 tube with 5 ml *S. typhimurium* antigen
1 tube with 10 ml physiological saline solution (PSS)
9 12 x 75 mm (Kahn) tubes
1 test tube rack
31 ml pipettes
37°C water bath
Centrifuge

LABORATORY PROCEDURES

Part 1
Known cultures: Each pair of students will be provided with cultures of *E. coli, Salmonella typhi, K. pneumoniae, Shigella dysenteriae,* and *P. vulgaris.* With each of these, except in Step 1, carry out the following:
1. Gram stain one species and microscopically examine. (Microscopically the enteric bacteria appear similar, therefore the morphology of one species is typical of most (Photo 8-1, 8-2.)
2. Transfer each species except *P. vulgaris* to ½ of a standard plate of the following media. Place *P. vulgaris* by itself on the third plate of each. Streak all for isolation, then incubate at 35°C for 24-48 hours. (Note: Differential properties usually best seen at 18-24 hours.)
    a. L-Eosin Methylene Blue agar
    b. MacConkey agar
    c. Hektoen Enteric agar
    d. *Shigella-Salmonella* agar
    e. Bismuth Sulfite agar
3. Inoculate the following media with each stock culture:
    a. TSI agar
    b. Christensen urea agar
    c. MIO medium
    d. Two tubes MR-VP medium (1 tube contains 0.5 ml; the other contains 2.5 ml)
    e. Simmons citrate

f. Arginine dihydrolase (overlay with one-half inch depth sterile mineral oil unless in a screw-capped tube. If the latter, tighten cap securely).
g. Lysine decarboxylase (same procedure as for arginine dihydrolase.)
h. Phenylalanine agar (use heavy inoculum.)
i. Glucose broth
j. Arabinose broth
k. Dulcitol broth
l. Lactose broth
m. Maltose broth
n. Mannitol broth
o. Mucate broth
p. Rhamnose broth
q. Sucrose broth
r. Trehalose broth
s. Xylose broth

Part 2
A. Previously inoculated media:
1. From *Part 1-2*: Describe and compare characteristics of isolated colonies on plates. Also, note inhibition of growth of certain species with types of media.
2. From *Part 1-3*:
    a. Read TSI agar tube reactions for the presence of acid, gas, and H_2S production. These should be read at 18-24 hours, and if necessary, again at 48 hours.
    b. Look for the presence of urease production. Recall that for strong producers of this enzyme, such as *Proteus* spp., the urea test may be positive within 2 to 4 hours.
    c. Motility-indole-ornithine medium is read in 18-24 hours as described in Exercise 8, *Part 2A-2* (page 134) (2).
    d. Incubate both tubes of MR-VP medium for 18-24 hours, though the VP test may require 48 hours. Test the tube containing 2.5 ml for acetoin (VP test) by adding 0.6 ml α-naphthol, shaking, then adding 0.2 ml KOH. If a red color develops within 15 minutes, the test is positive (13).

    The other tube containing 0.5 ml broth should be tested with methyl red reagent. Development of a red color after addition of one drop shows a positive test; an orange or yellow color is a negative test (13).

e. Is citrate used? What is responsible for the blue color reaction? Incubate negative tests up to 48 hours.

f. Lysine and arginine broths should be examined for the presence of a purple (positive reaction) or yellow (negative test) up to 48 hours (Photo 9-1). This shows the organism's capability to produce enzymes that will decarboxylate these amino acids. Take care in interpretation if read before 24 hours of incubation since, as with ornithine decarboxylation, a yellow color due to acid formation derived from glucose fermentation may occur early and be mistaken for a negative assay. Additional time may be necessary for enzyme activity to release alkaline products that will cause the medium to turn purple (13).

g. Phenylalanine agar is used to detect the production of phenylpyruvic acid after incubating for 18-24 hours. This is done by allowing 5 drops of 10% ferric chloride solution to run across the surface growth. A green color develops within 5 minutes in a positive test.

h. ONPG disks detect the capacity of the organism to degrade o-nitrophenyl-β-D-galactopyranoside by their producing the enzyme β-galactosidase. Its presence is detected by suspending a loopful of organisms in 0.2 ml physiological saline solution (PSS) in a tube, then dropping in one ONPG disk. Incubate for up to four hours at 37°C. A positive test is seen by a yellowing of the solution due to the release of o-nitrophenol.

i. Observe all fermentation tubes for the presence of acid, and in glucose broth, for the presence of gas.

j. Determine catalase and oxidase reaction for each species.

k. Tabulate results on Data Tables 1-6 provided. Compare results with Tables 8-4 through 8-7 or other published sources and discuss. Note that most sources give data based upon a maximum of 48 hours incubation. In order for your data to be comparable based upon this parameter, longer incubations are unnecessary.

B. Unknown samples: Each student will be given a small amount of fecal matter containing one or more species of the family *Enterobacteriaceae*. You are to make an identification of the correct organism(s) present, including at least one species of *Salmonella* or *Shigella*. Start by placing approximately one gram of unknown into GN or other type of enrichment broth. Also, inoculate your sample directly on to plating media provided. After 4-18 hours, depending on the type of enrichment broth, also streak the enriched culture on to fresh plating media. As previously emphasized, proper streaking technique is an absolute necessity. Typical colony characteristics important in the preliminary grouping of genera will not be observed on differential media lacking isolation.

Continue identifying steps with the aid of Figure 8-1, and Tables 8-5, 8-6, and 8-7. Following completion of laboratory identification of your unknown organisms, identify them using those tables, or other sources of information in a standard analysis. *After completion of your standard analysis, verify the identification using the computer and MICRIDX program.* Instructions concerning the use of the latter are given in Exercise 2, page 38. However, here your "ORGANISM NAME file" is ENT-ORG, your "TEST NAME file" ENT-TEST, and your "PROBABILITY DATA file" ENT-DATA. Use the information obtained by computer analysis in the overall rationalization of your identification. If your own analysis disagrees with that of the computer, you must determine the reason for the discrepancy. Remember, MICRIDX is to be used to verify *your* analysis, and not the other way around. Do not fall into the trap of letting the computer possibly misleading you to a faulty conclusion by not doing the standard analysis first.

Part 3

A. Unknown cultures: Continue identification of your unknown cultures by procedures outlined in *Part 1* and *2A*. Don't forget to do a Gram stain and microscopic observation of your isolate from TSI agar. In addition, a commercially-available miniaturized assay system will be made available for your use.

When you have completed your work, tabulate all results and submit a report including (1) Purpose; (2) Procedure; (3) Results; (4) Discussion; (5) Conclusions; and (6) References. Don't forget to include the unknown's code number.

B. Use the commercially-available identification system made available to you. Although it can be used to help in the identification (or perhaps in your case, verification of an identification) of one isolate from your unknown, the main purpose is to provide insight into their use, and their advantages and disadvantages. Be sure to follow the manufacturer's instructions concerning its use. Your instructor will advise you as to whether the information obtained from this kit also should be used in your unknown report.

Part 4

As discussed previously, culture identification methods can be greatly enhanced by use of antigens and antibodies. This may require the use of known antigen to identify the presence of an antibody response in the serum from a patient. Alternately, a known antiserum may be used to identify or serotype an unknown isolate. Examples of how these are accomplished is the subject of this section.

A. The tube agglutination test: Each pair of students will be provided with a killed suspension of *Salmonella typhimurium* and 0.25 ml anti-*S. typhimurium* serum. Using these materials carry out an agglutination titration by the following procedures and that shown in Figure 9-1:

1. Set up ten 12 x 75 mm tubes in a row, with the first tube containing the 0.25 ml of antiserum. Number from 1 through 10.
2. Add 0.5 ml physiological saline solution (PSS) to each tube, except for No. 1, with a 1 ml pipette.
3. To tube No. 1 add 0.75 ml PSS. (What dilution of serum does this give?)
4. Using the same pipette gently aspirate contents of Tube No. 1, then transfer 0.5 ml diluted serum to tube No. 2. Mix by gentle aspiration. (Note: Proper technique and accuracy require the use of separate pipettes for each transfer in a quantitative

dilution series. A qualitative procedure is being used here as a supply expediency.)
5. Again using the same pipette, transfer 0.5 ml from tube No. 2 to No. 3. Mix as previously.
6. Continue this procedure until you have made serial dilutions to tube No. 9. Discard 0.5 ml from this last tube after mixing. (What is the final serum dilution?) All tubes should now contain 0.5 ml.
7. Next, add 0.5 ml *S. typhimurium* antigen to each tube, including No. 10, which is the control tube, giving a final volume of 1 ml in all tubes.
8. Incubate at 37°C (in a water bath) for 15 minutes. Agitate contents in tubes by gently shaking entire rack. Incubate for an additional 15 minutes. Observe for clumping of the organisms.
9. Centrifuge tubes in a clinical centrifuge for 5 minutes at a speed of about 1000 rpm. Place tubes back into the tube rack, then gently shake the rack to resuspend the bacteria. Compare all tubes with the control. Determine the endpoint (i. e. titer) and record.

B. Serotyping:

Serotyping is frequently a helpful step in the identification of a species within the *Enterobacteriaceae*. This demonstration will involve suspending a pure culture of *S. typhi* or other salmonellae in PSS. The serological group of this organism will then be determined by the slide agglutination test using commercially-available polyvalent grouping antiserum. A negative control consisting of normal serum, saline, or a grouping serum known not to contain antibodies against any epitopes of the test organism is required.

C. Demonstration: Direct Fluorescent Antibody Test (14).

A commonly used procedure for serological detection of antigen is the fluorescent antibody (FA) method. In medical microbiology it has found application as a useful adjunct to the detection and identification of viruses, rickettsia, fungi, protozoa, and bacteria, including members of the *Enterobacteriaceae*.

Fluorescent antibody is prepared by conjugating appropriately prepared immunoglobulin (Ig) specific for the desired antigen with a

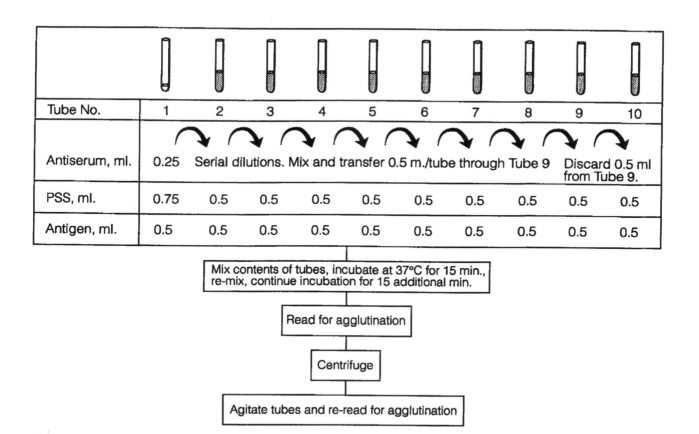

Tube No.	1	2	3	4	5	6	7	8	9	10
Antiserum, ml.	0.25	Serial dilutions. Mix and transfer 0.5 m./tube through Tube 9							Discard 0.5 ml from Tube 9.	
PSS, ml.	0.75	0.5	0.5	0.5	0.5	0.5	0.5	0.5	0.5	0.5
Antigen, ml.	0.5	0.5	0.5	0.5	0.5	0.5	0.5	0.5	0.5	0.5

Mix contents of tubes, incubate at 37°C for 15 min., re-mix, continue incubation for 15 additional min.

Read for agglutination

Centrifuge

Agitate tubes and re-read for agglutination

Figure 9-1: The tube agglutination test.

fluorescing compound, usually fluorescein isothiocyanate. In the direct test, an outline of which is shown in Figure 9-2, the antigen is placed on a microscope slide, fixed, then stained with fluorescent antibody for 10 to 60 minutes. Unbound FA is removed by washing, and the preparation mounted in buffered glycerol. If FA has reacted with the antigen, and the specimen observed in a microscope having a light source emitting the proper wavelength of light (for fluorescein isothiocyanate-labeled Ig this is 350-450 nm), a positive test is seen as a yellow-green fluorescent organism in a dark field (an example seen in Photo 3-5). Best results are obtained using a dark-field microscope equipped with a light source that emits in the ultraviolet to blue spectrum.

Variations in the fluorescent antibody procedure expand its usefulness. One of these is the indirect test, or sandwich technique. Here unlabeled antibody (Ig), which can be a patient serum specimen, is first applied to known antigen (Ag). The preparation is rinsed to remove unattached Ig, then fluorescent-labeled anti-immunoglobulin (FA-anti-Ig) is applied. The remainder of the procedure is the same as the direct test. Only if Ig reacts with Ag can the FA-anti-Ig attach to the complex, and therefore fluorescence seen. An example of an application of this assay is the fluorescent treponema antibody (FTA) test that is described in Exercise 14.

The demonstration available for observation here is the direct test. The organism being used is a *Salmonella* Subgroup 1

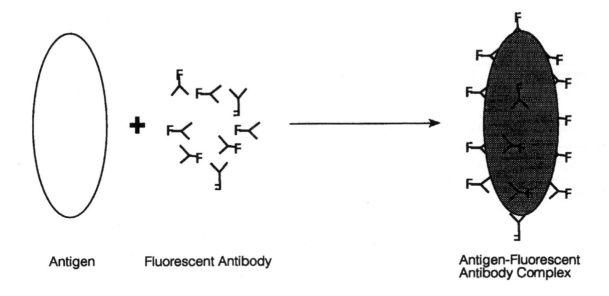

Antigen   Fluorescent Antibody   Antigen-Fluorescent Antibody Complex

Figure 9-2: The direct fluorecent antibody assay.

organism. It will be stained with FA-anti-*Salmonella* panvalent serum (Difco Laboratories), an antiserum that is capable of detecting all *Salmonella* species. A control preparation will consist of a non-salmonellae stained in the same manner with this antiserum. Observe and record your results. Can you readily differentiate which preparation contains the homologous antigen-antibody complex?

Also compare differences between the fluorescent microscope and the ordinary light microscope. Especially note the special light source and extensive filter system of the latter. Why is the filter system required? What is the purpose of each filter?

QUESTIONS

1. Give the primary substrate(s) and product(s) responsible for positive tests in each of the following. Also explain how the reactions become visible in each instance. (Note: See especially references 10 and 13):
   a. Citrate test
   b. Indole test
   c. Lysine and ornithine decarboxylase tests
   d. Arginine dihydrolase test
   e. Voges-Proskauer test
   f. Mucate fermentation test
   g. Phenylalanine test
2. Compare the genus *Klebsiella* with the *Enterobacter* on the basis of:
   a. Kinds of infections produced in humans and in animals;
   b. Distribution;
   c. Physiology, cytology, and morphological characteristics.
3. List the bacterial genera one is most likely to find in the normal gastrointestinal tract of the human.
4. Aside from the genera of the family *Enterobacteriaceae*, name those that are most likely to cause gastrointestinal disease.

REFERENCES

1. DuPont, H. L. 1990. Shigella species (bacillary dysentery), p. 1716-1722. *In* G. L. Mandell, R. G. Douglas, Jr., and J. E. Bennett (ed.), Principles and practices of infectious diseases, 3rd ed. Churchill Livingstone, New York.

2. Ederer, G. M., and M. Clark. 1970. Motility-indole-ornithine medium. Appl. Microbiol. **20**:849-850.

3. Eisenstein, B. I. 1990. Enterobacteriaceae, p. 1658-1672. *In* G. L. Mandell, R. G. Douglas, Jr., and J. E. Bennett (ed.), Principles and practices of infectious diseases, 3rd ed. Churchill Livingstone, New York.

4. Ewing, W. H. 1986. Edward and Ewing's identification of Enterobacteriaceae, 4th ed. Elsevier Science Publishing Co., Inc. p. 73-91, 181-318.

5. Farmer, J. J. III, and M. T. Kelly. 1991. *Enterobacteriaceae*, p. 360-383. *In* A. Balows, W. J. Hausler, Jr., K. L. Herrmann, H. D. Isenberg, and H. J. Shadomy (ed.), Manual of clinical microbiology, 5th ed. American Society for Microbiology, Washington, D. C.

6. Hickman-Brenner, F. W., A. D. Stubbs, and J. J. Farmer III. 1991. Phage typing of *Salmonella enteritidis* in the United States. J. Clin. Microbiol **29**:2817-2823.

7. Holland, R. E. 1990. Some infectious causes of diarrhea in young farm animals. Clin. Microbiol. Rev. 3:345-375.

8. Hook, E. W. 1990. Salmonella species (including typhoid fever), p. 1700-1716. *In* G. L. Mandell, R. G. Douglas, Jr., and J. E. Bennett (ed.), Principles and practices of infectious diseases, 3rd ed. Churchill Livingstone, New York.

9. Kauffmann, F. 1966. The bacteriology of Enterobacteriaceae. The Williams & Wilkins Co, Baltimore. 400 p.

10. Koneman, E. W., S. D. Allen, W. M. Janda, P. C. Schreckenberger, and W. C. Winn, Jr. 1992. Color atlas and textbook of diagnostic microbiology, 4th ed. J. B. Lippincott Co., Philadelphia. p. 105-184.

11. Le Minor, L. 1984. *Salmonella* Lignières 1900, p. 427-458. *In* N. R. Krieg, and J. G. Holt (ed.), Bergey's manual of systematic bacteriology, Vol. 1. Williams & Wilkins, Baltimore.

12. Le Minor, L., M. Y. Popoff, and J. Bockemühl. 1990. Supplement 1989 (no. 33) to the Kauffman-White scheme. Res. Microbiol. **141**:1173-1177.

13. MacFaddin, J. F. 1980. Biochemical tests for identification of medical bacteria, 2nd ed. Williams & Wilkins, Baltimore. p. 78-93; 209-214; 308-320.

14. Rosebrock, J. A. 1991. Labeled-antibody techniques: fluorescent, radioisotopic, immunochemical, p. 79-86. *In* A. Balows, A., W. J. Hausler, Jr., K. L. Herrmann, H. D. Isenberg, and H. J. Shadomy (ed.), Manual of clinical microbiology, 5th ed. American Society for Microbiology, Washington, D. C.

15. Sommerfelt, H., H. M. S. Grewal, W. Gaastra, A.-M. Svennerholm, and M. K. Bhan. 1992. Use of nonradioactive DNA probe hybridization for identification of enterotoxigenic *Escherichia coli* harboring genes for colonization factor antigen I, coli surface antigen 4, or putative colonization factor O166. J. Clin. Microbiol. **30**:1823-1828.

16. Thaller, M. C., B. Dainelli, F. Berlutti, S. Schippa, C. Fontana, and R. Pezzi. 1992. Double sugar-tyrosine medium improves O-1 phage *Salmonella* screening. J. Clin. Microbiol. **30**:533-534.

Exercise 9
Table 1: Results for Known Enteric: _____

		Culture	Characteristics on:					
		Age	EMB[a]	Mac	HE	SS	BiS	Other
Colony Size and Form	mm							
	Punctiform							
	Irregular							
	Circular							
	Rhizoid							
	Filamentous							
	Other							
Colony Surface	Flat							
	Raised							
	Convex							
	Pulvinate							
	Other							
Colony Margin	Entire							
	Undulate							
	Lobate							
	Erose							
	Other							
Colony Consistency	Butyrous							
	Viscid							
	Membranous							
	Brittle							
	Other							
Optical Character	Opaque							
	Translucent							
	Dull							
	Glistening							
	Other							
Surface	Smooth							
	Rough							
	Other							
TSI Agar[b]	Slant							
	Butt							
	Gas							
	H$_2$S							
Urea								

[a] L-EMB = Levine Eosin Methylene Blue; Mac = MacConkey; HE = Hektoen Enteric; SS = *Shigella-Salmonella*; BiS = Bismuth Sulfite agars.
[b] Usual designations: A = acid reaction; K = alkaline reaction.

Exercise 9
Table 2: Results for Known Enteric: _____

		Culture Age	Characteristics on:					
			EMB[a]	Mac	HE	SS	BiS	Other
Colony Size and Form	mm							
	Punctiform							
	Irregular							
	Circular							
	Rhizoid							
	Filamentous							
	Other							
Colony Surface	Flat							
	Raised							
	Convex							
	Pulvinate							
	Other							
Colony Margin	Entire							
	Undulate							
	Lobate							
	Erose							
	Other							
Colony Consistency	Butyrous							
	Viscid							
	Membranous							
	Brittle							
	Other							
Optical Character	Opaque							
	Translucent							
	Dull							
	Glistening							
	Other							
Surface	Smooth							
	Rough							
	Other							
TSI Agar[b]	Slant							
	Butt							
	Gas							
	H$_2$S							
Urea								

[a] L-EMB = Levine Eosin Methylene Blue; Mac = MacConkey; HE = Hektoen Enteric; SS = *Shigella-Salmonella*; BiS = Bismuth Sulfite agars.

[b] Usual designations: A = acid reaction; K = alkaline reaction.

Exercise 9

Table 3: Results for Known Enteric: _____

		Culture	Characteristics on:					
		Age	EMB*a*	Mac	HE	SS	BiS	Other
Colony Size and Form	mm							
	Punctiform							
	Irregular							
	Circular							
	Rhizoid							
	Filamentous							
	Other							
Colony Surface	Flat							
	Raised							
	Convex							
	Pulvinate							
	Other							
Colony Margin	Entire							
	Undulate							
	Lobate							
	Erose							
	Other							
Colony Consistency	Butyrous							
	Viscid							
	Membranous							
	Brittle							
	Other							
Optical Character	Opaque							
	Translucent							
	Dull							
	Glistening							
	Other							
Surface	Smooth							
	Rough							
	Other							
TSI Agar*b*	Slant							
	Butt							
	Gas							
	H$_2$S							
Urea								

a L-EMB = Levine Eosin Methylene Blue; Mac = MacConkey; HE = Hektoen Enteric; SS = *Shigella-Salmonella*; BiS = Bismuth Sulfite agars.

b Usual designations: A = acid reaction; K = alkaline reaction.

Exercise 9
Table 4: Results for Known Enteric: _____

		Culture	Characteristics on:					
		Age	EMB[a]	Mac	HE	SS	BiS	Other
Colony Size and Form	mm							
	Punctiform							
	Irregular							
	Circular							
	Rhizoid							
	Filamentous							
	Other							
Colony Surface	Flat							
	Raised							
	Convex							
	Pulvinate							
	Other							
Colony Margin	Entire							
	Undulate							
	Lobate							
	Erose							
	Other							
Colony Consistency	Butyrous							
	Viscid							
	Membranous							
	Brittle							
	Other							
Optical Character	Opaque							
	Translucent							
	Dull							
	Glistening							
	Other							
Surface	Smooth							
	Rough							
	Other							
TSI Agar[b]	Slant							
	Butt							
	Gas							
	H_2S							
Urea								

[a] L-EMB = Levine Eosin Methylene Blue; Mac = MacConkey; HE = Hektoen Enteric; SS = *Shigella-Salmonella*; BiS = Bismuth Sulfite agars.

[b] Usual designations: A = acid reaction; K = alkaline reaction.

Exercise 9

Table 5: Results for Known Enteric: _____

		Culture	Characteristics on:					
		Age	EMB[a]	Mac	HE	SS	BiS	Other
Colony Size	mm							
and Form	Punctiform							
	Irregular							
	Circular							
	Rhizoid							
	Filamentous							
	Other							
Colony	Flat							
Surface	Raised							
	Convex							
	Pulvinate							
	Other							
Colony	Entire							
Margin	Undulate							
	Lobate							
	Erose							
	Other							
Colony	Butyrous							
Consistency	Viscid							
	Membranous							
	Brittle							
	Other							
Optical	Opaque							
Character	Translucent							
	Dull							
	Glistening							
	Other							
Surface	Smooth							
	Rough							
	Other							
TSI Agar[b]	Slant							
	Butt							
	Gas							
	H_2S							
Urea								

[a] L-EMB = Levine Eosin Methylene Blue; Mac = MacConkey; HE = Hektoen Enteric; SS = *Shigella-Salmonella*; BiS = Bismuth Sulfite agars.

[b] Usual designations: A = acid reaction; K = alkaline reaction.

Exercise 9
Table 6: Results for Known Enteric Bacteria

		Culture Age	Code or Name of Bacteria				
Catalase test	Culture Source:						
Oxidase test	Culture Source:						
Gram stain Culture Source:	Reaction						
	Morphology						
	Arrangement						
MIO	Motility						
	Indole						
	Ornithine decarboxylase						
MR-VP	Methyl Red						
	Voges Proskauer						
Citrate							
Arginine							
Lysine							
Phenylalanine							
ONPG							
Fermentations	Glucose Acid						
	Gas						
	Arabinose						
	Dulcitol						
	Lactose						
	Maltose						
	Mannitol						
	Mucate						
	Rhamnose						
	Sucrose						
	Trehalose						
	Xylose						
Other							

**Exercise 9
Table A: Unknown Enteric Bacteria Results**

		Culture Age	Isolate characteristics on (name of medium)[a]:					
			Isolate No. _____		Isolate No. _____		Isolate No. _____	
Colony Size and Form	mm							
	Punctiform							
	Irregular							
	Circular							
	Rhizoid							
	Filamentous							
	Other							
Colony Surface	Flat							
	Raised							
	Convex							
	Pulvinate							
	Other							
Colony Margin	Entire							
	Undulate							
	Lobate							
	Erose							
	Other							
Colony Consistency	Butyrous							
	Viscid							
	Membranous							
	Brittle							
	Other							
Optical Character	Opaque							
	Translucent							
	Dull							
	Glistening							
	Other							
Surface	Smooth							
	Rough							
	Other							
TSI Agar[b]	Slant							
	Butt							
	Gas							
	H_2S							
Urea								

[a] L-EMB = Levine Eosin Methylene Blue; Mac = MacConkey; HE = Hektoen Enteric; SS = *Shigella-Salmonella*; BiS = Bismuth Sulfite agars.

[b] Usual designations: A = acid reaction; K = alkaline reaction.

Exercise 9
Table B: Unknown Enteric Bacteria Results

		Culture Age	Isolate characteristics on (name of medium)[a]:					
			Isolate No. _____		Isolate No. _____		Isolate No. _____	
Colony Size and Form	mm							
	Punctiform							
	Irregular							
	Circular							
	Rhizoid							
	Filamentous							
	Other							
Colony Surface	Flat							
	Raised							
	Convex							
	Pulvinate							
	Other							
Colony Margin	Entire							
	Undulate							
	Lobate							
	Erose							
	Other							
Colony Consistency	Butyrous							
	Viscid							
	Membranous							
	Brittle							
	Other							
Optical Character	Opaque							
	Translucent							
	Dull							
	Glistening							
	Other							
Surface	Smooth							
	Rough							
	Other							
TSI Agar[b]	Slant							
	Butt							
	Gas							
	H_2S							
Urea								

[a] L-EMB = Levine Eosin Methylene Blue; Mac = MacConkey; HE = Hektoen Enteric; SS = *Shigella-Salmonella*; BiS = Bismuth Sulfite agars.

[b] Usual designations: A = acid reaction; K = alkaline reaction.

Exercise 9
Table C: Unknown Enteric Bacteria Results

		Culture Age	Unknown Bacterial Isolate Code:					
Catalase test[a]								
Oxidase test[a]								
Gram stain[a]	Reaction							
	Morphology							
	Arrangement							
MIO	Motility							
	Indole							
	Ornithine decarboxylase							
MR-VP	Methyl Red							
	Voges Proskauer							
Citrate								
Arginine								
Lysine								
Ornithine								
Phenylalanine								
Motility								
ONPG[a]								
Fermentations	Glucose Acid							
	Gas							
	Adonitol							
	Arabinose							
	Dulcitol							
	Inositol							
	Lactose							
	Maltose							
	Mannitol							
	Mucate							
	Raffinose							
	Rhamnose							
	Salicin							
	Sorbitol							
	Sucrose							
	Trehalose							
	Xylose							
Other								

[a] Culture sources for these tests to be listed in Table D.

Exercise 9
Table D: Unknown Enteric Bacteria Results
Sources of Culture for Assays in Table C

Name of Assay	Unknown Isolate	Source of Culture
Catalase		
Oxidase		
Gram stain		
ONPG		

Exercise 9: Enteric Bacteria
Other Laboratory Data

Part 4

A. Tube Agglutination Test:

B. Demonstration: Typing *Salmonella* by the Slide Agglutination Test.

C. Demonstration: Direct Fluorescent Antibody Test.

Exercise 9: Enteric Bacteria
LABORATORY NOTES

EXERCISE 10
The Family *Vibrionaceae*

Important members of the family *Vibrionaceae* from a clinical view are *Vibrio, Aeromonas,* and *Plesiomonas* (one other genus, *Photobacterium,* is also contained in this family according to the current Bergey's Manual (2)). They all have the common properties of being able to produce gastrointestinal illness, although other clinical entities are produced. All members of the family are primarily located in the aquatic environment.

The *Vibrionaceae* are Gram-negative, straight to curving rods, that are catalase positive and ferment glucose. They may readily be distinguished from the evolutionarily-related *Enterobacteriaceae* by the fact that (i) most are oxidase positive, and (ii) they are motile by means of polar flagella (2, 16). Other distinguishing characteristics of clinically significant members are given in Table 10-1.

Despite these phenotypic similarities, changes have been suggested in the organization of the family. For example, it has been proposed that the genus *Aeromonas* be placed into its own family, the *Aeromonadaceae* (7). Also, new genera for the *Vibrionaceae* have been suggested. These include the addition of *Listonella, Shewanella* (20), and *Allomonas* (14). Finally, *Plesiomonas* is more closely related to the family *Enterobacteriaceae,* leading to the proposal to move it there (20). Except for *Allomonas,* which represents a group of previously unrecognized organisms, the changes are primarily based on molecular genetic relationships.

Vibrio: Of all species, *Vibrio cholerae* Serovar 01 (i. e. contains O antigen, serotype 1) has had the greatest worldwide impact due to its elaboration of cholera toxin (CT). It is the causative agent of Asiatic cholera, a severe diarrheal disease capable of occurring in epidemics and pandemics. The World Health Organization (26), as an example, reported 69,361 new cases of this disease in 1990. More than 99% of these occurred in Africa and Asia. In the United States, however, it continues to be an infrequent infection, with only 7 reported cases, and most of these were imported (i.e. originally contracted outside the U. S.). Although there were no outbreaks reported from South and Central America that year, the disease is now epidemic in several countries (6) following an outbreak in Peru in early 1991 (5). The number of cases in Latin America exceeded 340,000 by the end of November, 1991 (6). This shows the capacity of this organism to distribute quickly under circumstances of poor sanitary treatment of water and sewage. Unfortunately, it is expected that cholera will now remain endemic in this region for many years (10).

In the U. S., although cholera due to *Vibrio cholerae* 01 is of concern, gastrointestinal disease due to other strains or species of *Vibrio* occur more often. Gastroenteritis attributable to *Vibrio cholerae* non-01 (that is, strains not agglutinated by anti-01 serum) and *V. parahaemolyticus* after eating raw or improperly cooked or stored marine shellfish is not uncommon. In developed countries, the latter is the most common *Vibrio* associated with infection (24). Also, these and other species have been isolated from extraintestinal specimens. *V. parahaemolyticus* and *V. alginolyticus,* for example, occasionally cause eye, ear, and wound infections, and *V. vulnificus* can be associated with soft tissue wounds and septicemia.

This brief background concerning *Vibrio* suggests that clinical specimens most likely to bear these organisms are stools. Other types cannot, however, be excluded. As is usual, it is preferable to plate the organism immediately on collection of the sample. If transport is required, Cary and Blair medium (see Exercise 1, page 4) is satisfactory. Be aware that most of these organisms are halophilic; only *V. cholerae* and *V. mimicus* grow without any NaCl (Table 10-1). All grow satisfactorily at 1% concentration of this salt in the medium, as they will on MacConkey agar and on blood agar. However, if a *Vibrio* sp. is suspected the preferred isolation medium is thiosulfate-citrate-bile salts-sucrose (TCBS) medium (16). It is differential for *Vibrio* based upon fermentation of sucrose. Those fermenting this carbohydrate, including *Vibrio cholerae* form yellow colonies (Photo 10-1); others that do not, as *V. parahaemolyticus,* form green to blue colonies (8). Following isolation, identifying assays listed in Table 10-1 are done, some of which will be further described in the actual exercise protocol.

V. cholerae can be further subclassified into two biotypes, El Tor (or eltor) and "classical," the former being responsible for the current pandemic. Furthermore, serotype 01 exists as three subtypes based on the three kinds of O factors present on the cell detectable with anti-O serum. These "subtypes" are named Ogawa, Inaba, and Hikojima (16) and have epidemiological significance. For example, domestically acquired U. S. cases of cholera have been *V. cholerae*, serotype 01, biotype El Tor, subtype Inaba (13). From Peru, the initially analyzed cases were of this biovar-serovar (5), although the classical biovar appears to be reemerging (13).

The most commonly isolated members of *Vibrio* are usually identifiable using commercially-available kits. It should be remembered that inoculation suspensions are to be prepared in solutions supplemented with 1% NaCl (16). Evaluations show, however, that rapid identification systems provide variable rates of accuracy in speciating members of *Vibrionaceae* (13, 22). Furthermore, the data base for the various kits require expansion to be more useful when identifying members of this family (13).

Although serology is not done in this laboratory exercise, it should be apparent that it is critical to find whether a *V. cholerae* is an 01 type or a non-01 type. This is accomplished using the slide agglutination test, similar to that demonstrated in Exercise 9, page 148. An oxidase-positive Gram-negative rod that forms yellow colonies on TCBS and agglutinates with anti-*V. cholerae* 01 serum can presumptively be identified as *V. cholerae* (16). (But, yellow colonies should not be taken for use in an oxidase test. Why?) Non-01 *V. cholerae* and *V. parahaemolyticus* also may be serotyped.

Other approaches are being taken to find a more direct route to *V. cholerae* identification. An example of one method is the use of an enzyme-linked immunoassay in which anti-cholera toxin is adsorbed on to latex beads to detect cholera toxin directly in patient stools. This rapid and simple detection of toxin gives an 85% correlation with culture done on the same samples (23) suggesting at least its value as a screening assay. Also, detection of the cholera toxin gene is being investigated. A DNA oligonucleotide probe can detect as few as 10^3 cholera toxin-producing organisms from stools of volunteers. Its 100% specificity for CT-producing environmental strains

suggests its applicability to not only patient specimen testing, but also to environmental monitoring for pathogenic strains (27). Finally, PCR for detection of the CT gene in serotype 01 is being applied epidemiologically (9) on culture isolates from patients, food, and water. It yields 100% concordance with an ELISA method, but gave results in 4 hours compared to several days for the serologic assay.

Aeromonas: Aeromonads are commonly inhabitants of water, whether fresh, brackish, sewage, or in fish tanks. They are also found in food and in soil. There are 8 phenotype species (25), although hybridization studies show a total of 13 groups (12).

While it has been known for many years that *Aeromonas* spp. could be opportunistic agents of disease (21), only recently has definitive data become available of its potential. The annual number of cases in California, in its first year as a reportable disease agent, was 219. Over 70% of these were isolated from stools. Other types included wound, blood, etc. (4). Generally, it has been found that in the U. S. and Europe *A. caviae* most commonly cause diarrhea. In Australia, Bangladesh, and Thailand *A. hydrophilia* and *A. sobria* predominate (25).

Aeromonads associated with clinical samples generally grow well on commonly used enteric differential and selective media (as MacConkey agar), and blood agar, though TCBS should not be used (25). Therefore, isolation usually does not present special problems, although speciation may (1). Attempts have been made to define appropriate biochemical panels to identify *Aeromonas* at the species level (1, 15). Further study is required, however.

Plesiomonas: There is only a single species of *Plesiomonas*, *P. shigelloides*. Its habitat is similar to that described for *Aeromonas*, although it also may be found in marine waters during warm times of the year. Furthermore, isolation and characterization is similar to that described for the aeromonads.

P. shigelloides is a probable agent of gastroenteritis, although it has occasionally been found in a variety of other extra-intestinal diseases. It is also an agent occurring in the immunocompromised (21).

Table 10-1
Reactions Given by Some Clinically Important Members
of the Family *Vibrionaceae*[a] (16, 17, 19)

Genus-species	V-P	Cit[b]	0/129 Sensitivity 150µg[c]	String Test	Growth in NaCl, % Concentration:					Arg Dihydr[b]	Lys Decarb	Orn Decarb	PA	ONPG	Gas from Glucose	Acid From:				
					0	1	6	8	10							Arab	Inos	Lac	Sal	Suc
Vibrio[d] (16)																				
alginolyticus	+	−	V−	+	−	+	+	+	V	−	+	V	−	−	−	−	−	−	−	+
cholerae[e]	V+	+	+	+	+	+	V[f]	−	−	−	+	+	−	+	−	−	−	−	−	+
mimicus	−	+	+	+	+	+	V	−	−	−	+	+	−	+	−	−	−	V−	−	−
parahaemolyticus	−	−	V−	V	−	+	+	V+	−	−	+	+	−	−	−	V+	−	−	−	−
vulnificus	−	V+	+	+	−	+	V	−	−	−	+	V	V	V+[f]	−	−	−	V+	+	V−
Aeromonas (19, 25)[d]																				
caviae	−	+	[−]							[+]	−	−	V		−	+	−	V−	+	+
hydrophilia	V	+	[−]							[+]	+	−	V		V+	V	−	V	V+	V+
sobria	+	+	[−]							[+]	+	−	V+		V+	−	−	V	−	+
Plesiomonas (11, 17)[d]																				
shigelloides[a]	−	−	[+]		+	+	−[f]			+	+	+	−	+	−	−	+	V+	−	−

[a] Not shown in table is that all members of the family *Vibrionaceae* found in human specimens ferment glucose, except for *V. carchariae*, which is variable; all reduce nitrate to nitrite, and are oxidase-positive, except *V. metschnikovii*, which is negative for these (16, 19, 25).

[b] Abbreviations: VP = Voges-Proskauer (with 1% NaCl for *Vibrio*); Cit = Simmons citrate; 0/129 = 2, 4-diamino-6, 7-diisopropylpteridine phosphate; Arg Dihydr = arginine dihydrolase (with 1% NaCl for *Vibrio*); Lysine decarb = lysine decarboxylase (with 1% NaCl for *Vibrio*); ornithine decarb = ornithine decarboxylase (with 1% NaCl for *Vibrio*); PA = phenylalanine deaminase; ONPG = o-nitrophenyl-β-D-galacto-pyanoside; Arab = arabinose; Inos = *myo*-Inositol; Lac = lactose; Sal = salicin; and Suc = sucrose.

[c] 0/129 sensitivity is positive when any zone of inhibition noted around disks containing this compound.

[d] *Vibrio* contains over 30 species (13); *Aeromonas* has 8 species (25); and *Plesiomonas* consists of a single species.

[e] Reactions similar for both *V. cholerae* 01 and non-01, but biovar El Tor is VP+, while classical strain is VP−. Others differences also found, but are not shown.

[f] + = 90% or greater positive; V+ = 70-89% positive; V = 31-69% positive; V− = 11-30% positive; and − = 10% or less positive; [+] = usually positive; and [−] = usually negative.

MATERIALS

Part 1

Per pair of students:

1 slant culture each of *Vibrio cholerae* Serovar 0:1, *V. parahaemolyticus*, and *A. caviae*.

1 Thiosulfate-citrate-bile salts-sucrose (TCBS) agar "Y" plate

1 MacConkey agar "Y" plate

1 Sheep blood agar (SBA) "Y" plate

3 0/129 (2,4-diamino-6,7-diisopropylpteridine phosphate) impregnated (150µg) filter paper disks

3 tubes each of:
Peptone broth without NaCl
Peptone broth with 6% NaCl

Arabinose fermentation broth
Sucrose fermentation broth
Petri dish
Catalase and oxidase reagents
0.5% sodium desoxycholate reagent

Part 2

Per bench:

3-ONPG disks and 3 tubes PSS, 0.2 ml/12 x 75 mm tubes

1 peptone broth culture of *Enterobacter cloacae*
Flagella stain supplies:
Rhu staining solution
New microscope slide
Coplin jar containing acetone
Coplin jar only

PROCEDURE

Part 1

Each pair of students will be provided with slant cultures of *Vibrio cholerae* Serovar O:1, *V. parahaemolyticus* and *A caviae*. With these, carry out the following:

1. Prepare a Gram stain and observe microscopically. Despite its typically curved form, *Vibrio* may have other types of morphology as straight rods and swollen forms (16). Are these found in your preparation?

2. Streak each for isolation onto one-third of a TCBS, a MacConkey, and a SBA "Y" plate. Place a disk containing 0/129 in a heavily-streaked area of the SBA plate only.

3. Inoculate each organism into the following tube media:
   a. Peptone broth without NaCl.
   b. Peptone broth containing 6% NaCl.
   c. Arabinose and sucrose fermentation broths.

4. Incubate all cultures at 35-37°C for 48 hours.

5. Do a "string test" by the following method:
   a. Place three separate drops of 0.5% sodium desoxycholate solution into an empty petri dish.
   b. Suspend a loopful of one organism into one of the drops of sodium desoxycholate solution.
   c. After one minute, touch the loop to the drop and slowly draw it away. If a mucoid "string" forms between the drop and the loop, the test is considered positive.
   d. Repeat this procedure by placing each remaining species into one of the other drops of solution. Do your results correspond with that shown in Table 10-1?

6. Do a catalase test with each organism, removing them from the culture and testing in the petri dish that had been used for the string test. Following completion of this, the dish with its spent assays can be disposed of in the proper container.

7. Finally, use the stock culture slants to do an oxidase test. Discard after the results have been read.

8. Record all of your results and discuss.

Part 2

A. Known cultures:

1. TCBS agar: Note the colony form and color, and the relative amounts of growth of *V. cholerae*, *V. parahaemolyticus*, and *A. caviae* on this selective and differential medium. To record the latter, the following can be used: +4 to +1 = maximum to minimal growth, respectively; - = no growth. Compare these characteristics to that on MacConkey agar.

2. Sheep blood agar: Note the difference, if any, in the zone of inhibition due to O/129 on this plate. Measure the zone diameter to the nearest millimeter and record. Any inhibition due to this vibriostatic agent is considered positive. Also, observe whether any of the organisms are hemolytic. If so, note the type.

3. Read the results of your tube tests. Is there a difference in growth (i.e. turbidity) in the peptone broth containing 0% NaCl as compared to that containing 6% NaCl? Which organism is halophilic? Are arabinose and sucrose fermented?

4. Find whether these organisms produce β-galactosidase by doing the ONPG disk test (procedures in Exercise 9, **page 147**).

5. Prepare a wet mount of *V. cholerae* from peptone broth and observe by phase contrast microscopy. Compare this with a peptone broth culture of *Enterobacter cloacae* provided for this purpose. Can you establish the motility of these bacteria?

6. Prepare a flagella stain of *V. cholerae* and *E. cloacae* using the method of Kodaka et al. (18) as follows.
   a. Use an isolated colony of bacteria grown on a sugar-free medium (e.g. sheep blood agar) that is in its logarithmic or early stationary phase of growth.
   b. Obtain two new slides. Briefly dip these into a Coplin jar containing acetone to remove any surface oil that may be present. On removal, tilt the slide to drain and evaporate dry, or quickly wipe with tissue to dry.
   c. Place two small drops of distilled water on the cleaned microscope slide.
   d. Pick a *small* amount of bacteria from a colony with an inoculating *needle*, being careful not to touch the agar. Usually,

just touching the tip of the needle to the top of the colony will provide adequate concentrations of organisms. Transfer the bacteria to the drops of water by lightly touching (not dipping or stirring) the tip of the needle to each in consecutive order. Use care not to dislodge the flagella.

e. Allow the drops to air-dry. Do not attempt to hasten by heating. Do not heat fix.

f. Flood the slide with Rhu staining solution and allow to remain 5 minutes.

g. Wash the slide with a gentle stream of tap water for 2-3 minutes. This can be accomplished by connecting one end of a rubber tubing to a water tap, then placing the other end in the bottom of a coplin jar placed in a sink. Allow the water to flow gently from bottom to top and around the immersed slide.

h. Allow the slide to air-dry, then examine microscopically. Begin your observations near the periphery of the stained drop, since bacteria with characteristic flagella are usually found in greatest numbers here.

i. Note your findings. Count the number of flagella per cell. Also, describe their arrangement on the bacteria. *V. cholerae* is typically polar and monotrichous (3) (Photo 10-2). What is the expected finding for *E. cloacae*?

7. Tabulate your results. Discuss.

B. Demonstration of the Kanagawa Reaction: Observe *V. parahaemolyticus* on Wagatsuma blood agar. Does it present a positive Kanagawa reaction (beta hemolysis)? There is a strong association of a positive Kanagawa reaction with recent isolation of this organism from human disease, while environmental isolates are negative 99% of the time. Therefore, this assay is important in associating an isolate with gastroenteritis (13, 16).

QUESTIONS

1. Despite the explosive epidemics of cholera that can occur, this is not the expectation in the United States. Why?

2. Give the expected TSI agar fermentation results for each species used in the above exercise. Base these upon fermentation patterns given in Table 10-1.

3. Show the minimum number of tests required to differentiate the genera *Vibrio, Aeromonas,* and *Plesiomonas* shown in Table 10-1.

REFERENCES

1. Abbott, S. L., W. K. W. Cheung, S. Kroske-Bystrom, T. Malekzadeh, and J. M. Janda. 1992. Identification of *Aeromonas* strains to the genospecies level in the clinical laboratory. J. Clin. Microbiol. **30**:1262-1266.

2. Baumann, P., and R. H. W. Schubert. 1984. *Vibrionaceae* Veron 1965, p. 516-517. *In* N. R. Krieg, and J. G. Holt (ed.), Bergey's manual of systematic bacteriology, Vol. 1. Williams & Wilkins, Baltimore.

3. Baumann, P., A. L. Furniss, and J. V. Lee. 1984. *Vibrio* Pacini 1854, p. 518-538. *In* N. R. Krieg, and J. G. Holt (ed.), Bergey's manual of systematic bacteriology, Vol. 1. Williams & Wilkins, Baltimore.

4. California Department of Health Services. 1990. Results of the first population-based study of *Aeromonas* infection. Calif. Morbid. **25/26**.

5. Centers for Disease Control. 1991. Cholera-Peru, 1991. MMWR **40**:108-110.

6. Centers for Disease Control. 1991. Update: Cholera-Western hemisphere, 1991. MMWR **40**:860.

7. Colwell, R. R., M. T. MacDonell, and J. De Ley. 1986. Proposal to recognize the family *Aeromonadaceae* fam. nov. Int. J. Syst. Bacteriol. **36**:473-477.

8. Difco Laboratories. 1984. Difco Manual, 10th ed. Difco Laboratories, Inc., Detroit, MI, p. 930-932.

9. Fields, P. I., T. Popovic, K. Wachsmuth, and Ø. Olsvik. 1992. Use of polymerase chain reaction for detection of toxigenic *Vibrio cholerae* O1 strains from the Latin American cholera epidemic. J. Clin. Microbiol. **30**:2118-2121.

10. Glass, R. I., M. Libel, and A. D. Brandling-Bennett. 1992. Epidemic cholera in the Americas. Science **256**:1524-1525.

11. Janda, J. M. 1987. *Aeromonas* and *Plesiomonas* infections, p. 37-44. *In* B. B. Wentworth (ed.), Diagnostic procedures for bacterial infections, 7th ed. American Public Health Association, Inc., Washington, D. C.

12. Janda, J. M. 1991. Recent advances in the study of the taxonomy, pathogenicity, and infectious syndromes associated with the genus *Aeromonas*. Clin. Microbiol. Rev. **4**:397-410.

13. Janda, J. M., C. Powers, R. G. Bryant, and S. L. Abbott. 1988. Current perspectives on the epidemiology and pathogenesis of clinically significant *Vibrio* spp. Clin. Microbiol. Rev. **1**:245-267.

14. Kalina, G. P., A. G. Somova, V. A. Nikonova, T. P. Turova, T. I. Grafova, L. S. Podosinnikova, M. I. Lapenkov, and I. M. Badalova. 1983. Allomonads-a new group of microorganisms in the *Vibrionaceae* family. J. Hyg. Epidemiol. Microbiol. Immunol. **27**:271-279.

15. Kämpfer, P., and M. Altwegg. 1992. Numerical classification and identification of *Aeromonas* genospecies. J. App. Bacteriol. **72**:341-351.

16. Kelly, M. T., F. W. Hickman-Brenner, and J. J. Farmer III. 1991. *Vibrio*, p. 384-395. *In* A. Balows, W. J. Hausler, Jr., K. L. Herrmann, H. D. Isenberg, and H. J. Shadomy (ed.), Manual of clinical microbiology, 5th ed. American Society for Microbiology, Washington, D. C.

17. Kelly, M. T., and K. C. Kain. 1991. Biochemical characteristics and plasmids of clinical and environmental *Plesiomonas shigelloides*. Experimentia **47**:439-441.

18. Kodaka, H., A. Y. Armfield, G. L. Lombard, and V. R. Dowell, Jr. 1982. Practical procedure for demonstrating bacterial flagella. J. Clin. Microbiol. **16**:948-952.

19. Kuijper, E. J., A. G. Steigerwalt, B. S. C. I. M. Schoenmakers, M. F. Peeters, H. C. Zanen, and D. J. Brenner. 1989. Phenotypic characterization and DNA relatedness in human fecal isolates of *Aeromonas* spp. J. Clin. Microbiol. **27**:132-138.

20. MacDonell, M. T., and R. R. Colwell. 1985. Phylogeny of the *Vibrionaceae*, and recommendation for two new genera, *Listonella* and *Shewanella*. Syst. Appl. Microbiol. **6**:171-182.

21. McGowen, J. E., Jr., and C. Del Rio. 1990. Other Gram-negative bacilli, p. 1782-1793. *In* G. L. Mandell, R. G. Douglas, Jr., and J. E. Bennett (ed.), Principles and practices of infectious diseases, 3rd ed. Churchill Livingstone, New York.

22. Overman, T. L., J. F. Kessler, and J. P. Seabolt. 1985. Comparison of API 20E, API Rapid E, and API rapid NFT for identification of members of the family *Vibrionaceae*. J. Clin. Microbiol. **22**:778-781.

23. Ramamurthy, T., S. K. Bhattacharya, Y. Uesaka, K. Horigome, M. Paul, D. Sen, S. C. Pal, T. Takeda, Y. Takeda, and G. B. Nair. 1992. Evaluation of the bead enzyme-linked immunosorbent assay for detection of cholera toxin directly from stool specimens. J. Clin. Microbiol. **30**:1783-1786.

24. Tison, D. L. 1987. *Vibrio* infections, p. 599-611. *In* B. B. Wentworth (ed.), Diagnostic procedures for bacterial infections, 7th ed. American Public Health Association, Inc., Washington, D. C.

25. von Graevenitz, A., and M. Altwegg. 1991. *Aeromonas* and *Plesiomonas*, p. 396-401. *In* A. Balows, W. J. Hausler, Jr., K. L. Herrmann, H. D. Isenberg, and H. J. Shadomy (ed.), Manual of clinical microbiology, 5th ed. American Society for Microbiology, Washington, D. C.

26. World Health Organization. 1991 Cholera in 1990. Week. Epidemiol. Rec. **66**:133-140.

27. Wright, A. C., Y. Guo, J. A. Johnson, J. P. Nataro. and J. G. Morris, Jr. 1992. Development and testing of a nonradioactive DNA oligonucleotide probe that is specific for *Vibrio cholerae* cholera toxin. J. Clin. Microbiol. **30**:2302-2306.

Exercise 10
Data Table 1: *Vibrio* and *Aeromonas* Results

		Culture Age	V. cholerae				V. parahaemolyticus				A. caviae			
			TCBS[a]	Mac	SBA	Other	TCBS[a]	Mac	SBA	Other	TCBS[a]	Mac	SBA	Other
Growth	Relative amounts[b]													
Colony size and Colony Form	mm													
	Punctiform													
	Irregular													
	Circular													
	Rhizoid													
	Filamentous													
	Other													
Colony Surface	Flat													
	Raised													
	Convex													
	Pulvinate													
	Other													
Colony Margin	Entire													
	Undulate													
	Lobate													
	Erose													
	Other													
Colony Consistency	Butyrous													
	Viscid													
	Membranous													
	Brittle													
	Other													
Optical Character	Opaque													
	Translucent													
	Dull													
	Glistening													
	Other													
Surface	Smooth													
	Rough													
	Other													
Hemolysis	Type													
Wagatsuma agar	Kanagawa Reaction													
0/129	Inhibition zone													

[a] TCBS = Thiosulfate citrate bile sucrose agar; Mac = MacConkey agar; and SBA = Sheep blood agar.

[b] Use +4 growth = maximum to +1 = minimum growth; − = no growth.

Exercise 10
Data Table 2: *Vibrio* and *Aeromonas* Results

		Culture Age	Vibrio cholerae	Vibrio parahaemolyticus	Aeromonas caviae	Enterobacter cloacae
Catalase test						
Oxidase test						
Gram stain	Reaction					
	Morphology					
	Arrangement					
Flagella	Number/cell					
stain	Arrangement					
Wet mount	Motility					
0% NaCl Broth	Growth					
6% NaCl Broth	Growth					
ONPG						
String test						
Fermentations	Arabinose					
	Sucrose					
Other						

Other Laboratory Notes

EXERCISE 11
Campylobacter and *Helicobacter*

Campylobacter species were formerly classified as members of the family *Spirillaceae* (22). These were then separated from this family and became unaffiliated with any family, being grouped with other unaffiliated helical and vibrioid (curved) Gram-negative bacteria. (23). It has now been proposed that these be placed in their own family, the *Campylobacteraceae* (28). Besides *Campylobacter*, the family also would include *Helicobacter, Wollinella, Arcobacter,* and "Flexibacteria." This grouping is based upon their phenotypic and genotypic similarities. They are all Gram-negative organisms, morphologically curved, S-shaped or spiral rods. All members are motile by means of a polar flagellum at one or both ends of the cell. Metabolically, they are neither oxidative nor fermentive, but they are oxidase-positive. DNA-rRNA hybridization studies reflect their family relationship. Whether such a taxonomic scheme as this stands the test of time will, however, be determined by usage (or lack of it). In any case, the genera of interest in this exercise are *Campylobacter* and *Helicobacter*.

Campylobacter itself continues to develop in its taxonomy at the genus and species level. Some of these, as seen below, can be potentially confusing. For example, *Helicobacter pylori* was formerly *C. pylori* (9). Several others are proposed to be included in this new genus *Helicobacter*, so it would include 4 other species. As noted below, *H. pylori* will be of most immediate interest to us here. The remaining campylobacteria include 13 species, within which there are 4 subspecies and 3 biotypes (28). Of these, *C. jejuni* subsp. *jejuni* (formerly *C. fetus* subsp. *jejuni*) is the predominant human pathogen (17, 21).

Campylobacter may be placed into three general groups (17). The thermophilic group, as shown in Table 11-1, includes those that grow well at 42°C, but not at 25°C, are true campylobacteria and all cause human gastroenteritis. The second group also consists of true campylobacteria, but will not grow at 42°C, although they do at 25°C. These are less prevalent in human infection, although *C. fetus* subsp. *fetus* (formerly subsp. *intestinalis*) can cause diarrheal-associated disease. It is, however, more widely recognized for its

occasional extraintestinal infections, as vascular disease, bacteremia, abortions, etc. *C. sputorum* biovar sputorum, a non-pathogen also contained in this group, is a normal flora organism of the mouth and intestinal tract (1, 17). However, excepting the latter, the members of this group are more significant in lower animals. For example, *C. fetus* subsp. *fetus* produces abortion in sheep and occasionally in cattle; *C. fetus* subsp. *venerealis* (formerly *C. fetus* subsp. *fetus*) causes infertility and abortion in cattle; and *C. sputorum* biovar mucoralis causes necrotic enteritis and intestinal adenomatosis in pigs (27).

The last group of *Campylobacter* is the cryophilic group, which grows best at less than 37°C, and include *C. butzleri* (14), *C. nitrofigilis,* and *C. cryaerophilia*. The last two of these, at least, may not be true campylobacteria based on rRNA homology differences. This led to the proposal that those be placed in a new genus, *Arcobacter* (28). In any case, *C. cryaerophilia* has been isolated from human diarrhea (17), as has the recently proposed new species *C. butzleri* (14). *C. nitrofigilis* is an environment organism not associated with human disease.

Helicobacter pylori has been subject to a high level of investigation in recent years. This is primarily due to findings that it is very likely responsible for Type B (antral) gastritis. It also may be responsible for other conditions as duodenal ulcers. Its usual habitat is the human stomach and duodenum and can be found in about 10% of non-symptomatic adults less than 30 years old, and nearly 60% of those over 60. Interestingly, it is susceptible to acid, but is protected from this in the stomach by the gastric mucosa (2, 4, 18).

Diagnosis of *H. pylori* has generally included tissue examination using a biopsy sample and culture. Tissue examination includes histological staining and microscopic examination. The preferred stains are the Warthin-Starry silver stain, Giemsa, and hematoxylin and eosin (17). Because *H. pylori* is a strong urease-producing bacterium, biopsy material has also been used directly for determination of the presence of this enzyme. One procedure, for example, merely involves placing a small amount of tissue in urea solution and incubating (12). A non-invasive breath test has also been developed to detect *in situ* urease production. This involves ingestion of ^{13}C- or ^{14}C-labeled urea by the patient followed by a determination of the level of radiolabeled CO_2 measured from a breath sample (20).

For the microbiologist, the problem is how best to handle and identify this group of organisms. The nature of the problem can be exemplified in that *Campylobacter* causes more cases of gastroenteritis in the U. S. than either *Salmonella* or *Shigella*, and more than both combined in England (1). The number of cases per year in England continues to rise (21). Yet, it was not until the 1970's that the importance of these organisms in gastroenteritis began to become known (10). The probability is that then, as now, the organisms were present, but awareness and methodology were deficient. In terms of the latter, usual methods for isolation of Gram-negative bacteria, as the *Enterobacteriaceae*, fail to provide conditions for isolation of *Campylobacter*. Thus, even today the continuing increase in England is attributed, not to an increasing number of cases of disease, but to detection of a greater proportion of cases that actually exist (21).

Thus, several conditions for optimal isolation of *Campylobacter* and *Helicobacter* need to be met. These include a microaerophilic environment and a proper isolation medium, especially for stool samples. Furthermore, although not required, for most *C. jejuni* and others of the thermophilic group, an optimal growth temperature of 42°C is very useful. However, as noted in Table 11-1, all grow at 37°C.

Transport of *Campylobacter*-containing specimens can readily be done in pH 8.5 thioglycollate broth, alkaline peptone water with reducing agents, Stuart's transport medium, or by the specimen alone. It is important, though, that in the latter two cases that they are kept refrigerated (3, 24). Enrichment is usually unnecessary for these organism because of their large numbers, especially in a stool specimen (1).

Several different types of selective media have been developed that have markedly contributed to success enjoyed today in isolation of the campylobacteria. These include Skirrow's, Butzler, and Campy-BAP. These all contain blood, which is probably useful in reducing concentrations of toxic oxygen end products, and several antimicrobials to provide the selective environment (10). Recently, charcoal-containing (rather than blood) selective agar has been used with promising results (8).

H. pylori also can be isolated on Skirrow's medium. However, the content of the antimicrobial compounds needs modification to allow growth of this organism. Other types developed for it are also available (17, 25). For example, an IsovitaleX, urea-containing non-blood agar (5) has been described where rapid urease production by *H. pylori* aids in its separation from other slower urease producing organisms. Because some strains of both *H. pylori* and *Campylobacter* fail to grow on all media, a combination of two isolation agar types is recommended (8, 25).

It should be noted that filtration of samples through 0.3 to 0.6 μm pore diameter filters may improve chances of *Campylobacter* isolation. In stool specimens, for example, these organisms are sufficiently small in width to allow their passage while other organisms are retained on the filter. The filtrate then can be cultivated on nonselective media, as chocolate agar (1). However, a disadvantage of this method is that if a sample contains small numbers of campylobacteria, they may not be detected following filtration. Conversely, some strains are sensitive to antimicrobials contained in selective media, and in these instances such a method allows their isolation without the use of these inhibiting factors (10).

Providing the proper atmosphere has also added to the improved success in *Helicobacter* and *Campylobacter* isolation. Although some strains will tolerate atmospheric concentrations of oxygen, they are all classified as microaerophilic. Fortunately, the need for the correct atmosphere can be met quite readily. For *C. jejuni*, a candle extinction jar will usually suffice (1). However, best success for all species comes with providing an atmosphere containing 5-10% O_2 and some H_2, the latter enhancing the growth of some strains. This can be supplied by using commercially-available gas-generating packets in closed containers with the cultures (Photo 16-1) (as, for example, the BBL® Campy Pouch™ and the Bio-Bag™ Environmental Chamber (Type Cfj). Also, evacuated bottles or chambers in which proper gas mixtures are used to replace the original atmospheric content are an alternative. An example of this is evacuating ⅔ of the air from a container containing the cultures, then refilling to atmos-

Table 11-1
Some Characteristics of *Campylobacter* Species Associated With Humans[a], and *H. pylori*[b] (1, 17, 28)

Taxon	Catalase Reaction	H₂S in TSI	Urease	Reduction of: NO₃	Reduction of: NO₂	Hydrolysis of: Hippurate	Hydrolysis of: Indoxyl Acetate	Growth at: 15°C	Growth at: 25°C	Growth at: 37°C	Growth at: 42°C	Growth in 1% Glycine	Susceptible to 30µg: Nalidixic acid	Susceptible to 30µg: Cephalothin
Campylobacter														
The Thermophilic Group														
C. jejuni subsp. jejuni	+c	−	−	+	−	+	+	−	−	+	+	+	+	−
C. jejuni subsp. doylei	V	−	−	−	−	Vc	+	−	−	+	−	+	+	+
C. coli	+	−	−	+	−	−	+	−	−	+	+	+	+	−
C. laridis (or C. lari)	+	−	V	+	−	−	−	−	−	+	+	+	−	−
C. upsaliensis	W	−	−	+	−	−	+	−	−	+	+	V	+	+
Other true *Campylobacter* that are not thermophilic														
C. fetus subsp. fetus	+	−	−	+	−	−	−	−	+	+	−	+	−	+
C. hyointestinalis	+	+	−	+	−	−	−	−	+	+	+	+	−	+
C. sputorum subsp. sputorum	−	+	−	+	+	−	−	−	−	+	+	+	+	+
Psycrophilic group														
C. butzleri (14)	V	−	−	+	−	−	+	+	+	+	−	+	V	+
C. cryoaerophilia (or														
C. cryoaerophilus)	+	−	−	+	−	−	+	+	+	+	−	−	V	−
Helicobacter														
H. pylori	+	−	+	−		−	−		−	+	V		+	−

[a] Not shown: All species given on this table are motile with polar flagella, are oxidative, and are non-fermentive.
[b] Eight of 14 species of *Campylobacter*, and one of four established species of *Helicobacter* shown.
c + = usually positive; − = usually negative; V = variable; and W = weak reaction.

pheric pressure with a mixture of 80% N₂, 10% CO₂, and 10% H₂ (10). The growth of *Campylobacter* usually requires 48 hours or longer; *H. pylori* grows more slowly and should be incubated up to 7 days (4).

Following isolation, *Campylobacter* and *Helicobacter* can be identified using assays listed in Table 11-1 or other references (e.g. 1, 17, 28). Recall that *H. pylori* is strongly positive for urease, and this may be determined in the absence of culture. Also, it should be reemphasized that *C. jejuni* is the predominant isolate of the genus, especially from stool specimens. Stains and wet mounts should not be neglected, and done as early as possible in the identification procedure. Their curving, S- and gull-wing shapes, spiral morphology and darting motility, along with a positive oxidase test can provide tentative diagnosis of the genus (17).

Finally, rapid assays can be used, especially the non-biochemically based types, for identification of *Campylobacter* and *Helicobacter*. Latex agglutination kits (Campyslide™ and Meritec™-

Campy *jcl*) for culture confirmation of campylobacteria and *Helicobacter* are available. An Accuprobe™ Campylobacter Identification Test for identification of *C. jejuni*, *C. coli*, and *C. laridis* also can be obtained from Gen-Probe Inc. (see Exercise 3 for further information on genetic probes and the Gen-Probe system). In one study, this assay showed 100% accuracy in identification. However, it does not distinguish between the species that it detects (26). The PCR (polymerase chain reaction), though not commercially available, appears promising for identification of *H. pylori* in culture confirmation or directly from stomach biopsy (6, 11). In both cases, this procedure can detect and identify the species with 100 cells or less.

In *H. pylori* infection, it has been found that assay of patient IgG antibody response can be useful in diagnosis (2, 29). A non-automated Pyloragen™ *Helicobacter pylori* Test kit, semi-automated indirect enzyme-linked immunosorbent (ELISA) assays (Premier™ *H. pylori*; Pyloristat Rapid EIA), and an indirect fluorescent antibody (IFA) test (PyloriFiax®) are commercially available. As previously cautioned, the use of these or other commercially-produced assays should be thoroughly investigated for sensitivity, specificity, and appropriateness for the needs of a particular laboratory. In this case, there appears to be a need to improve the specificity and sensitivity of some commercially available kits designed to detect anti-*H. pylori* from infected patients (13).

MATERIALS

Part 1
Per pair of students:
1 culture each of *Campylobacter jejuni* and *C. fetus* subsp. *fetus*, 48 hours old and grown on sheep blood agar.
1 *Campylobacter* Blood Agar Plate (10% sheep blood agar with the antimicrobials vancomycin, trimethoprim, polymyxin B, and cephalothin)
4 Triple Sugar Iron (TSI) agar tubes
2 30 μg nalidixic acid and cephalothin-containing disks

Per bench:
Gram stain reagents
Flagella stain supplies:
  Rhu staining solution
  Acetone in Coplin jar
  Coplin jar
  New microscope slide
Container for incubating cultures in microaerophilic atmosphere
Commercially-available gas-generating system

For class:
42°C air incubator

Part 2
Per pair of students:
2 Hippurate containing disks and 12 x 75 mm tubes, each containing 0.1 ml sterile distilled water
2 Indoxyl acetate-containing disks, 2.5 mg/disk
1 Petri dish

Per bench:
1 Dropper bottle with sterile distilled water
Oxidase and catalase reagents

LABORATORY PROCEDURES

Part 1
Each pair of students will be provided with a stock culture of *Campylobacter jejuni* subsp. *jejuni* and *C. fetus* subsp. *fetus*. Carry out the following with these:
A. Determine their morphological characteristics.
  1. Prepare a Gram stain of *C. jejuni* and *C. fetus* and observe. Note its curving morphology. Can you observe "gull-wing" and "S" forms?
  2. Observe *C. jejuni* by wet mount under phase contrast microscopy. Describe its motility. Also compare this to that seen with *Vibrio cholerae* and *Enterobacter cloacae* seen in Exercise 10, *Part 2A-5*.
  3. Do a flagella stain on *C. jejuni* by the method described in Exercise 10, *Part 2A-6*, page 178. Describe the type of flagella seen. Is it polar? How many flagella are there per cell?
B. Inoculate the following with each organism:
  1. One-half of a Campy BAP. Streak for isolation, then place a 30 μg nalidixic acid and 30μg cephalothin disk in the heavily streaked area of each organism. Locate disks as far apart as possible within this area.
  2. Two TSI agar tubes each (stab butt and streak surface).
  3. Label all tubes and the plate. Incubate one pair of TSI agar tubes inoculated with each organism and the plate for 48 hours in the presence of a microaerophilic atmosphere at 37°C. The required atmosphere is most conveniently provided by use of a commercially-available generating system. Incubate the remaining two TSI agar tubes at 42°C in the same atmosphere.

Part 2
A. Read the cultures inoculated above.
  1. Campy BAP: Note the colony size and morphology of *C. jejuni* subsp. *jejuni* and *C. fetus* subsp. *fetus*. Is either organism hemolytic? (If the culture has failed to grow, reincubate for an additional three days in a microaerophilic atmosphere, and then observe.)
  2. Is either *Campylobacter* spp. sensitive to 30 μg nalidixic acid and/or cephalothin?

Measure the zone of inhibition, if any, and record.

3. Observe the TSI agar tubes incubated at 37°C and at 42°C. Describe your results. Is acid produced in either the butt or on the slant? Did both organisms grow at these temperatures? At which temperature did each species show optimal growth? Grade these on a scale of +4 (maximal growth) to +1 (minimal growth), or - (no growth). Is H_2S detected in the agar of those with maximum growth?

B. After reading the above results do the following for each species:
1. Carry out the sodium hippurate hydrolysis test (procedure described in Exercise 2, *Part3* A-5, page 34). You should begin this assay early in the period because of the 2-hour incubation period that is required.
2. Test for the capacity of indoxyl acetate hydrolysis (15, 16) by these species using the disk test. Place two disks into an empty petri dish (or other disposable container). Remove a loopful of *C. jejuni* from a TSI agar slant. Place this on to one disk, then add a drop of sterile distilled water. Repeat with *C. fetus* on the second disk. Replace the dish cover and observe for up to 10 minutes. A positive test is noted by the development of a dark blue color (19). (What is the compound responsible for this blue color?) (Note: See reference 7)
3. Find the catalase and oxidase reactions for both organisms. This can be done directly on the cultures that you have available, or by use of the filter paper method.

C. Record your data. Compare your results with the data shown in Table 11-1. Are they similar? Discuss.

Part 3
Demonstration:

Examine the chocolate agar plate containing *H. pylori*. One plate is available for each bench. These cultures were streaked for isolation on the date written on the plate, and 30 μg nalidixic acid and cephalothin-containing disks placed on the heavily streaked areas, as done in your work in *Part 1* B above. They were then incubated at 37°C in a microaerophilic atmosphere. With the plate for your bench:

1. Examine the isolated colony forms of *H. pylori*.
2. Determine sensitivity of this organism to nalidixic acid and cephalothin.
3. Prepare a wet mount and microscopically observe using phase contrast optics.
4. Do the catalase and oxidase tests.
5. Record and discuss your results. Compare these with those obtained from your study of *Campylobacter*.

QUESTIONS

1. As discussed in the introduction to this exercise, patient antibody against *H. pylori* can be assayed by the indirect ELISA and indirect fluorescent antibody (IFA) assays. for these:
   a. What is the source of antigen?
   b. What is the primary antibody directed against, and what is its source?
   c. Give the possible source of the secondary antibody for both types of tests, and the antigen it is directed against.
   d. Name a possible label that could be used on the secondary antibody for the ELISA and for the IFA test.
2. Describe the indoxyl acetate hydrolysis reaction. (Note: See reference 7.)
3. Although the reaction data in Table 11-1 readily distinguish *Campylobacter* spp. from *H. pylori*, a major clue providing tentative separation even before culture is not included there. What is it?

REFERENCES

1. Blaser, M. J. 1990. Campylobacter species, p. 1649-1658. *In* G. L. Mandell, R. G. Douglas, Jr., and J. E. Bennett (ed.), Principles and practices of infectious diseases, 3rd ed. Churchill Livingstone, New York.
2. Blaser, M. J. 1990. *Helicobacter pylori* and the pathogenesis of gastroduodenal inflammation. J. Infect. Dis. **161**:626-633.
3. Blaser, M. J., and W. L. Wang. 1987. *Campylobacter* infections, p. 195-211. *In* B. B. Wentworth (ed.), Diagnostic procedures for bacterial infections, 7th ed. American Public Health Association, Inc., Washington, D. C.
4. Buck, G. E. 1990. *Campylobacter pylori* and gastroduodenal disease. Clin. Microbiol. Rev. 3:1-12.
5. Cellini, L., N. Allocati, R. Piccolomini, E. Di Campli, and B. Dainelli. 1992. New plate medium for growth and detection of urease activity of *Helicobacter pylori*. J. Clin. Microbiol. 30:1351-1353.
6. Clayton, C. L., H. Kleanthous, P. J. Coates, D. D. Morgan, and S. Tabaqchali. 1992. Sensitive detection of *Helicobacter pylori* by using polymerase chain reaction. J. Clin. Microbiol. **30**:192-200.

7. Dealler, S. F., P. M. Hawkey and M. R. Millar. 1988. Enzymatic degradation of urinary indoxyl sulfate by *Providencia stuartii* and *Klebsiella pneumoniae* causes the purple urine bag syndrome. J. Clin. Microbiol. **26**:2152-2156.

8. Endtz, H. P., G. J. H. M. Ruijs, A. H. Zwinderman, T. van der Reijden, M. Bierver, and R. P. Mouton. 1991. Comparison of six media, including a semisolid agar, for isolation of various *Campylobacter* species from stool specimens. J. Clin. Microbiol. **29**:1007-1010.

9. Goodwin, C. S., J. A. Armstrong, T. Chilvers, M. Peters, M. D. Collins, L. Sly, W. McConnell, and W. E. S. Harper. 1989. Transfer of *Campylobacter pylori* and *Campylobacter mustelae* to *Helicobacter* gen. nov. as *Helicobacter pylori* comb. nov. and *Helicobacter mustelae* comb. nov., respectively. Int. J. Syst. Bacteriol. **39**:397-405.

10. Griffiths, P. L., and R. W. A. Park. 1990. Campylobacters associated with human diarrhoeal disease. J. Appl. Bacteriol. **69**:281-301.

11. Hammar, M., T. Tyszliewicz, T. Wadström, and P. W. O'Toole. 1992. Rapid detection of *Helicobacter pylori* in gastric biopsy material by polymerase chain reaction. J. Clin. Microbiol. **30**:54-58.

12. Hazell, S. L., T. J. Borody, A. Gal, and A. Lee. 1987. *Campylobacter pyloridis* gastritis I. Detection of urease as a marker of bacterial colonization and gastritis. Am. J. Gastroenterol. **82**:292-295.

13. Hoek, F. J., L. A. Noach, E. A. J. Rauws, and G. N. J. Tytgat. 1992. Evaluation of the performance of commercial test kits for detection of *Helicobacter pylori* antibodies in serum. J. Clin. Microbiol. **30**:1525-1528.

14. Kiehlbauch, J. A., D. J. Brenner, M. A. Nicholson, C. N. Baker, C. M. Patton, A. G. Steigerwalt, and I. K. Wachsmuth. 1991. *Campylobacter butzleri* sp. nov. isolated from humans and animals with diarrheal illness. J. Clin. Microbiol. **29**:376-385.

15. Mills, C. K., and R. L. Gherna. 1987. Hydrolysis of indoxyl acetate by *Campylobacter* species. J. Clin. Microbiol. **25**:1560-1561.

16. On, S. L. W., and B. Holmes. 1992. Asssessment of enzyme detection tests useful in identification of campylobacteria. J. Clin. Microbiol. **30**:746-749.

17. Penner, J. L. 1991. *Campylobacter, Helicobacter,* and related spiral bacteria, p. 402-409. *In* A. Balows, W. J. Hausler, Jr., K. L. Herrmann, H. D. Isenberg, and H. J. Shadomy (ed.), Manual of clinical microbiology, 5th ed. American Society for Microbiology, Washington, D. C.

18. Peterson, W. L. 1991. *Helicobacter pylori* and peptic ulcer disease. N. Eng. J. Med. **324**: 1043-1048.

19. Popovic-Uroic, T., C. M. Patton, M. A. Nicholson, and J. A. Kiehlbauch. 1990. Evaluation of the indoxyl acetate hydrolysis test for rapid differentiation of *Campylobacter, Helicobacter,* and *Wolinella* species. J. Clin. Microbiol. **28**:2335-2339.

20. Rauws, E. A. J. 1989. Detecting *Campylobacter pylori* with the ^{13}C- and ^{14}C-urea breath test. Scan. J. Gastroenterol. **24**(Suppl. 160):25-26.

21. Skirrow, M. B. 1990. Campylobacter. Lancet **336**:921-923.

22. Smibert, R. M. 1974. *Campylobacter* Sebold and Véron 1963, p. 207-212. *In* R. E. Buchanan, and N. E. Gibbons (ed.), Bergey's manual of determinative bacteriology, 8th ed. The Williams & Wilkins Co., Baltimore.

23. Smibert, R. M. 1984. *Campylobacter* Sebold and Véron 1963, p. 111-118. *In* N. R. Krieg, and J. G. Holt (ed.), Bergey's manual of systematic bacteriology, Vol. 1. Williams & Wilkins, Baltimore.

24. Soltesz, V., B. Zeeberg, and T. Wadström. 1992. Optimal survival of *Helicobacter pylori* under various transport conditions. J. Clin. Microbiol. **30**:1453-1456.

25. Tee, W., S. Fairley, R. Smallwood, and B. Dwyer. 1991. Comparative. evaluation of three selective media and a non-selective medium for culture of *Helicobacter pylori* from gastric biopsies. J. Clin. Microbiol. **29**:2587-2589.

26. Tenover, F. C., L. Carlson, S. Barbagallo, and I. Nachamkin. 1990. DNA probe culture confirmation assay for identification of thermophilic *Campylobacter* species. J. Clin. Microbiol. **28**: 1284-1287.

27. Timoney, J. F., J. H. Gillespie, F. W. Scott, and J. E. Barlough. 1988. Hagan and Bruner's microbiology and infectious diseases of domestic animals, 8th ed.. p. 153-160. Comstock Publishing Associates, Ithica, NY

28. Vandamme, P., and J. De Ley. 1991. Proposal for a new family, *Campylobacteraceae*. Int. J. Syst. Bacteriol. **41**:451-455.

29. Wyatt, J. I., and B. J. Rathbone. 1989. The role of serology in the diagnosis of *Campylobacter pylori* infection. Scand. J. Gastroenterol. **24**(Suppl. 160):27-34.

Exercise 11
Data Table 1: *Campylobacter* and *Helicobacter pylori* Results

		Culture Age	*C. jejuni* subsp. *jejuni*		*C. fetus* subsp. *fetus*		*H. pylori*	
			Campy BAP	Other	Campy BAP	Other	Campy BAP	Other
Colony size and Colony Form	mm							
	Punctiform							
	Irregular							
	Circular							
	Rhizoid							
	Filamentous							
	Other							
Colony Surface	Flat							
	Raised							
	Convex							
	Pulvinate							
	Other							
Colony Margin	Entire							
	Undulate							
	Lobate							
	Erose							
	Other							
Colony Consistency	Butyrous							
	Viscid							
	Membranous							
	Brittle							
	Other							
Optical Character	Opaque							
	Translucent							
	Dull							
	Glistening							
	Other							
Surface	Smooth							
	Rough							
	Other							
Hemolysis	Type						■	
Nalidixic acid, 30 μg	Inhibition							
Cephalothin, 30 μg	Inhibition							

Exercise 11
Data Table 2: *Campylobacter* and *Helicobacter pylori* Results

		Culture Age	*C. jejuni* subsp. *jejuni*	*C. fetus* subsp. *fetus*	*H. pylori*
Gram stain	Reaction				
Culture	Morphology				
source:	Arrangement				
Wet Mount	Motility				
Flagella	No./cell				
	Arrangement				
TSI agar (37°C	Slant Reaction				
Incubation)	Butt Reaction				
	H$_2$S in agar				
	Gas				
TSI agar (42°C	Slant Reaction				
Incubation)	Butt Reaction				
	H$_2$S in agar				
	Gas				
TSI agar	37°C				
Growth[a]	42°C				
Hippurate	Hydrolysis				
Indoxyl acetate	Hydrolysis				
Catalase test					
Oxidase test					
Other					

[a] Grade growth rate based on scale of +1 to +4 or −.

Laboratory Notes:

EXERCISE 12
Pseudomonas of the Family *Pseudomonadaceae*

In the 1984 Bergey's Manual of Systematic Bacteriology (6) the family *Pseudomonadaceae* included four genera, *Pseudomonas, Xanthomonas, Frateuria,* and *Zoogloea.* At that time, only *Pseudomonas* contained species that are pathogenic to humans and lower animals, the subject of this exercise. However, many plant pathogens are contained in both this genus and in *Xanthomonas.* All are Gram-negative, aerobic, straight to curving rods that are catalase positive, and motile by means of polar flagella.

As might be expected, the genus *Pseudomonas* has and is undergoing significant taxonomic change. However, because most do not impact on the common isolates from clinical samples, except in one case, these modifications will not be discussed here. The exception is that *P. maltophilia,* a human disease agent, has been reclassified as *Xanthomonas maltophilia* based upon genotypic an phenotypic data (11). A summary of other changes may be found in Gilardi (3).

Despite the large number of species (80 listed in Bergey's Manual (7)) in the genus *Pseudomonas* only a few have been frequently implicated in human infection. Almost all are opportunistic agents, their usual habitat being soil, water, and other areas of the environment.

P. aeruginosa is the most frequently isolated organism of the genus. In fact, it is among the leading causes of nosocomial infections (3, 8) accounting for about 70% of non-fermenting bacterial isolates (3). Furthermore, it is exceedingly versatile, causing a broad spectrum of disease including pneumonia, urinary tract infection, septicemia, wound infections, endocarditis, otitis media, meningitis, and corneal ulcers, to name a few. It is also a significant factor in the morbidity and mortality (but not the underlying cause) of cystic fibrosis (5). Although this organism is susceptible to many of the more recently developed antimicrobials (3), infections due to it have historically been difficult to manage.

Others of the pseudomonads that are isolated, but much less frequently than *P. aeruginosa,* include *P. fluorescens, P. paucimobilis, P. putida, P. stutzeri, X. maltophilia (or P. maltophilia),* and *P. cepacia.* These also may be associated with a variety of opportunistic infections, however the latter is increasing in its frequency in patients with cystic fibrosis (10). There are two other species that cause primary infections in healthy individuals (i.e. do not require opportunistic conditions). These are *P. pseudomallei,* the agent of melioidosis, and *P. mallei,* which causes glanders (9, 10). Melioidosis is seen in a variety of forms, but usually is an acute pneumonia, and less so as a septicemia or a suppurative infection (3). While it rarely occurs in the U. S., it is in the soil and an endemic disease in humans and lower animals in Southeast Asia, Papua New Guinea, and Northern Australia. The organism is probably endemic in the soil of other areas of the world as well (2). Glanders is primarily a disease of equines, from which it is rarely transmitted to humans. Its manifestations are highly variable, but usually similar to melioidosis. It is epidemiologically restricted to Asia and parts of Africa and the Middle East (3).

Certain laboratory characteristics of the pseudomonads should be emphasized. They will, for example, readily grow on many common isolation media used for the enteric bacteria, as MacConkey and EMB agars. You will recall, however, that pseudomonads are non-fermenting Gram-negative bacteria (NFB) (Photo 12-1), and strict aerobes (see the "Introduction to Anaerobic Bacteria and Facultative Anaerobic Rods," page 63 and Table 5-1, page 95). Furthermore, all produce catalase, and except *X. maltophilia,* all of the most common clinical isolates, as those shown in Table 12-1, are oxidase-positive. Thus, several important clues are available within 24 hours following streaking these organisms on isolation media, including the distinctive "grape-like" odor and pigmentation of the most common isolate, *P. aeruginosa* (Photo 12-2). However, take care not to confuse these with the many other genera of oxidative, oxidase-positive bacteria, such as *Moraxella,* discussed in Exercise 4.

Table 12-1
Some Characteristics of Selected Clinically Significant *Pseudomonas* Species (1, 3, 7)

Pseudomonas species	Oxidase	O-F Medium[b] Acid			Pigment Produced		Growth at 42°C	Decarboxylase		Arginine Dihydrolase	Nitrate to gas	Motility	Number of polar flagella
		Glucose	Maltose	Lactose	Pyocyanin[c]	Pyoverdin[c]		Lysine	Ornithine				
P. aeruginosa	+[a]	+	−	−	+	+	+	−	−	+	V	+	1
P. cepacia	+	+	+	+	−	−[d]	V	+	V	−	−	+	3-8
P. fluorescens	+	+	−	V	−	+	−	−	−	+	−	+	>1
P. mallei	+	+	D+	+	−	−	−			+ or D+	−	−	0
X. maltophilia (or P. maltophilia)	−	+	+	V	−	−[e]	V	+	−	−	−	+	1-6
P. pseudomallei	+	+	+	+	−	−	+			+	+	+	>1
P. paucimobilis	+	+	+	+	−	−[f]	−	−	−	−	−	+& −	1[f]
P. putida	+	+	−	V	−	V	−	−	−	+	−	+	>1
P. stutzeri	+	+	+	−	−	−	+	−	−	−	+	+	1

[a] + = 90% or more positive; − = 10% or less positive; V = 11-89% positive; D+ = delayed reaction. All reactions usually occur within 48 hours.
[b] Oxidation-fermentation medium exposed to air.
[c] Pyocyanin is a chloroform and water soluble blue-green pigment; pyoverdin is a fluorescent yellow-green pigment insoluble in chloroform, but water soluble.
[d] P. cepacia may form colonies with yellow to yellow-green diffusible, but non-fluorescent pigments.
[e] X. maltophilia may form a slight yellow pigmentation on nutrient agar. Also, colonies emit an ammonia-like odor.
[f] P. paucimobilis form colonies with yellow non-diffusible pigment at 30°C; also, motility may be difficult to show as few cells in population motile.

Beyond this, the oxidative nature of these bacteria must be determined using O-F media. Many other assays are available to distinguish species within the pseudomonads, some of which are given in Table 12-1. Commercially-available assays can be applied to the pseudomonads as discussed in Exercise 4, **page 87**.

The following brief exercise will provide some added insight into this group of organisms.

MATERIALS

Part 1
Per pair of students:
- 1 Stock culture each of *Pseudomonas aeruginosa* and of *P. fluorescens* on nutrient agar slants
- 1 MacConkey agar plate
- 4 tubes OF glucose
- 4 tubes OF maltose
- 1 tube sterile petrolatum (7 ml)
- 2 tubes nitrate broth (with Durham tubes)
- 2 tubes lysine broth
- 2 tubes arginine broth

Part 2
Reagents for catalase, oxidase (0.5% tetra-methyl-*p*-phenylenediamine dihydrochloride) and nitrate tests
Strips of Whatman No. 1 filter paper
60°C water bath

LABORATORY PROCEDURES

Part 1
Each pair of students do the following steps:
A. Inoculate *P. aeruginosa* and *P. fluorescens* to:
  1. One-half of a MacConkey agar plate. Streak for isolation.
  2. Paired tubes of oxidation-fermentation (OF) medium containing glucose and maltose. Overlay one of each of these with melted petrolatum. (See Exercise 4, *Part 1-4*, page 89 for instruction on the use of this medium.) If needed, the petrolatum can be melted in a 60°C water bath.
  3. Nitrate broth.
  4. Lysine decarboxylase and arginine dihydrolase broths.

Incubate all cultures at 35-37°C and observe as often as necessary for up to 48 hours. If growth of *P. fluorescens* has not occurred within 24 hours, place at room temperature and continue incubation up to 4 additional days.

B. Using the stock cultures of each species, each pair of students now do the following steps:

1. Prepare a Gram stain, wet mount, and flagella stain (procedure for latter in Exercise 10, *Part 2* A-6, page 178. Observe each of these, recalling that wet mounts are best observed using phase contrast microscopy. Compare the numbers of polar flagella present on *P. aeruginosa* and *P. fluorescens*, and these with the data given in Table 12-1.

2. Observe and note the colony and agar pigmentation on and in the stock cultures, if any. Also determine the odor emitted by each organism. Both pyocyanin pigmentation and aminoacetophenone are unique to *P. aeruginosa*. The blue-green color of pyocyanin combined with pyoverdin, a yellow fluorescent pigment (Table 12-1) are responsible for the characteristic green to blue-green color of the agar. The fact that the agar becomes colored attests to the water soluble nature of both. Aminoacetophenone is responsible for the unique odor (3).

3. Finally, again using the stock cultures, find their catalase and oxidase reactions. For the latter, place a small amount of colony growth on a strip of Whatman No. 1 filter paper contained in a petri dish. Wet the strip with 0.5% tetramethyl-*p*-phenylenediamine dihydrochloride (Appendix 3) and observe for reaction.

4. Record your data. Following these steps the stock cultures may be discarded.

Part 2

A. Observe and compare growth and/or reaction of *P. aeruginosa* and *P. fluorescens* on the media inoculated above. Record the following:

1. Colony characteristics on MacConkey agar. Particularly note its color.
2. Acid formation in carbohydrate-containing broths exposed to and shielded from air.
3. Reactions in lysine decarboxylase and arginine dihydrolase broths.
4. Nitrate reduction. Also observe for the presence of gas production after 48 hours,

or after good growth in the case of *P. fluorescens*.

Part 3
Demonstration

This demonstration consists of *P. cepacia* grown 48 hours on PC agar, OF-maltose, lysine decarboxylase and arginine dihydrolase broths. PC agar (4) is selective for this organism. To show this, one half of this plate has been streaked with *P. aeruginosa*, the other half with *P. cepacia*. (Note: Another selective and differential medium called "OFPBL" (12) is also available for isolation of *P. cepacia*.

Compare the amount of growth of *P. cepacia* with *P. aeruginosa* on PC agar. Prepare colony descriptions of the former on this medium also. Read results of *P. cepacia* on O-F maltose, lysine decarboxylase and arginine dihydrolase broths. Is there sufficient data to distinguish this organism from *P. aeruginosa* and from *P. fluorescens* studied earlier? If so, what are those distinguishing characteristics?

QUESTIONS

1. An organism from a clinical specimen has been streaked for isolation on a MacConkey agar plate. After 18 hours at 35°C growth occurred. Assume the isolate to be a Gram-negative rod and belonged to one of the following: *Pseudomonas, Enterobacteriaceae, Vibrionaceae, Campylobacter, Acinetobacter,* or *Kingella*.

   For this situation, distinguish between the taxa named based upon a few key characteristics. Use standard laboratory assays, excluding serology, and do so using the fewest tests possible.

2. *P. aeruginosa* has been regarded by some to be identical with *P. polycolor*, a plant pathogen. If this were true, postulate how a single organism might be able to cause infection in both plants and animals. (Or, placing it another way, why is it that more organisms cannot produce infections in both?)

3. Infections due to *Pseudomonas* spp. are a good example (but, certainly not the only ones) of bacteria that were once considered of little importance in human disease. Obviously, this is no longer the case. What is the reason for this increased role of such organisms in infection?

REFERENCES

1. Baron, E. J., L. R. Peterson, and S. M. Finegold. 1994. Bailey & Scott's diagnostic microbiology, 9th ed. Mosby-Year Book, Inc., St. Louis. p. 386-405.

2. Dance, D. A. B. 1991. Melioidosis: the tip of the iceberg? Clin. Microbiol. Rev. 4:52-60.

3. Gilardi, G. L. 1991. *Pseudomonas* and related genera, p. 429-441. *In* A. Balows, W. J. Hausler, Jr., K. L. Herrmann, H. D. Isenberg, and H. J. Shadomy (ed.), Manual of clinical microbiology, 5th ed. American Society for Microbiology, Washington, D. C.

4. Gilligan, P. H., P. A. Gage, L. M. Bradshaw, D. V. Schidlow, and B. T. DeCicco. 1985. Isolation medium for recovery of *Pseudomonas cepacia* from respiratory secretions of patients with cystic fibrosis. J. Clin. Microbiol. 22:5-8.

5. May, T. B., D. Shinabarger, R. Maharaj, J. Kato, L. Chu, J. D. DeVault, S. Roychoudhury, N. A. Zielinski, A. Berry, R. K. Rothmel, T. K. Misra, and A. M. Chakrabarty. 1991. Alginate synthesis by *Pseudomonas aeruginosa*: a key pathogenic factor in chronic pulmonary infections of cystic fibrosis patients. Clin. Microbiol. Rev. 4:191-206.

6. Palleroni, N. J. 1984. *Pseudomonadaceae* Winslow, Broadhurst, Buchanan, Krumwiede, Rogers and Smith, 1917, p. 141. *In* N. R. Krieg, and J. G. Holt (ed.), Bergey's manual of systematic bacteriology, Vol. 1. Williams & Wilkins, Baltimore.

7. Palleroni, N. J. 1984. *Pseudomonas* Migula 1894, p. 141-199. *In* N. R. Krieg, and J. G. Holt (ed.), Bergey's manual of systematic bacteriology, Vol. 1. Williams & Wilkins, Baltimore.

8. Pollack, M. 1990. Pseudomonas aeruginosa, p. 1673-1691. *In* G. L. Mandell, R. G. Douglas, Jr., and J. E. Bennett (ed.), Principles and practices of infectious diseases, 3rd ed. Churchill Livingstone, New York.

9. Ryan, K. J. 1990. *Pseudomonas* and other opportunistic Gram-negative bacilli, p. 393-400. *In* J. C. Sherris (ed.), Medical microbiology: an introduction to infectious diseases, 2nd ed. Elsevier Science Publishing Co., Inc. New York.

10. Sanford, J. P. 1990. Pseudomonas species (including melioidosis and glanders), p. 1692-1696. *In* G. L. Mandell, R. G. Douglas, Jr., and J. E. Bennett (ed.), Principles and practices of infectious diseases, 3rd ed. Churchill Livingstone, New York.

11. Swings, J., P. De Vos, M. Van den Mooter, and J. De Ley. 1983. Transfer of *Pseudomonas maltophilia* Hugh 1981 to the genus *Xanthomonas* as *Xanthomonas maltophilia* (Hugh 1981) comb. nov. Int. J. System. Bacteriol. 33:409-413.

12. Welch, D. F., M. J. Muszynski, C. H. Pai, M. J. Marcon, M. M. Hribar, P. H. Gilligan, J. M. Matsen, P. A. Ahlin, B. C. Hilman, and S. A. Chartrand. 1987. Selective and differential medium for recovery of *Pseudomonas cepacia* from the respiratory tract of patients with cystic fibrosis. J. Clin. Microbiol. 25:1730-1734.

Exercise 12
Data Table 1: *Pseudomonas* Results

		Culture Age	P. aeruginosa		P. fluorescens		P. cepacia	
			MacConkey	Other	MacConkey	Other	MacConkey	Other
Colony size and Colony Form	mm							
	Punctiform							
	Irregular							
	Circular							
	Rhizoid							
	Filamentous							
	Other							
Colony Surface	Flat							
	Raised							
	Convex							
	Pulvinate							
	Other							
Colony Margin	Entire							
	Undulate							
	Lobate							
	Erose							
	Other							
Colony Consistency	Butyrous							
	Viscid							
	Membranous							
	Brittle							
	Other							
Optical Character	Opaque							
	Translucent							
	Dull							
	Glistening							
	Other							
Surface	Smooth							
	Rough							
	Other							
Colony Color								
PC agar	Relative growth[a]		▇▇▇		▇▇▇			
Nutrient Agar slant	Pigment						▇▇▇	▇▇▇
	Odor							

[a] Use +4 growth = maximum to +1 = minimum growth; − = no growth

Exercise 12
Data Table 2: *Pseudomonas* Results

		Culture		*Pseudomonas aeruginosa*	*Pseudomonas fluorescens*	*Pseudomonas cepetia*
		Source	Age			
Catalase test						
Oxidase test						
Gram stain	Reaction					
	Morphology					
	Arrangement					
Wet mount	Motility					
OF, Acid from	Open					
Glucose	Sealed					
Maltose	Open					
	Sealed					
Lysine	Decarboxylase					
Arginine	Dihydrolase					
Nitrate	Reduction					
	Gas					
Flagella stain	No. of Flagella					
Other						

Laboratory Notes:

EXERCISE 13
Legionella and the Family *Legionellaceae*

Legionella pneumophilia, is one of several species (and the most important from a disease standpoint) in the family *Legionellaceae* that can cause legionellosis. Since its discovery as the agent of Legionnaires' disease in 1976, the genus has grown to over 30 species (14). There are over 50 serotypes distributed within these, including 14 in *Legionella pneumophilia*. Although at least 19 species have been implicated in pneumonia (10), many others have been isolated from the environment (12). It has been proposed that several organisms in the genus be placed in newly developed taxa, the *Tatlockia* and *Fluoribacter*, based upon unique genetic and chemical differences of these (6). Although not universally agreed upon, the proposed names will be given here along with the *Legionella* sp. name when appropriate.

Legionellosis most commonly occurs in two clinical forms: Legionnaires' disease and Pontiac fever. The former has a 1-5% attack rate and is typically a pneumonia. It can be fatal in up to 20% of cases. Conversely, Pontiac fever has up to a 95% attack rate, is flu-like, does not include pneumonia, and is not fatal. The reason for the occurrence of two seemingly separate clinical entities in unknown (12, 14). *L. pneumophilia* accounts for 90% of all legionellae infections, and serogroups 1, 4, and 6 are most frequently involved. Of the other species *Legionella* [or *Tatlockia*] *micdadei* ranks second in frequency, followed by *Legionella* [or *Fluoribacter*] *bozemanii*, *L.* [*F.*] *dumoffii*, *L. longbeachae*, and others (5). The clinical symptoms are similar for all of the legionellae. It should be noted that these organisms cause nosocomial as well as community-acquired infections, and legionellosis also can occur as non-pulmonary infections.

Besides clinical specimens containing legionellae bacteria, which obviously are primarily of pulmonary origin, other types of samples may require processing. Since these organisms naturally occur in the environment, suspected samples could be soil and especially water. Of particular concern has been the presence of the bacteria in water supplies of hospitals and large buildings, both in hot and cold water supplies. Also, water cooling towers and their aerosols are implicated as sources of infection (5, 12, 14). Interestingly, strains of *L. pneumophilia* vary between water supplies of buildings, even when the reservoir source is the same (2). Thus, when an outbreak of legionellosis does occur, an identification of the causative clinical agent is needed, not only from the patient source, but also from the environmental source.

Despite its capacity to survive in a wide range of environmental conditions, legionellae have quite strict growth requirements. They will not, for example, grow on sheep blood agar (8). The most successful isolation medium has been buffered charcoal yeast extract supplemented with iron, L-cysteine, and α-ketoglutarate (BCYEα or BCYEA). L-cysteine is an absolute requirement, and comparing growth with and without this in the medium can be useful as a diagnostic tool (12) (Photo 13-1). Several variations of this basic medium can be used. For example, it can be made more selective by addition of antimicrobial agents. Also, the addition of bromcresol purple and bromthymol blue can aid in differentiation of legionellae from other genera (12, 14). Because some strains of *Legionella* are inhibited by selective agents, non-selective BCYEα should always be included (12).

Although cultivation is the definitive procedure for diagnosis of legionellosis with a specificity of 100%, its sensitivity is only 70-75% (10, 12). Furthermore, complete speciation by standard culture testing can be difficult for the general laboratory due to phenotype similarity (12, 13). Because of this, identification methods employing serology and DNA probes have been developed. However, recall that all species and serotypes cause similar clinical symptoms, therefore therapeutic measures are also normally similar. Thus, identification to the genus level is most critical and should be possible by most laboratories. Furthermore, as mentioned earlier, *L. pneumophilia* and *L.* [*T.*] *micdadei* represent over 90% of cause of legionellosis. Differentiation of these, as shown in Table 13-1 is straightforward. However, speciation and serogrouping is most important from an epidemiological view.

Table 13-1
Selected Characteristics of Some Members of the Family *Legionellaceae*[b] (8, 12)

Genus-species	Oxidase	Beta Lactamase	Hippurate Hydrolysis	Motility	Blue-white Fluorescence[b]	Browning of agar[c]	Gelatinase
L pneumophilia[d]	V[e,f]	+	+	+	−	+	+
L micdadei (or *Tatlockia micdadei*)	+	−	−	+	−	−	−
L bozemanii (or *Fluoribacter bozemanii*)	V	V	−	+	+	+	+
L dumoffii (or *Fluoribacter dumoffii*)	−	+	−	+	+	V	+
L longbeachae	+	V	−	+	−	+[f]	+

[a] Species shown are most commonly implicated in infection (5) out of 19 isolated from humans. There are over 30 species total (10); it has been proposed that *L. micdadei* be renamed *Tatlockia micdadei*. Also, *L. bozemanii* and *L. dumoffii* proposed to be placed in the genus *Fluoribacter* (6).
[b] Colony fluorescence using long wavelength UV light (366 nM).
[c] Browning in tyrosine-containing agar.
[d] *L pneumophilia* consists of 3 subspecies and 14 serogroups.
[e] + = usually positive; − = usually negative; V = varies between strains.
[f] Environmental isolates of *L. pneumophilia* may give negative oxidase reaction.

Characteristically, *Legionella* are Gram-negative rods. They counterstain poorly with safranin, therefore carbol fuchsin is used in its place. They are non-fermentive and non-oxidative for carbohydrates. Clinically-important species all show weak catalase and peroxidase activity, and variable oxidase reaction. Except for *L. oakridgensis*, they are motile by polar or near-polar flagella. Some differential characteristics of species most frequently involved in Legionnaires' disease and Pontiac fever are given in Table 13-1.

The most widely accepted tool for diagnosis besides culture is the direct fluorescent antibody (DFA) assay. When properly done and controlled, this method is over 99% specific and up to 77% sensitive. The low sensitivity is due to the need for 10^4 to 10^5 cells to be able to detect them microscopically. It has the advantage though, of being rapid compared to culture, and it can be used directly on tissue or sputum (12). Labeled *Legionella* antibody for DFA (Photo 13-2) is commercially available from several sources, as are indirect fluorescent antibody assay reagents.

Radioimmunoassay (RIA), latex agglutination (LA) tests, microagglutination and ELISA have also been developed (e.g. 3, 4, 9). Pro-Lab's LA panel is used for culture confirmation. An RIA kit (Equate® Legionella Antigen kit) to detect antigen in urine is commercially available and has been shown to be 100% specific and 93% sensitive (1) for detection of *L. pneumophilia* serogroup 1 antigenuria. Others, which are not used nor fully evaluated for routine use, may detect soluble antigen in urine and from other sources (12).

Gen-Probe supplies an isotopically-labeled nucleic acid probe kit, the Gen-Probe® Rapid Diagnostic System for *Legionella*. Although the sensitivity of this test is reported to be similar, and could be used as a replacement for the DFA assay, it has the advantage of being able to detect all species of *Legionella* and its serogroups (11, 12). Culture confirmation is still required, however.

PCR technology is now available commercially for the detection of the *Legionella* genus, and for *L. pneumophilia* from environmental water samples (EnvironAmp™ Legionella kit). This assay is based upon principles discussed in Exercise 3, Section 2, p. 75 in which the identification kit is integrated with the GenAmp™ Instrument System to provide sample preparation, amplification, and detection of legionellae within five hours.

Serological determination of patient antibody responses to legionellae infection is also diagnostically useful, with a four-fold increase in titer to 1:128 being significant (12, 14). To find this, an indirect fluorescent antibody test is used. Dilutions of patient serum are applied to slides containing killed organisms, and anti-legionellae, if present, is detected with fluorescent-labeled anti-immunoglobulin (12). (The principles of this type of assay are discussed in Exercise 14.)

Legionella identification, then, can be accomplished by culture, usually in combination with probe, PCR, or antigen-detection methods. Full identification, at this time at least, requires serological, fatty acid, and/or further genetic analysis (12). In this exercise, we will examine only some methods used in culture identification of *Legionella* and species separation of the two most commonly isolated clinically-important species.

MATERIALS

Part 1

Per pair of students
1 Buffered charcoal yeast extract with α-ketoglutarate slant (BCYEα) cultures of:
 L. pneumophilia
 L. [or *T.*] *micdadei*
1 BCYEα agar plate
1 Charcoal yeast extract (CYE) without supplements agar plate
1 Sheep blood agar plate
2 *Legionella* differentiation disks
2 Tubes hippurate broth, 0.4 ml in screw-capped 13 x 100 mm tubes

Part 2

Per pair of students
1 Petri dish
4 Filter paper strips
2 tubes hippurate broth
2 β-lactamase detection disks
Per bench:
 Carbol fuchsin
 Catalase reagent
 Oxidase reagent
 Dropper bottle with distilled water
 Dropper bottle with ninhydrin reagent
Per class:
 UV lamp that emits at 360 nM

LABORATORY PROCEDURES

(Also outlined in Figure 13-1):
(Note: All transfer and open culture procedures must be done in the biohazard hood.)

Part 1

Each pair of students carry out the following:
 1. Transfer a large inoculum of *L. pneumophilia* and *L.* [*T.*] *micdadei* from the stock culture slant, each to one-half BCYEα, CYE and sheep blood agar plate. Streak each for isolation.
 2. Aseptically place a *Legionella* differentiation disk on to the heavily streaked segment of each organism on the CYE plate only.

3. Incubate all plate cultures at 35°C until good growth occurs on the BCYEα plate. This may take from 2 to 5 days.
4. Inoculate hippurate reagent tubes each with a loopful of one legionellae species. Emulsify to give a heavy, dispersed suspension. Incubate at 35°C for 18-20 hours (7).
5. Prepare heat-fixed smears of the stock organisms. Stain by the usual Gram stain procedure, except that carbol fuchsin should be applied for 60 seconds in the place of the usual safranin. Microscopically examine and record your results. Do the species appear similar? Are they of uniform width and length? If not, what kinds of variation do you see?

Part 2

(Remember! Use the biohazard hood for all open culture steps.)
 1. Observe the growth of *L. pneumophilia* and *L.* [*T.*] *micdadei* on BCYEα, CYE, and sheep blood agars. Record the relative amounts of growth on each, and if isolated colony growth is present, note the relative colony size and appearance on each medium. On BCYEα agar pinpoint colonies appear in 2-3 days, growing to 3-4 mm in diameter. They are convex, circular, with entire margins, and gray in color in 5 days. When examined in a dissecting microscope, colonies also exhibit a "cut glass" appearance (23). Is growth observable on sheep blood agar? If so, what should be the interpretation with respect to the identification of these organisms (or any other *Legionella* spp.)?
 2. Examine the CYE plate for the presence of satellite growth around the *Legionella* differentiation disk. Based upon the results of this, the requirement for L-cysteine by these organisms should be evident.
 3. Place the BCYEα plate under a UV lamp that emits 366nM. Is fluorescence produced? If present, note its color. This will most readily be seen in an area where growth is heavy. (Note: Use appropriate precautions using UV light.) Although those species given in Table 13-1 either lack fluorescence or fluoresce blue-white, others may produce a red or yellow-green fluorescence (12.)

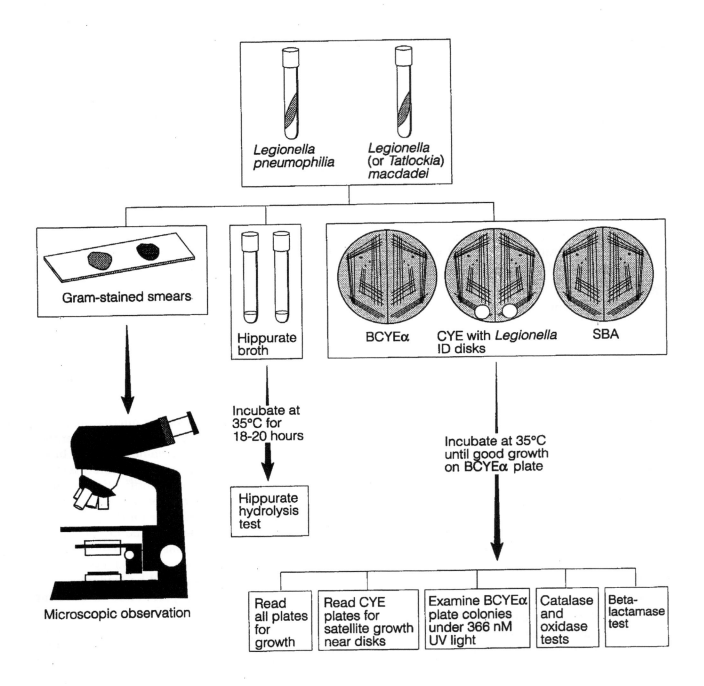

Figure 13-1: Procedural outline of laboratory examination of *L. pneumophilia* and *L. (or Tatlockia) macdadei*.

4. Carry out the β-lactamase disk assay. Use the same procedure described in Exercise 1, *Part* 2C, page 12. (How does the purpose of β-lactamase detection differ here as compared to that of Exercise 1 when *Staphylococcus aureus* was tested?)

5. Complete the hippurate tube test by adding 0.2 ml ninhydrin reagent to each tube. Tighten caps, then agitate well. Incubate at 35°C for 10 minutes, then read for color development occurring within 20 minutes (7).

6. Place a filter paper strip into a petri dish, then wet with oxidase reagent. Remove some growth from the BCYEα agar plate and rub it onto the reagent-containing strip. Are they oxidase positive?

7. Test the growth on the BCYEα agar plate for catalase production. Use a loop or needle to disturb the growth within the drop of H_2O_2. Bubbles should be observed within 30 seconds. (Are you working within a biohazard hood?)

8. Record your results and discuss them. Especially draw out differential characters of *L. pneumophilia* and *L. [T.] micdadei*. Also, give characteristics that are unique to *Legionella* compared to other Gram-negative rods thus far studied.

QUESTIONS

1. *Legionella* species have complex media requirements for their *in vitro* growth. Yet, they have been isolated from water and soil, sources that are usually nutritionally poor. How can this be explained? (Hint: See reference 12 or 14.)

2. The antimicrobial sensitivity of legionellae is broad when tested *in vitro*. However, this sensitivity may not be reflected *in vivo*. Why? And, what is the connection between this and the answer in Question 1, above?

REFERENCES

1. Aguero-Rosenfeld, M. E., and P. H. Edelstein. 1988. Retrospective evaluation of the Du Pont radioimmunoassay kit for detection of *Legionella pneumophilia* serogroup 1 antigenuria in humans. J. Clin. Microbiol. **26**: 1775-1778.

2. Bezanson, G., S. Burbridge, D. Haldane, C. Yoell, and T. Marrie. 1992. Diverse populations of *Legionella pneumophilia* present in the water of geographically clustered institutions served by the same water reservoir. J. Clin. Microbiol. **30**:570-576.

3. Birtles, R. J., T. G. Harrison, D. Samuel, and A. G. Taylor. 1990. Evaluation of urinary antigen ELISA for diagnosing *Legionella pneumophilia* serogroup 1 infection. J. Clin. Pathol. **43**:685-690.

4. Constantine, C. E., and T. G. Wreghitt. 1991. A rapid micro-agglutination technique for the detection of antibody to *Legionella pneumophilia* serogroup 5. J. Med. Microbiol. **34**:29-31.

5. Fang, G.-D., and V. L. Yu. 1990. Other Legionella species, p. 1774-1782. *In* G. L. Mandell, R. G. Douglas, Jr., and J. E. Bennett (ed.), Principles and practices of infectious diseases, 3rd ed. Churchill Livingstone, New York.

6. Garrity, G. M., A. Brown, and R. M. Vickers. 1980. *Tatlockia* and *Fluoribacter*: two new genera of organisms resembling *Legionella pneumophilia*. Int. J. Syst. Bacteriol. **30**:609-614.

7. Hébert, G. A. 1981. Hippurate hydrolysis by *Legionella pneumophilia*. J. Clin. Microbiol. **13**:240-242.

8. Koneman, E. W., S. D. Allen, W. M. Janda, P. C. Schreckenberger, and W. C. Winn, Jr. 1992. Color atlas and textbook of diagnostic microbiology, 4th ed. J. B. Lippincott Co., Philadelphia. p. 351-368.

9. Leland, D. S., and R. B. Kohler. 1991. Evaluation of the L-Clone *Legionella pneumophilia* serogroup 1 urine antigen latex test. J. Clin. Microbiol. **29**:2220-2223.

10. Nguyen, M. L. T., and V. L. Yu. 1991. *Legionella* infection. Clin. Chest Med. **12**:257-268.

11. Pasculle, A. W., G. E. Veto, S. Krystofiak, K. McKelvey, and K. Vrsalovic. 1989. Laboratory and clinical evaluation of a commercial DNA probe for detection of *Legionella* spp. J. Clin. Microbiol. **27**:2350-2358.

12. Rodgers, F. G., and A. W. Pasculle. 1991. *Legionella*, p. 442-453. *In* A. Balows, W. J. Hausler, Jr., K. L. Herrmann, H. D. Isenberg, and H. J. Shadomy (ed.), Manual of clinical microbiology, 5th ed. American Society for Microbiology, Washington, D. C.

13. Vesey, G., P. J. Dennis, J. V. Lee, and A. A. West. 1988. Further development of simple tests to differentiate the legionellas. J. Appl. Bacteriol. **65**:339-345.

14. Yu, V. L. 1990. Legionella pneumophilia (Legionnaires' disease), p. 1764-1774. *In* G. L. Mandell, R. G. Douglas, Jr., and J. E. Bennett (ed.), Principles and practices of infectious diseases, 3rd ed. Churchill Livingstone, New York.

**Exercise 13
Data Table 1: *Legionella* Results**

		Culture	*Legionella pneumophilia*				*Legionella* (or *Tatlockia*) *micdadei*			
		Age	BCYEα[a]	CYE Agar	SBA	Other	BCYEα[a]	CYE Agar	SBA	Other
Amount of growth[b]										
Colony size and Colony Form	mm									
	Punctiform									
	Irregular									
	Circular									
	Rhizoid									
	Filamentous									
	Other									
Colony Surface	Flat									
	Raised									
	Convex									
	Pulvinate									
	Other									
Colony Margin	Entire									
	Undulate									
	Lobate									
	Erose									
	Other									
Colony Consistency	Butyrous									
	Viscid									
	Membranous									
	Brittle									
	Other									
Optical Character	Opaque									
	Translucent									
	Dull									
	Glistening									
	Other									
Surface	Smooth									
	Rough									
	Other									
Colony Color and Hemolysis	Without UV									
	With UV									
	Type									

[a] BCYEα agar = Buffered yeast extract agar with α-ketoglutarate; CYE = charcoal yeast extract agar; SBA = sheep blood agar.

[b] Record as +4 for maximum growth to +1 for minimal growth, and − for no growth.

Exercise 13
Data Table 2: *Legionella* Results

		Culture		*L. pneumophilia*	*L. (T.) micdadei*
		Source	Age		
Catalase test					
Oxidase test					
Gram stain	Reaction				
	Morphology				
	Arrangement				
Hippurate	Hydrolysis				
β-lactamase	Produced				
Other					

Laboratory Notes

D. THE SPIROCHETES

INTRODUCTION TO EXERCISES 14 AND 15

The spirochetes encompass a group of non-sporulating, motile (by rotation or undulation, due to periplasmic flagella) helical bacteria. They are widely distributed in our environment; some species are pathogenic for humans. When these bacteria can be stained by the Gram method, they are Gram-negative. Taxonomically they are classified in the order *Spirochaetales* that consists of two families, *Spirochaetaceae* and *Leptospiraceae* (6). While the latter consists of a single genus, *Leptospira* (15, 16), the *Spirochaetaceae* includes four genera. These are *Spirochaeta* (free-living organisms usually found in H_2S-containing mud, sewage, and polluted waters); *Cristispira* (commensals, especially of univalve and bivalve mollusks); *Treponema*, and *Borrelia* (6). Exercises 14 and 15 will provide further information and practical laboratory methodology concerning those genera most important in human disease, namely *Treponema*, *Borrelia*, and *Leptospira*. However, it would be useful to note some general characteristics of these species here.

There are some notable differences between the three genera containing pathogenic species, as seen in Table 14-1. For example, *Borrelia*, because they have a greater width, can be seen by conventional microscopy. Conversely, *Leptospira* and *Treponema* pathogenic for humans require the higher resolution of a phase contrast microscope, or best, a dark field microscope. Furthermore, *Leptospira* cells curve or hook over at one or both ends, a feature not seen with the other two genera. Morphologically, coiling of *Treponema* and *Leptospira* is "tighter" than that of *Borrelia*. The importance of these and other characteristics will be drawn out in the next two exercises.

Table 14-1
Comparison of Selected Characteristics of *Borrelia, Leptospira,* and *Treponema* Pathogenic for Humans (1, 3, 12, 17, 25)

Character	Genus		
	Treponema	*Borrelia*	*Leptospira*
Size, μm	0.1-0.2 x 6-20	0.2-0.5 x 5-25	0.1 x 6-20
Number of coils	5-18	4-30	18 or more
Coiling	Regular, tight	Irregular, loose	Tight
Appearance at ends	Pointed ends	Pointed ends	Hooked at one or both ends
No. of periplasmic flagella	6-10	30-44	2
O_2 relationships	Microaerophilic and anaerobic	Microaerophilic	Strict aerobe

EXERCISE 14
Treponema

The genus *Treponema* consists of anaerobic to microaerophilic, tightly-spiraled, thin rods. Both pathogenic and non-pathogenic forms are found among the thirteen recognized species, all of which are associated with humans or lower animals (25). *Treponema pallidum* subsp. *pallidum* (formerly *T. pallidum*, and still frequently called this) is the most significant disease agent of the genus in the U. S. as the agent of syphilis, a sexually transmitted disease. Organisms that cannot be morphologically or serologically distinguished from this agent of venereal syphilis, but induce diseases that differ in symptoms and epidemiology have been given different species and subspecies designations. *T. pallidum* subsp. *endemicus* (25), for example, causes non-venereal, endemic syphilis, or bejel, in foci of populations of Western Asia, Africa, and Australia (10); *T. pallidum* subsp. *pertenue* (formerly *T. pertenue)* (24) and *T. carateum*, agents of yaws (Frambesia) and pinta, respectively, are also non-venereal diseases. These occur in tropical Africa and India (yaws) or Central and South America (pinta). None of these organisms have been successfully cultured *in vitro*, except *T. pallidum* subsp. *pallidum* (11). However, even this organism shows very limited growth outside the intact animal, and culture for diagnostic purposes remains an unfulfilled hope. In any event, these essentially non-cultivatable organisms form one group within the genus *Treponema* causing the human treponematoses.

The second group of treponemes consists of cultivatable bacteria. Several of these species of *Treponema* are found in the normal oral cavity of humans. Some include *T. denticola, T. socranskii, T. pectinovorum, T. skoliodontum,* and *T. vincentii* (26). Some of these appear to be involved, with fusobacteria, in producing acute necrotizing gingivitis (Vincent's angina, Trench mouth). *T. denticola,* for example, has been implicated as a factor in the severity of this disease (23). One species of this cultivatable group, *T. hyodysenteriae,* has veterinary significance causing swine dysentery or bloody scours (27).

Of the various diseases caused by the treponemes, syphilis requires the most attention by the diagnostic microbiologist. This is primarily because its incidence is epidemic in the U. S. where in 1990 there were over 48,800 cases of primary and secondary syphilis. During the years 1985-1990 the number of reported cases increased by 75% (7).

Many problems confront the microbiologist in detecting the presence of this disease, including that culture is not an option. The organisms are not visible by Gram or other commonly used microbiological staining techniques. This has led to greater dependency on laboratory tests that show the organism under dark-field microscopy, or detection of the presence of infection by serological procedures. However, these are complicated by the complex nature of the disease, and by the nature of the assays.

Venereal syphilis traditionally has been classified into three clinical stages, primary, secondary, and tertiary. The primary stage always occurs, and starts at the time of infection. After a period of 3 days to 3 months, a painless, indurated ulcer, the chancre, occurs, then heals after 3-6 weeks completing the primary infection. If untreated, the secondary stage may occur, showing itself in an average of 6 weeks. The most common symptoms occurring here are mainly skin rash and constitutional evidence of fever and malaise. Again, symptoms eventually subside signaling the end of this stage. Following this, relapses may occur or late or tertiary syphilis develop. The latter is an inflammatory disease and may not display itself for several years after the end of the secondary stage. Symptoms include gummas (granulomatous lesions, particularly of the skin and bones), and central nervous system and cardiovascular symptom effects, which can be irreversible (22, 28).

Symptoms of the primary, secondary, and tertiary stages do not occur in a continuous sequence. Rather, there are periods when no symptoms occur, but the disease is still present, the latent periods. Finally, as another clinical group, *in utero* fetal infection can occur leading to congenital syphilis.

More recent categorizations of syphilis have provided for other clinical groupings of noncongenital types (8, 9). Early syphilis is that of less than one year of duration, whether primary, secondary, or latent stages occur. Late syphilis is that stage that occurs after one year, including late latency, and symptoms associated with tertiary syphilis. During early syphilis, including latency, the disease continues to be transmissible. This is not true during the late latency period (22).

Laboratory Diagnosis of Treponematoses

Although our major concern is laboratory diagnosis of syphilis, the treponemes that cause it, bejel, yaws, or pinta are microscopically indistinguishable. Also, they induce antibody responses that are all detectable by the same serologic assays (10, 12). Thus, the following discussion is applicable to all forms of human treponematoses.

Microscopic Observation

Direct microscopic examination using dark field optics continues to be a useful method for diagnosis of syphilis. Samples are obtained from syphilitic lesions, as the chancre of the primary stage. The finding of typically-shaped spirochetes (Table 14-1) makes diagnosis certain, assuming normal flora treponemes have not contaminated the sample, as from an oral lesion. False negative observations can occur, however, if the patient has been treated with antimicrobials before sampling (12, 19).

Unfortunately, successful direct observation of *T. pallidum* subsp. *pallidum* is frequently unsuccessful, or the patient may not have displayed lesions that could contain the bacteria. Therefore, serologic assays have been traditionally used to detect the presence of infection in suspected patients by showing whether anti-*T. pallidum* subsp. *pallidum* antibodies are present. Thus, syphilis diagnosis is frequently made without ever having directly seen the causative agent.

Serologic Tests for Syphilis (STS)

Many serological tests have been developed for the identification of syphilitic antibody with the hope that they could be made more sensitive and specific. They fall into two general categories, the treponemal and the nontreponemal types. Most of the older-developed tests are in the latter category and use antigens derived from sources other than treponemal organisms. They are of a flocculation or complement fixation (CF) type. The once popular Wasserman test, developed in 1906, was the first STS, and of the CF type (19).

All of the non-treponemal tests involve the reaction of the syphilitic antibody "reagin" (not to be confused with IgE allergic antibody of the same name) with a lipoid antigen. This is usually an alcoholic extract of beef heart to which cholesterol and lecithin have been added. The latter are not antigens, but cholesterol is necessary to form minute particles that are then coated by antigen and lecithin (2, 20).

Flocculation tests are based upon the aggregation of the soluble lipoid antigen-patient antibody precipitate yielding macroscopically and microscopically visible particles. Many types of flocculation tests have been developed. The Kahn test was among the earliest STS, but others such as Kline, Kolmer, Mazzini, Eagle, and Hinton have been used. Most laboratories presently use the VDRL (Venereal Disease Research Laboratory) test, and variations of it (20). Especially popular is the Rapid Plasma Reagin Card (RPRC) test (19). Each of these tests uses varying composition of antigen preparation due to attempts to develop a stable and sensitive antigen working solution. The VDRL test has been most successful in this regard, one reason for its popularity.

The flocculation test offers the distinct advantage of simplicity. The VDRL qualitative test on serum, as will be seen in doing the assay below, can be accomplished within 45 minutes. This includes the steps of heating serum at 56°C for 30 minutes, preparation of antigen, and doing the test. The RPRC test (Photo 14-2), which is commercially available, is done on a card instead of in tubes. The antigen suspension, which contains carbon particles or dyes to enhance macroscopic reading, is premixed and ready for use. Furthermore, it is unnecessary to heat the serum, nor to read microscopically as needed with the VDRL test. Therefore, this test can be done in 10 minutes or less. In addition, this test can be automated (the automated reagin test, ART).

Another variation of the non-treponemal test is a commercially available ELISA that uses a modified VDRL antigen (Visuwell® Reagin). It is reported to have greater sensitivity and equal specificity of flocculation tests (30).

Unfortunately, the flocculation procedures suffer from some non-sensitivity of reaction. That is, these tests may be falsely negative, especially in latent and tertiary syphilis (see Table 14-2). Conversely, they can be non-specific or positive when syphilis or other treponematosis is known

Table 14-2
Sensitivity of Some Serologic Tests for Syphilis[a]

Name of Assay[b]	Stage of Disease				
	Primary	Secondary	Latent	Tertiary	Congenital
Non-Treponemal:					
VDRL	70-80	100	75-90	62-75	88
RPR	~80	100	75-90	~75	100
Treponemal:					
FTA-ABS	85-92	100	97	97-100	100
TPHA	65-78	100	89-99	94-98	100
TPI	57	99	97	92	NA

[a] Percent rounded to nearest whole number.
[b] Abbreviations: VDRL = Veneral Disease Research Laboratory; RPR = Rapid plasma reagin; FTA-ABS = Fluorescent treponemal antibody-Absorbent; TPHA = *Treponema pallidum* hemagglutination assay; TPI = *Treponema pallidum* immobilization. (Reprinted as modified from C. Sheehan, Clinical Immunology: Principles and Laboratory Diagnosis. J.B. Lippincott Co., Philadelphia, © 1990, by permission of the publisher.)

not to be present, as in certain other types of infections or conditions. These are known as "biological false positive" or BFP reactions. Drug addiction, autoimmune diseases (especially lupus erythematosus), certain infectious diseases (as malaria, leprosy, tuberculosis, leptospirosis, and borreliosis), malignant tumors, and even aging may temporarily induce a positive non-treponemal antibody test (20, 28). Despite such disadvantages, the simplicity and speed of accomplishing VDRL and RPR tests have led to their extensive use for screening purposes. Also, their specificity is 99% or greater in tests on healthy individuals, or those with infectious diseases other than syphilis (19).

The specificity problem with non-treponemal tests has driven the development of the treponemal type tests. These use the treponemes themselves, or non-lipoidal antigens derived from them, and detect antibody specifically directed against *T. pallidum* subsp. *pallidum,* instead of the reagin-type antibody. The result has been a more sensitive assay, especially during the latent and tertiary stages of disease (Table 14-2).

The earliest of the treponemal tests to be developed was the *Treponema pallidum* immobilization (TPI) test in 1949. This assay measures the decrease in motility of freshly isolated *T. pallidum* subsp. *pallidum* when mixed with patient serum and complement compared to controls. It is a complex assay that requires the use of freshly isolated, viable spirochetes from the testicles of infected rabbits (one of the few methods for

cultivating this spirochete outside humans). This, as well as other factors, has made the test expensive to perform and, therefore, has been supplanted by other methods (19, 20).

In 1964, the fluorescent treponemal antibody test with the absorption modification (FTA-ABS) test was developed (14) and became popular. It first involves absorption of patient serum or plasma with non-pathogenic Reiter strain of *T. phagedenis* organisms to remove non-specific treponemal antibodies. Following this, the absorbed antiserum is applied to the Nichols strain of *T. pallidum* subsp. *pallidum* contained on a slide, then there is addition of fluorescent-tagged antiglobulin. If patients serum or plasma has syphilitic antibody, it reacts with the bacterium. This primary antibody, in turn acts as antigen to which secondary fluorescent antibody attaches. Examination of this preparation under the fluorescent microscope reveals the presence of fluorescing spirochetes. Table 14-2 shows that this test is at least as sensitive and specific as the TPI test, and becomes reactive 1-2 weeks before others (20). Also, it offers the distinct advantage of relative simplicity and economy compared to the TPI test. It is currently recommended by the World Health Organization for confirmation testing of positive non-treponemal test (31). Kits containing all components for doing the FTA-ABS test are commercially available.

Other types of treponemal assays based on hemagglutination and ELISA reactions are also currently available. The *Treponema pallidum* hemagglutination assay (TPHA), as the Hemagglutination Treponemal Test for Syphilis (HATTS) for the detection of specific treponemal antibody are becoming increasingly prominent. These make use of red cells that have been coated with *T. pallidum* subsp. *pallidum* antigens. In the presence of specific antibody, red cell agglutination occurs. Table 14-2 shows that this type of assay generally gives comparable results to the FTA-ABS test, though they may be less sensitive for detection of disease in patients with primary syphilis. However, they have the advantage of being more economical, faster, and technically less demanding than the FTA-ABS test.

ELISA assays also offer relative simplicity for a treponemal assay, as well as the capacity to be automated. Commercially-available kits for detection of IgM or IgG anti-*T. pallidum* antibodies are available (Syphilis-M and Syphilis-G Test kits). It should be noted that the presence of *T. pallidum* subsp. *pallidum* IgM antibodies correlate with early infection, reinfection, or congenital syphilis and reduction of these is related to successful therapy. The reason for these responses is that, as is true in a normal immune response, IgM appears early after exposure to an immunogen, but are non-persisting antibodies. IgG class antibodies appear soon after the appearance of IgM. However, unlike the latter, IgG levels continue to climb, in syphilis usually reaching its highest titer during the secondary stage. Reinfection can cause a reinduction of IgM; therapy leads to its decrease. In congenital syphilis, IgM antibody, unlike IgG, cannot cross the placenta due to its large molecular size. The presence of fetal IgM of any type, including treponemal antibodies, therefore reflects antibody production by the fetus and can be an indicator of infection (20, 21). This is not to imply that IgG type *T. pallidum* subsp. *pallidum* antibodies are not diagnostically important. It should be obvious that without IgM, no other indicator of infection may exist.

Experimental assays exploring the polymerase chain reaction on human specimens relevant to early and late syphilis and to congenital syphilis (4, 13) have been done, detecting as few as 10 organisms. While these results suggest potential usefulness, much development remains to be done. Western blot (WB) assays have also been investigated. This procedure involves electrophoretic banding of *T. pallidum* subsp. *pallidum* proteins on polyacrylamide gels. Following banding, these are electronically transferred (blotted) to nitrocellulose, then reacted with patient antibody. A positive test occurs when antibody can be demonstrated to have reacted with one or more protein bands from the spirochete. In an investigation of IgM antibodies in congenital syphilis (18) this method showed improved sensitivity and specificity over an FTA-ABS method for IgM. Similarly, sera from normal human donors, primary, secondary and latent syphilis, and biological false positive patients displayed at least equivalent sensitivity between FTA-ABS and WB. Specificity, however, appears to be better in the latter case (5). At this stage, therefore, WB appears promising as another tool in serologic confirmation of syphilis.

In this exercise, the morphology of *T. pallidum* subsp. *pallidum* will be demonstrated along with some serological procedures involved in the diagnosis of syphilis.

MATERIALS

Part 1A-1.
Per bench:

    VDRL antigen (Note: Store at room temperature)

1 1 ml pipette
1 5 ml pipette
1 30 ml screw-capped bottle with vinylite- or foil-lined cover
    Buffered saline solution

Part 1A-2.
Per pair of students:

    Positive and negative sera (heated at 56°C for 30 minutes)
    Antigen preparation from *Part 1*A-1

1 paraffin or ceramic ringed slide with ring diameter of about 14 mm
1 1 cc syringe with unbeveled 18 gauge needle
2 0.2 ml pipettes
    Slide rotator

Part 1B
Per pair of students:

    Positive and negative sera heated at 56°C for 30 minutes
    Paraffin or ceramic ringed slides (as in *Part 1*A-1)

1 1 cc syringe with unbeveled 19 gauge
   needle
1 0.2 ml pipette
1 13 x 100 mm tube with 0.7 ml of 0.9%
   saline
   Antigen preparation (from *Part 1* A-1)
1 1cc syringe with unbeveled 23 gauge needle
   Slide rotator

Part 2
Per Pair of students:
   Positive and negative sera (unheated or
   heated at 56°C for 30 minutes)
   Rapid plasma reagin (RPR) antigen in dis-
   penser bottle fitted with 20 gauge unbeveled needle (Note: Store in refrigerator)
1 Plastic-covered cards containing 18 mm
   diameter circles
2 0.05 ml capillary pipettes and capillary
   pipette bulb, or
2 0.1 ml serological pipettes
2 Stirrers
   Slide rotator

LABORATORY PROCEDURES

***Part 1* A:** The VDRL Slide Flocculation Test
(29)

All serologic tests for syphilis have been
carefully standardized to provide maximum sensitivity and reproducibility. Attention to detail is
important and must be followed. Complete
procedures on the VDRL and other types of STS
may be found in the National Centers for Disease
Control's "Manual of Tests for Syphilis" (29).
1. One pair of students at each bench prepare
   antigen for all other groups at that bench as
   follows:
   a. Deliver 0.4 ml buffered saline solution to
      the bottom of a round 30 ml screw-capped
      bottle (cap must be foil or vinylite-lined).
   b. While gently rotating the bottle on a flat
      surface add dropwise 0.5 ml VDRL antigen.
      Blow out last drop of antigen. Do not touch
      pipette to saline solution.
   c. Rotate bottle for 10 seconds after addition
      of antigen.
   d. Add 4.1 ml buffered saline, place top on
      bottle, then shake from top to bottom
      approximately 30 times in 10 seconds. The
      antigen is now ready for use. It may be used
      for 1 day, but gently mix before each use.

2. Each pair of students is to carry out the
   following slide test:
   a. Deliver 0.05 ml heated (56°C. for 30
      minutes) positive serum to one 14 mm
      diameter paraffin ring on a slide and control
      serum to the other. Each should completely
      cover the surface area of the ring.
   b. Add 1/60 ml (drop from an 18-gauge
      unbeveled needle held vertically) antigen to
      each ring.
   c. Rotate slides in a circle of ¾ inch diameter
      for 4 minutes on rotator set at 180 rpm.
      After this immediately read reaction with
      the aid of your microscope at 100X mag-
      nification. Use optimal lighting.
   d. Interpretation of test:
      i. No clumping to slight granularity: Non-
         reactive.
      ii. Small clumps: Weakly reactive.
      iii. Medium to large clumps: Reactive.
   e. Record results in your notebook as non-
      reactive, weakly reactive, or reactive.
   f. Any degree of reactivity should be further
      assayed by a quantitative slide test as
      outlined below.

***Part 1* B:** The VDRL Quantitative Slide Test.
Each pair of students having reactive serum as
determined in the above test carry out the
following steps (also see Figure 14-1):
   a. Add 0.1 ml of reactive or weakly reactive
      serum to 0.7 ml of 0.9% saline solution with
      a 0.2 ml pipette to give a 1:8 dilution.
   b. Using the same pipette, mix the diluted
      serum thoroughly, then transfer 0.04, 0.02,
      and 0.01 ml to each of 3 rings on a slide
      numbered 4, 5, and 6, respectively. These
      will eventually be dilutions of 1:8, 1:16, and
      1:32. Expel the remainder of liquid from
      pipette back into dilution tube.
   c. Using the same pipette, deliver 0.04, 0.02,
      and 0.01 ml of undiluted serum to paraffin
      rings marked 1, 2, and 3. These will be
      dilutions of 1:1, 1:2, and 1:4 when other
      components are finally added.
   d. Add 2 drops (0.01 ml/drop) of 0.9% saline
      to the 2nd and 5th rings, and 3 drops to the
      3rd and 6th rings with a 23 ga. unbeveled
      needle and syringe.
   e. Rotate slide by hand for 15 seconds to
      mix.

f. Add one drop (1/75 ml) of previously prepared antigen (*Part 1* A-1) with an unbeveled 19 ga. needle and syringe.

g. Proceed as with the qualitative test, *Part 1* A, Step 2-c above.

h. Report results in terms of the highest serum dilution giving a reactive test.

i. If all serum dilutions are reactive, dilute the 1:8 serum mixture to 1:64 (0.1 ml of serum diluted 1:8 added to 0.7 ml of 0.9% saline), then retested by the quantitative slide method.

j. Enter results in your notebook and discuss. What is the significance of a reactive VDRL test? Of a weakly reactive test?

Part 2 The Rapid Plasma Reagin (RPR) Card Test (29)
(Note: Several commercial sources of RPR card tests are available. The instructions provided with the one used should be followed.)

Each pair of students is to carry out the following test using serum samples provided to you.

1. If necessary, allow antigen and sera to warm to room temperature before using.

2. With separate 0.1 ml pipettes (or 0.05 ml capillary pipettes), dispense 0.05 ml of each serum sample into separate circles on the RPR card. Note that samples may be unheated or heated at 56°C for 30 minutes.

3. Using disposable stirrers, spread the contents of each circle to cover its entire area. Use separate, clean stirrers for each circle.

4. Add 1/60 ml (1 drop from a plastic bottle with a unbeveled 20 gauge needle) RPR antigen to each circle containing a serum sample. It is not necessary to stir.

5. Set card on mechanical rotator. Cover the card to reduce evaporation.

6. Rotate card at 100 rpm for 8 minutes.

7 Macroscopically read your results and report as:
Reactive (R): Small to large clumps.
Non-reactive (N): No clumps to a slight granularity.

Part 3

A. Dark-field demonstration of *Treponema pallidum* subsp. *pallidum*:

Although *T. pallidum* subsp. *pallidum* exhibits only limited growth *in vitro*, it may be grown in rabbit testicles. Such infections usually cause swelling and an inflammatory reaction in the scrotum (orchitis), but the animal spontaneously recovers within a month or so. Syphilitic antibody is formed in the process.

This demonstration will consist of spirochetes obtained from the testicles of an infected rabbit. The sample is obtained by mincing this organ in a small amount of phosphate buffered saline containing glucose and dithiothreitol. Some of this liquid is placed on a slide and mounted with a cover slip, then sealed with vaseline or vaspar.

Observe this preparation by dark-field microscopy and record your observations.

B. Dark-field observations of spirochetes from the oral cavity:

Prepare a wet mount as described above with material obtained by scraping between your teeth near the gum margin with a toothpick. Suspend the material in a small drop of saliva. Observe and describe. Particularly note the treponemes and compare with those observed in *Part 3*-A above. What other forms can you find? Describe them.

C. The hemagglutination assay for syphilitic antibody.

Observe the demonstration hemagglutination assay for treponemal antibody. It has been set up with a positive and a negative syphilitic serum, along with appropriate controls, using the specific manufacturer's protocol. Note the "spread" pattern of red cells that constitute a positive test, and "button" pattern of a negative test. (Why are these patterns formed in the presence and absence of antibody?) Give the purpose of each control test. Record your results and discuss.

QUESTIONS

1. What is the purpose of heating plasma or serum at 56°C for 30 minutes, as required in doing the VDRL test?

2. In the VDRL test, what is the quantitative difference between "reactive" and "weakly reactive" serum?

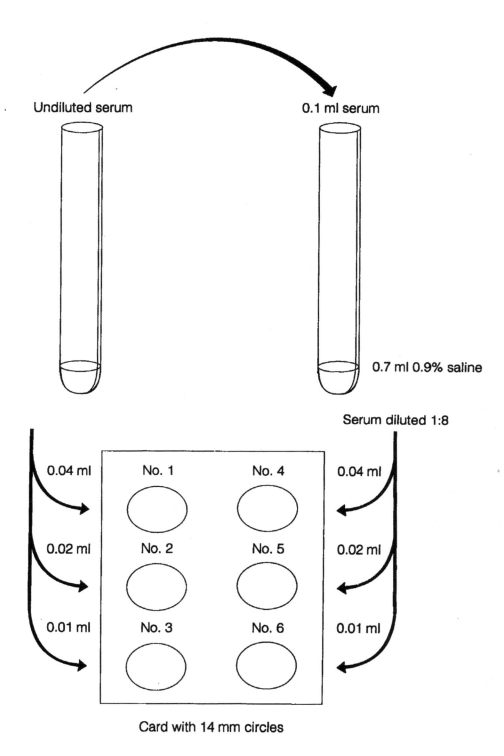

Figure 14-1: Diagram showing serum dilution and additions in VDRL quantitative slide test. This is then followed by additions of 0.9% saline, VDRL antigen, shaking, and reading of results.

REFERENCES

1. Alexander, A. D. 1991. *Leptospira*, p. 554-559. *In* A. Balows, W. J. Hausler, Jr., K. L. Herrmann, H. D. Isenberg, and H. J. Shadomy (ed.), Manual of clinical microbiology, 5th ed. American Society for Microbiology, Washington, D. C.

2. Baron, E. J., L. R. Peterson, and S. M. Finegold. 1994. Bailey & Scott's diagnostic microbiology, 9th ed. Mosby-Year Book, Inc., St. Louis. p. 157–167.

3. Burgdorfer, W., and T. G. Schwan. 1991. *Borrelia*, p. 560-566. *In* A. Balows, W. J. Hausler, Jr., K. L. Herrmann, H. D. Isenberg, and H. J. Shadomy (ed.), Manual of clinical microbiology, 5th ed. American Society for Microbiology, Washington, D. C.

4. Burstain, J. M., E. Grimprel, S. A. Lukehart, M. V. Norgard, and J. D. Radolf. 1991. Sensitive detection of *Treponema pallidum* by using the polymerase chain reaction. J. Clin. Microbiol. **29**:62-69.

5. Byrne, R. E., S. Laska, M. Bell, D. Larson, J. Phillips, and J. Todd. 1992. Evaluation of a *Treponema pallidum* Western immunoblot assay as a confirmatory test for syphilis. J. Clin. Microbiol. **30**:115-122.

6. Canale-Parola, E. 1984. *Spirochaetaceae* Swellengrebel 1907, p. 39-46. *In* N. R. Krieg, and J. G. Holt (ed.), Bergey's manual of systematic bacteriology, Vol. 1. Williams & Wilkins, Baltimore.

7. Centers for Disease Control. 1991. Primary and secondary syphilis-United States, 1981-1990. MMWR **40**:314-315, 321-323.

8. Centers for Disease Control. 1989. Sexually transmitted disease treatment guidelines. MMWR (Suppl.) **38**(S-8):5-15.

9. Centers for Disease Control. 1985. Syphilis. MMWR **34** (No. 4S):94S-99S.

10. Chulay, J. D. 1990. Treponema species (yaws, pinta, bejel), p. 1808-1812. *In* G. L. Mandell, R. G. Douglas, Jr., and J. E. Bennett (ed.), Principles and practices of infectious diseases, 3rd ed. Churchill Livingstone, New York.

11. Fieldsteel, A. H., D. L. Cox, and R. A. Moeckli. 1981. Cultivation of virulent *Treponema pallidum* in tissue culture. Infect. Imm. **32**:908-915.

12. Fitzgerald, T. J. 1991. *Treponema*, p. 567-571. *In* A. Balows, W. J. Hausler, Jr., K. L. Herrmann, H. D. Isenberg, and H. J. Shadomy (ed.), Manual of clinical microbiology, 5th ed. American Society for Microbiology, Washington, D. C.

13. Grimprel, E., P. J. Sanchez, G. D. Wendel, J. M. Burstain, G. H. McCracken, Jr., J. D. Radolf, and M. V. Norgard. 1991. Use of polymerase chain reaction and rabbit infectivity testing to detect *Treponema pallidum* in amniotic fluid, fetal and neofetal sera, and cerebrospinal fluid. J. Clin. Microbiol. **29**:1711-1718.

14. Hunter, E. F., W. E. Deacon, and P. E. Meyer. 1964. An improved FTA test for syphilis, the absorption procedure (FTA-ABS). Pub. Hlth Rep. **79**:410-412.

15. Johnson, R. C., and S. Faine. 1984. *Leptospira* Noguchi 1917, p. 62-67. *In* N. R. Krieg, and J. G. Holt (ed.), Bergey's manual of systematic bacteriology, Vol. 1. Williams & Wilkins, Baltimore.

16. Johnson, R. C., and S. Faine. 1984. *Leptospiraceae* Hovind-Hougen 1979, p. 62. *In* N. R. Krieg, and J. G. Holt (ed.), Bergey's manual of systematic bacteriology, Vol. 1. Williams & Wilkins, Baltimore.

17. Kelly, R. T. 1984. *Borrelia* Swellengrabel 1907, p. 57-62. *In* N. R. Krieg, and J. G. Holt (ed.), Bergey's manual of systematic bacteriology, Vol. 1. Williams & Wilkins, Baltimore.

18. Lewis, L. L., L. H. Tabor, and R. E. Baughn. 1990. Evaluation of immunoglobulin M Western blot analysis in the diagnosis of congenital syphilis. J. Clin. Microbiol. **28**:296-302.

19. Löwhagen, G. -B. 1990. Syphilis: test procedures and therapeutic strategies. Sem. Dermatol. **9**:152-159.

20. Luger, A. F. H. 1988. Serological diagnosis of syphilis: current methods, p. 249-274. *In* H. Young, and A. McMillan (ed.), Immunological diagnosis of sexually transmitted diseases. Marcel Dekker, Inc. New York.

21. Pederson, N. S., J. P. Sheller, A. V. Ratman, and S. K. Hira. 1989. Enzyme-linked immunosorbent assays for detection of immunoglobulin M to nontreponmemal and treponemal antigens for diagnosis of congenital syphilis. J. Clin. Microbiol. **27**:1835-1840.

22. Shulman, S. T., J. P. Phair, and H. M. Sommers. 1992. The biologic & clinical basis of infectious diseases, 4th ed. W. B. Saunders Co., Philadelphia, p. 238-268.

23. Simonson, L. G., C. H. Goodman, J. J. Bial, and H. E. Morton. 1988. Quantitative relationship of *Treponema denticola* to severity of periodontal disease. Infect. Imm. **56**:726-728.

24. Smibert, R. M. 1974. *Treponema* Schaudinn 1905, p. 175-184. *In* R. E. Buchanan, and N. E. Gibbons (ed.), Bergey's manual of determinative bacteriology, 8th ed. The Williams & Wilkins Co., Baltimore.

25. Smibert, R. M. 1984. *Treponema* Schaudin 1905, p. 49-57. *In* N. R. Krieg, and J. G. Holt (ed.), Bergey's manual of systematic bacteriology, Vol. 1. Williams & Wilkins, Baltimore.

26. Smibert, R. M. 1991. Anaerobic spirochetes, p. 572-578. *In* A. Balows, W. J. Hausler, Jr., K. L. Herrmann, H. D. Isenberg, and H. J. Shadomy (ed.), Manual of clinical microbiology, 5th ed. American Society for Microbiology, Washington, D. C.

27. Timoney, J. F. J. H. Gillespie, F. W. Scott, and J. E. Barlough. 1988. Hagan and Bruner's microbiology and infectious diseases of domestic animals, 8th ed. Comstock Publishing Associates, Ithica, NY, p. 45-60.

28. Tramont, E. C. 1990. Treponema pallidum (syphilis), p. 1794-1808. *In* G. L. Mandell, R. G. Douglas, Jr., and J. E. Bennett (ed.), Principles and practices of infectious diseases, 3rd ed. Churchill Livingstone, New York.

29. U. S. Department of Health, Education and Welfare, Public Health Service, National Communicable Disease Center Venereal Disease Program. 1969. Manual of tests for syphilis. Public Health Service Pub. No. 411. 81 p.

30. White, T. J., and S. A. Fuller. 1989. Visuwell reagin, a non-treponemal enzyme-linked immunosorbent assay for the serodiagnosis of syphilis. J. Clin. Microbiol. **27**:2300-2304.

31. World Health Organization. 1982. Treponemal infections, report of a WHO Scientific Group. Technical report Series No. 674, WHO, Geneva.

Exercise 14: *Treponema*
Laboratory Results

Part 1A: VDRL Slide Flocculation Test.

Positive Serum: _____

Negative Serum: _____

Part 1B: VDRL Quantitative Slide Test.

Positive Serum: _____

Negative Serum: _____

Part 2: RPR Card Test.

Positive Serum: _____

Negative Serum: _____

Part 3:

A. Dark-Field Demonstration of *T. pallidum.*
   Description:

B. Dark-Field Observations of Spirochetes from Oral Cavity.
   Description and comparison with *Part 3*A:

C. Hemagglutination Assay for Treponemal Antibody.

Laboratory Notes

EXERCISE 15
Leptospira and *Borrelia*

Leptospira

The genus *Leptospira* consists of only two species, *L. interrogans* and *L. biflexa*. Of these, the former is parasitic and pathogenic in lower animals and humans, and most pertinent for our discussion here. *L. biflexa* is a free-living organism, and can grow at a lower temperature (13°C) than *L. interrogans*. Also, in contrast to *L. interrogans*, this organism grows in the presence of 225 μg/ml 8-azoguanine. Otherwise they are morphologically (Table 14-1), culturally, and physiologically similar to one another (13). Differentiation of pathogenic and parasitic strains is not made on these criteria, however. Instead, it is largely done from antigenic make-up, which yields over 200 serovarieties in 23 serogroups (1). Unlike *Borrelia*, which are microaerophilic, the leptospires are strict aerobes (Table 14-1). They are also oxidase and catalase positive, and long chain (15 carbon or more) fatty acids are required as an energy and carbon source (13).

The disease produced by all *L. interrogans* serogroups is called leptospirosis, and is an acute, febrile, systemic infection. However, it may be referred to by other names such as Weil's disease (usually associated with *L. interrogans* serogroup Icterohaemorrhagiae), and canicola fever (due to serogroup Canicola). Infection is most commonly contracted by contact with soil or water contaminated with urine of infected animals that harbor the bacterium. While rats are a major source of infection worldwide, in the United States dogs, domestic livestock, cats, etc. serve as the most important reservoirs. From 50 to 100 cases of leptospirosis are reported in this country annually (9).

In human infection, this organism can best be isolated from the blood during the systemic stage in the first week of disease, then from urine following this period. Failing this, serological methods are used to detect patient antibody response to infection. Here, microscopic and macroscopic agglutination assays are common (1). Other types of assays used include complement fixation (especially used in Europe) and ELISA (1, 24). A leptospirosis indirect hemagglutination assay is also commercially available.

While not commercially available, other methods of identification of organisms are also being studied. These include DNA hybridization (23), PCR (21), and pulsed-field gel electrophoresis (PFGE) of leptospiral DNA (10). In the latter case, single endonuclease digestion of leptospiral DNA was subjected to PFGE, a technique that can resolve large and complex DNA molecules leading to fingerprint patterns, each spot or band representing a particular molecular weight of DNA. This, in turn, is determined by the restriction patterns of that DNA from each organism. In this instance, most organisms yielded distinct, reproducible restriction patterns, and the assay could be accomplished more rapidly than by serotyping methods.

Borrelia

The species of *Borrelia* are all parasitic and spread from their lower animal reservoirs by insect vectors. In the U. S., *B. turicatae*, and *B. hermsii* are mainly responsible for the classical type of human borreliosis, relapsing fever. These are both tick-borne (*Ornithodoros* spp.), as are the at least 12 other species that produce this disease world-wide. One species, *B. recurrentis*, is transmitted by the human body louse (*Pediculus humanus*), and has been associated with epidemics of relapsing fever. Historically, millions of people have died of this disease, usually occurring during famine, war, and other unfortunate circumstances of these types. However, it is also maintained endemically in parts of Africa and South America (5, 11).

Relapsing fever occurs in sporadic outbreaks in the United States. For example, 14 cases occurred in the summer of 1990 among employees and visitors to the Grand Canyon (7). Fortunately, it does not occur in large numbers, 219 cases being reported in the period of 1979-1989 (5). Clinically, as the name suggests, it is characterized by periods of fever and other symptoms. This is followed by normal temperature, after which relapse of fever and other symptoms again can occur. The number of relapses averages 3, but there may be as many as 13 cycles in tick-borne disease (11).

In laboratory diagnosis of relapsing fever, it is important to note that spirochaetemia occurs during the febrile periods and diagnosis in the majority of cases can be made at this time by observation of the organism in a blood specimen using dark field microscopy. The bacteria also stain with Romanowsky stains as Giemsa, Wright, etc., and these can used on blood smears. Typical forms will then be apparent by conventional light microscopy (5).

The relapsing fever agents are antigenic, and an immune response is induced during infection. Interestingly, however, serologic diagnosis has not been particularly successful (5, 11), though the indirect fluorescent antibody (IFA) assay and ELISA tests are applied (5).

In recent years, a new form of tick-borne borreliosis has attracted attention. Lyme disease, named after Lyme, Connecticut where it was first identified, was reported as a distinct entity in 1977 by Steere, Malawistam and Syndman (28). The bacterial agent was later identified as a borreliae by Burgdorfer (6), and named by others *Borrelia burgdorferi* (Photo 15-1) (14). Its reservoir includes *Peromyscus leucopus*, the whitefooted deer mouse, especially for tick nymphs and larvae, and deer for the adult tick vector. *Ixodes dammini* is most frequently found to transmit disease from the reservoirs to humans in the U. S. midwest and east, and *I. ricinus*, the European sheep tick, in Europe. Other ticks as *T. scapularis* can also spread it (Photo 15-2). *I. Pacificus* is common in the western U.S. (27). In 1990, about 8,000 cases of human disease were reported in this country (8).

Lyme disease occurs, like syphilis, in three stages. The earliest sign of disease is the occurrence of erythema chronicum migrans (ECM) that appears in 60%-80% of cases (8). This cutaneous lesion, characterized as a slowly enlarging rash, appears at the site of the tick bite within 3 to 32 days (27). A variety of symptoms can occur with this first stage, including those that are flu-like, arthralgia, muscle stiffness, etc. Second stage of disease encompasses cardiac, joint, nervous system, and skin symptoms, while the third stage especially involves arthritis. The latter, as well as skin lesions, may continue for many years (3, 27).

The observation of ECM, especially if 5 cm or more in diameter and following a tick bite, is the best clinical evidence for the presence of Lyme disease (3, 8). Unfortunately, it may not always be present, typical, or accompanying a previous tick bite, at least that the patient can recall. In its absence, (i) laboratory confirmation of disease, and observation of one or more characteristics of disease is required, or (ii) laboratory diagnosis is needed (8).

The current approach to laboratory diagnosis is either by culture identification or through detection of patient antibody. Unlike borreliae of relapsing fever, *B. burgdorferi* cannot be easily observed in the blood of infected patients (5). However, it can be cultivated using BSK II medium (2) from either infected ticks or the blood, CSF, or skin of infected patients. Serologically, the indirect fluorescent antibody (IFA) and enzyme-linked immunosorbent assay (ELISA) procedures are widely used (4, 5) although false negative and false positive reactions are both problems with these.

As in syphilis, IgM class antibodies arise early, followed by IgG antibodies. IgM antibodies decrease after 1 to 2 months, while IgG continues to rise (4) and remains for many years (17). False negative tests can occur early in the disease before an IgG response develops or because early treatment with antimicrobial agents has led to a lack of antibody response. Conversely, a false positive Lyme disease serological test can occur because of syphilis and other treponemal diseases, relapsing fever, as well as non-spirochetal diseases (4).

Because of problems with IFA and ELISA, other methods have or are being developed, primarily to serve as confirmatory tests. These include Western immunoblotting (15, 16, 29), but band patterns are complex due to changes in antibody specificity produced as the disease progresses (29). This, and other variations, make interpretation difficult (26). The polymerase chain reaction (PCR) (18, 20, 21) and DNA hybridization (19, 25) are also being investigated. Although highly sensitive, spirochetes must be present in a sample. Skin samples from Lyme disease patients, for example yield positive PCRs (20), but canine blood and urine samples from animals with evidence of disease were generally negative by this assay (18). In DNA hybridization, a probe has been described that specifically detects *B. burgdorferi*, excluding several other species of *Borrelia* (25). However, the diagnostic usefulness of such a test, as well as PCR, awaits further study.

Many commercial kits for serological diagnosis of Lyme disease are available to do all of the above assays except DNA hybridization and PCR. For example, immunofluorescent staining reagents can be obtained commercially, as can ELISA-based and immunoblot kits. Obviously, many choices can be made. Again, selection will depend on the needs of each user, as well as the demonstrated accuracy of the assay.

MATERIALS

Part 1

Per pair of students:
A. Stock culture of *L. interrogans* serogroup Canicola
   Tube of Fletcher's semisolid medium containing 5-fluorouracil or EMJH medium
B. Stock culture of *B. burgdorferi*
   Tube of BSK II medium
C. Prepared blood smears containing *B. recurrentis* or *B. burgdorferi*

LABORATORY PROCEDURES

Part 1

A. *Leptospira interrogans* serogroup Canicola:
   Each pair of students will be provided with a stock culture of *L. interrogans* serogroup Canicola.
   1. Inoculate a single tube of Fletcher's or EMJH (12, 22) medium. Recall that these organisms are strict aerobes. Therefore, take the inoculum from the disc of growth in the upper portion of your stock culture (see Figure 15-1). Inoculate it within the top ⅓ of your own culture tube.
   2. Incubate at 30°C for one week or more.
       Note that either Fletcher's or EMJH medium may be used for the growth of *Leptospira*. However, EMJH is better able to meet the complex growth requirements of these organisms (9), especially for isolation from clinical or other specimens (1).
B. Inoculate *B. burgdorferi* into the depths of a tube of BSK II medium (2). Incubate at 35°C in a candle jar for one week.
C. *Borrelia recurrentis* or *B. burgdorferi*:
   Each student examine a prepared blood smear containing either *B. recurrentis* or *B. burgdorferi* provided. Describe your observations.

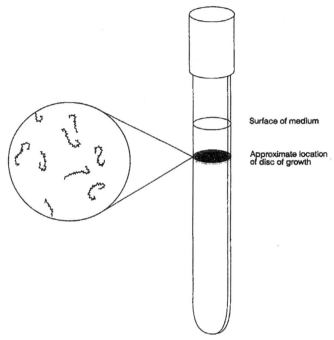

Surface of medium

Approximate location of disc of growth

Figure 15-1: Diagram showing location of growth of Leptospira interrogans in tube culture.

Part 2

A. With the culture of *L. interrogans* serogroup Canicola inoculated one week previously:
   1. Observe the amount and appearance of growth. This should appear as a disc of growth from 1-3 cm below the surface (Figure 15-1).
   2. Remove a small drop of growth from the culture tube. Place on a slide and mount with cover slip. Seal with vaspar, then observe with the phase-contrast or, preferably, dark field microscope. Describe your findings. Compare the morphology of this organism with *B. recurrentis* or *B. burgdorferi*, and *T. pallidum* subsp. *pallidum* examined earlier. Especially note the hooked forms, tightness of spirals, and the general width of the *Leptospira*. Describe the organism's motility.
B. With *B. burgdorferi* culture:
   1. Carry out growth and microscopic observations as done for *Leptospira* in *Part 2A* above. Here, however, use phase contrast microscopy for your wet mount observation.
   2. Prepare a Gram stain of this organism from your culture. Microscopically observe and record your findings.

Compare the morphological and motility characteristics of all the organisms you have examined here. Note their comparative sizes, coiling and character of their motility. From your own observations, show those characteristics that *you* would choose as most important in identification of whether *Leptospira*, *Borrelia*, or *Treponema* is present.

QUESTIONS

1. As mentioned earlier, serologic diagnosis of relapsing fever has not been particularly successful. This problem is related to the relapsing nature of the disease caused by *Borrelia*. What is it?
2. Give the purpose of adding 5-fluorouracil to Fletcher's medium for the culture of leptospires. Also, what components of EMJH medium provide the complex amino acids and fatty acid requirements used by this group of organisms?

REFERENCES

1. Alexander, A. D. 1991. *Leptospira*, p. 554-559. *In* A. Balows, W. J. Hausler, Jr., K. L. Herrmann, H. D. Isenberg, and H. J. Shadomy (ed.), Manual of clinical microbiology, 5th ed. American Society for Microbiology, Washington, D. C.
2. Barbour, A. G. 1984. Isolation and cultivation of Lyme disease spirochetes. Yale J. Biol. Med. 57:521-525.
3. Barbour, A. G. 1988. Laboratory aspects of Lyme borreliosis. Clin. Microbiol. Rev. 1:399-414.
4. Berg, D., K. G. Abson, and N. S. Prose. 1991. The laboratory diagnosis of Lyme disease. Arch. Dermatol. 127:866-870.
5. Burgdorfer, W., and T. G. Schwan. 1991. *Borrelia*, p. 560-566. *In* A. Balows, W. J. Hausler, Jr., K. L. Herrmann, H. D. Isenberg, and H. J. Shadomy (ed.), Manual of clinical microbiology, 5th ed. American Society for Microbiology, Washington, D. C.
6. Burgdorfer, W., A. G. Barbour, S. F. Hayes, J. L. Benach, E. Grunwaldt, and J. P. Davis. 1982. Lyme disease - a tick-borne spirochetosis? Science 216:1317-1319.
7. Centers for Disease Control. 1991. Outbreak of relapsing fever - Grand Canyon National Park, Arizona, 1990. MMWR 40:296-297, 303.
8. Centers for Disease Control. 1991. Lyme disease surveillance - United States, 1989-1990. MMWR 40:417-421.
9. Farrar, W. E. 1990. Leptospira species (leptospirosis), p. 1813-1816. *In* G. L. Mandell, R. G. Douglas, Jr., and J. E. Bennett (ed.), Principles and practices of infectious diseases, 3rd ed. Churchill Livingstone, New York.
10. Herrmann, J. L., E. Bellenger, P. Perolat, G. Baranton, and I. Saint Girons. 1992. Pulsed-field gel electrophoresis of *Not*I digests of leptospiral DNA: a new rapid method of serovar identification. J. Clin. Microbiol. 30:1696-1702.
11. Johnson, W. D., Jr. 1990. Borrelia species (relapsing fever), p. 1816-1819. *In* G. L. Mandell, R. G. Douglas, Jr., and J. E. Bennett (ed.), Principles and practices of infectious diseases, 3rd ed. Churchill Livingstone, New York.
12. Johnson, R. C., and V. G. Harris. 1967. Differentiation of pathogenic and saprophytic leptospires I. Growth at low temperatures. J. Bacteriol. 94:27-31.
13. Johnson, R. C., and S. Faine. 1984. *Leptospira* Noguchi 1917, p. 62-67. *In* N. R. Krieg, and J. G. Holt (ed.), Bergey's manual of systematic bacteriology, Vol. 1. Williams & Wilkins, Baltimore.
14. Johnson, R. C., G. P. Schmid, F. W. Hyde, A. G. Steigerwalt, and D. J. Brenner. 1984. *Borrelia burgdorferi* sp. nov.: etiologic agent of Lyme disease. Int. J. System. Bacteriol. 34:496-497.
15. Karlsson, M. 1990. Western immunoblot and flagellum enzyme-linked immunosorbent assay for serodiagnosis of Lyme borreliosis. J. Clin. Microbiol. 28:2148-2150.
16. Ma, B., B. Christen, D. Leung, and C. Vigo-Pelfrey. 1992. Serodiagnosis of Lyme borreliosis by Western immunoblot: reactivity of various significant antibodies against *Borrelia burgdorferi*. J. Clin. Microbiol. 30:370-376.
17. Magnarelli, L. A. 1989. Laboratory diagnosis of Lyme disease. Rheumatic Dis. Clin. N. Amer. 15:735-745.
18. Malloy, D. C., R. K. Nauman, and H. Paxton. 1990. Detection of *Borrelia burgdorferi* using the polymerase chain reaction. J. Clin. Microbiol. 28:1089-1093.
19. Marconi, R. T., L. Lubke, W. Hauglum, and C. F. Garon. 1992. Species-specific identification of and distinction between *Borrelia burgdorferi* genomic groups by using 16S rRNA-directed oligonucleotide probes. J. Clin. Microbiol. 30:628-632.
20. Melchers, W., J. Meis, P. Rosa, E. Claas, L. Nohlmans, R. Koopman, A. Horrevorts, and J. Galama. 1991. Amplification of *Borrelia burgdorferi* DNA in skin biopsies from patients with Lyme disease. J. Clin. Microbiol. 29:2410-2406.
21. Mérien, F., P. Amouriaux, P. Perolat, G. Baranton, and I. Saint Girons. 1992. Polymerase chain reaction for detection of *Leptospira* spp. in clinical samples. J. Clin. Microbiol. 30:2219-2224.
22. Nash, P., and M. M. Krenz. 1991. Culture media, p. 1226-1288. *In* A. Balows, W. J. Hausler, Jr., K. L. Herrmann, H. D. Isenberg, and H. J. Shadomy (ed.), Manual of clinical microbiology, 5th ed. American Society for Microbiology, Washington, D. C.
23. Pacciarini, M. L., M. L. Savio, S. Tagliabue, and C. Rossi. 1992. Repetitive sequences cloned from *Leptospira interrogans* serovar hardjo genotype hardjoprajitno and their application to serovar identification. J. Clin. Microbiol. 30:1243-1249.
24. Palmer, M. F. 1988. Laboratory diagnosis of leptospirosis. Med. Lab. Sci. 45:174-78.
25. Schwan, T. G., W. J. Simpson, M. E. Schrumpf, and R. H. Karstens. 1989. Identification of *Borrelia burgdorferi* and *B. hermsii* using DNA hybridization probes. J. Clin. Microbiol. 27:1734-1738.
26. Stanek, G. 1991. Laboratory diagnosis and seroepidemiology of Lyme borreliosis. Infection 19:263-266.
27. Steere, A. C. 1990. Borrelia burgdorferi (Lyme disease, Lyme borreliosis), p. 1819-1827. *In* G. L. Mandell, R. G. Douglas, Jr., and J. E. Bennett (ed.), Principles and practices of infectious diseases, 3rd ed. Churchill Livingstone, New York.
28. Steere, A. C., S. E. Malawista, D. R. Syndman, R. E. Shope, E. A. Andiman, M. R. Ross, and F. M. Steele. 1977. Lyme arthritis: an epidemic of oligoarticular arthritis in children and adults in three Connecticut communities. Arthritis Rheum. 20:7-17.
29. Zöller, L., S. Burkard, and H. Schäfer. 1991. Validity of Western immunoblot band patterns in the serodiagnosis of Lyme borreliosis. J. Clin. Microbiol. 29:174-182.

Exercise 15
Leptospira* and *Borrelia
Results

Leptospira interrogans serogroup *Canicola*

Date: _____ Culture age: _____

Culture Medium: _____

Culture Appearance:

Description of microscopic appearance and motility from wet mount:

Type of optics used: _____

Magnification: _____

Borrelia burgdorferi culture:
Date: _____ Culture age: _____

Culture appearance:

Description of microscopic appearance and motility from wet mount:

Type of optics used: _____

Magnification: _____

Borrelia burgdorferi culture:
Description of Gram stain:

Prepared microscope slides of *Borrelia recurrentis* or *B. burgdorferi*
Description:

Other Laboratory Notes

E. ANAEROBIC BACTERIA

AN INTRODUCTION TO EXERCISES 16 AND 17

Most of the bacteria studied in this manual are aerobic, microaerophilic, or facultatively anaerobic. There is also a group of infectious organisms that are anaerobic, the subject of Exercises 16 and 17.

Although superficially it may seem obvious what anaerobic bacteria are, a true definition is elusive (8). One that is widely accepted is that most anaerobic bacteria are those that will not grow in air or 10% CO_2, but will at reduced oxygen tensions (3, 8, 24). (You will note, therefore, that the atmosphere of candle jars is not adequate for the growth of anaerobic bacteria.) These can be further divided into moderate anaerobes and strict anaerobes. The former group can form surface growth at 2% to 8% oxygen concentrations, while strict anaerobes require 0.5% or less O_2 to do this. In practice, it is fortunate that most infectious anaerobes are of the moderate type because more flexibility is provided in their handling. Thus, because they, unlike strict anaerobes, can survive moderate periods of atmospheric exposure (e.g. 80-100 minutes) (12) brief periods of open bench handling are allowed.

Of course, the anaerobic bacteria have a formal taxonomic classification. A summary of the more significant genera are presented in Table 16-1. Many changes have occurred since the recommendations of the last editions of Bergey's Manual (11, 20), especially in the genus *Bacteroides*. A proposal has been made to transfer mildly saccharolytic members of the this genus to the new genus *Prevotella* (17); the assacharolytic members of *Bacteroides* are now in the genus *Porphyromonas* (18). The remainder of the original genus includes *B. fragilis* and similar species and are highly saccharolytic and usually inhabitants of the intestinal tract.

Among all those given in Table 16-1, excluding *Treponema*, the *Bacteroides fragilis* group is the most commonly implicated in infection (13). Most of the genera in the table are also common normal flora bacteria in areas of the body shown in Table 16-2. Other characteristics of many of these will be covered in subsequent exercises. However, it is important to note at this point that anaerobic infections are usually due to endogenous normal flora. It is therefore useful to become acquainted with the type of anaerobes one can normally expect to find at various body sites (10, 13).

Microbiologists have recognized the importance of disease-causing anaerobic bacteria for many years. One need only recall that, for example, Kitasato obtained pure cultures of *Clostridium tetani*, the agent of tetanus, in the late 1800s. Also, the agent of gas gangrene was described during this period. In fact, methods for isolation and identification of clostridial agents, organisms that form endospores, have been available to the medical microbiologist for most of this century (26). It is probable that since these organisms form highly resistant spores, restrictive conditions required for routine growth of non-sporing anaerobes were eased.

It has only been relatively recently that general interest developed in non-spore forming anaerobes as disease agents. That these bacteria could play an important role in disease is logical considering: (i) they range from equal in concentration to 1000 times greater in number than aerobes (3); and (ii) their role as disease agents were well documented (3, 26). Bartlett (3) ascribes the increased interest to three major factors. These are the development of the GasPak type anaerobic system; the transfer of technology and information from research laboratories to broader applicability in diagnostic situations; and clarification of the taxonomy of this group of organisms.

With the improvement in the technical aspects of isolation of anaerobic bacteria, increasing numbers among the non-sporing anaerobes are identified from infection. It is now evident, for instance, that they are the major cause of aspiration pneumonia, lung abscess, peritonitis, brain abscess, periodontal abscesses, and female genital tract abscesses (10, 13). Also, such infections are usually polymicrobic, reflecting the mixed populations of our normal flora. Therefore, it is important that proper procedures are employed in the laboratory to encourage the growth of all organisms, aerobic, facultatively anaerobic, and anaerobic species. Highlights of such procedures follow in subsequent sections. More thorough treatment will be found in references (2) and (23).

Table 16-1
Classification of Some Major Groups of Anaerobic Bacteria

Gram-Reaction and Morphology	Family	Genus	Notes
Gram-negative			
Rods	*Bacteroidaceae*[a]	*Bacteroides*[b]	Highly saccharolytic
		Prevotella[c]	Mildly saccharolytic, pigmented and non-pigmented
		Porphyromonas[d]	Assacharolytic, pigmented colonies
		Fusobacterium	Rods with pointed ends
Cocci	*Veillonellaceae*[a]	*Veillonella*	Small cocci, arranged in pairs, short chains, clusters
Spiral	*Spirochaetaceae*	*Treponema*	
Gram-positive[e]			
Non-sporeforming Rods		*Actinomyces*	Branched, filamentous forms
		Propionibacterium	Pleomorphic, diphtheroid arrangements[f]
		Bifidobacterium	Pleomorphic, club shapes
		Lactobacillus	
		Eubacterium	
Cocci		*Peptostreptococcus*	
Sporeforming rods		*Clostridium*	Endospores formed to give swollen cell

[a] Reference 11, [b] Reference 19; [c] Reference 17. Both *Prevotella* and *Porphyromonas* were formerly classified as *Bacteroides*; [d] Reference 18, [e] Reference 20; [f] See Exercise 20.

Specimens

There are several clues that can be observed that will suggest the presence of infection due to anaerobic bacteria. Samples with foul odor; those from abscesses, necrosis, animal bites, lesions with gas formation; or those next to locations usually inhabited by normal flora anaerobic bacteria, as shown in Table 16-2, should be suspect. Furthermore, microscopic observations may suggest their presence, as can failure of an isolation culture to grow aerobically from a sample where there is a strong suspicion of the presence of infection. Of course, such samples should be cultured anaerobically.

Conversely, some parts of the body are inappropriate for the collection of specimens for anaerobic culture. Throat, gingival, and nasopharyngeal swabs, for example, will generally not provide useful diagnostic information. Other examples include stools, except for certain clostridia; catheterized and voided urine; swabs of the cervix and vagina; sputum, whether obtained by suction or expectorated; and others (7, 13, 22). This is because of the large number of anaerobes indigenous to those locations that probably will be isolated and their significance is problematic. It generally leads to a wasted effort by the laboratory staff and an unneeded expense for the patient. It was not uncommon, in 1990, for example, for the cost of culture analysis of a sample containing a mixed flora to be $500 to $1000 (9).

Specimen Collection and Transport

The method of specimen collection and transport is important to the success of isolation and identification of any microorganism. However, because of the added sensitivity of anaerobic bacteria to oxygen, care is necessary since methods used for aerobes or facultative anaerobes can lead to the loss of strict anaerobes. This is undoubtedly one reason that non-spore forming anaerobes remained as the "invisible" disease agent for many years.

If purulent specimens of at least 2 ml volumes are obtained, these will yield most anaerobes for at least 24 hours, even if held under aerobic conditions (4). Also, if a maximum transport time of 30 minutes can be maintained, collection of the sample in a needle and syringe from which all air is expelled has been found effective. By this method, air is temporarily excluded from the needle by inserting its point into a sterile rubber stopper. However, if longer transport times are needed, the content of the syringe should be injected into an air-free anaerobic transport tube (10). Swabs may be used, though they are less desirable than some other methods (13). They must be kept under anaerobic conditions before use, and immediately placed back into an oxygen-free container after the specimen is collected (22). Small pieces of tissue should be placed in an anaerobic atmosphere, with or without transport medium (10, 13, 22). Large tissue pieces, however, can be transported in the presence of atmospheric oxygen since anaerobes are protected by the tissue itself. Any specimen to be used for anaerobic culture should not be refrigerated (16).

Several commercially-available systems are available for these steps of sample collection and transport (10, 13). Anaerobic transport medium with or without swabs is available, as are systems for generating anaerobic atmospheres in portable plastic bags or jars.

Isolation of anaerobes from blood specimens is done in the usual manner (22), although it should be done only if the presence of an anaerobic organism is suspected. Drawn blood is immediately placed into blood culture liquid media, usually in a ratio of 1:10 to 1:20 (blood:broth). Samples also

Table 16-2
Anaerobic Bacteria Most Frequently Implicated in Human Infection and Their Primary Residence as Normal Flora

Group or Genus	Important Normal Flora Locations[a] (10, 22)
Gram negative rods:	
Bacteroides fragilis group	Colon, mouth, upper respiratory tract (URT), genital tract
Prevotella melaninogenica (*B. melaninogenicus*)	Mouth, URT, female genital tract
Other *Bacteroides*	Female genital tract, mouth, URT (13)
Porphyromonas	Mouth, URT, female genital tract
Fusobacterium	Mouth, URT, urethra, external genitalia
Gram-positive cocci:	
Peptostreptococcus	Intestinal tract, mouth, vagina, skin, URT, external genitalia
Gram-positive non-sporing rods:	
Actinomyces	Upper respiratory tract, mouth
Propionibacterium	Skin, upper respiratory tract, vagina
Eubacterium	Intestinal tract
Bifidobacterium	Mouth, intestinal tract
Gram-positive spore-forming rods:	
Clostridium	Intestinal tract (some potential disease clostridia also commonly found in environment)

[a] Based on organisms either being commonly present or present in large numbers at locations shown.

may be cultivated in pour plates. Which ever method is employed, it is advantageous to inoculate bottles or plates in pairs. One container is then incubated aerobically, the other anaerobically.

Pre-culture Examination of Samples

As with most other types of organisms, early examination directly from the sample can be very informative, although culture confirmation is still required (7, 13). For example, microscopic examination of smears may reveal the presence of spore-forming bacteria typical of clostridia (e.g. Photo 17-1 through 17-4). Furthermore, Gram-positive, branched filaments strongly suggest *Actinomyces*, and long, thin, Gram-negative bacteria with pointed ends are recognizable as *Fusobacterium* (Photo 16-7). Fluorescent antibodies may be used for direct staining of organism, that for detection of *B. fragilis* and *B. melaninogenicus* being commercially available. An enzyme-linked immunosorbent assay is also marketed for detection of Toxin A of *C. difficile*. Gas liquid chromatography, it has been reported (21), can be applied to early analysis of purulent and blood samples.

Producing Anaerobic Environments for Microbial Cultures

Many procedures have been developed for culturing anaerobic organisms. The objective of all these is to reduce oxygen tension, or reduce its access to the organisms such that they can initiate growth. Once they have begun to grow in broth, for example, anaerobes can maintain their own reduced atmosphere, and cause it to become even more anaerobic.

Measurement of a reducing atmosphere is usually given in terms of Eh (oxidation-reduction potential, or re-dox potential). This is a measure of the tendency for a compound to accept (be reduced) or donate (be oxidized) electrons. Most anaerobes require an Eh of at least -100 mV to initiate growth. Color indicators are frequently employed to tell whether adequate reducing levels are present in a medium, or in the immediate environment. Resazurin and methylene blue are commonly employed. These are colorless in the reduced form at an Eh of about -110 and -49 mV, respectively (5). However, low Eh alone may not predict successful culture; oxygen concentrations also must be reduced because of its direct inhibiting effects on these organisms (25). Some commonly used methods of providing the required conditions for initiating anaerobic growth are as follows.

1. Liquid media that may be incubated under aerobic conditions:

Broths containing sodium thioglycollate, as enriched thioglycollate broth, or cooked meat glucose (CMG) maintains an adequately reduced environment for initiation of growth by anaerobic bacteria. Dithiothreitol, cysteine hydrochloride, sodium sulfite, etc. also may be used to provide lowered Eh (5). Cooked meat medium contains relatively large amounts of unsaturated fatty acids that take up oxygen and keep it from penetrating into the depths of the tube. Also, -SH (sulfhydryl) groups aid in maintaining a reduced environment (27). Before using cooked meat-containing broths, they should be heated in a boiling water bath for 10 minutes before use to drive off dissolved oxygen. These are then quickly cooled and inoculated near the bottom. Thioglycollate-containing media should be heated only after the indicator (if any) shows oxidation at greater than ⅓ the tube depth and they should not be heated more than once. (Why?)

A more recently developed method is the use of a commercially available product, Oxyrase™ Enzyme. This sterile oxygen-absorbing enzyme is prepared from *Escherichia coli*, and can be used in either plates or broths. When added to media it enzymatically removes oxygen by reducing it directly to water in the presence of proper hydrogen donors (6). Although its relative cost and effectiveness for the growth of anaerobes and other organisms compared to other procedures is still to be broadly determined, there are studies to suggest its effectiveness for their growth (for example, references 1, 6, 28). In a comparison of rapid methods for isolation and counting of *C. perfringens* from meat, for example, Oxyrase Enzyme was at least as effective as the use of the GasPak, a method discussed below. Also, it was easy to use since cultivation steps can be accomplished aerobically. Conversely, it was comparatively costly, and less effective than a double tube method that was also used (1).

2. Chemical methods:

Chemical reactions can be used to generate anaerobic environments. The BBL® GasPak System (Photo 16-1) provides an example as one of several commercially-available types that give a simple means for growing anaerobic bacteria. Here, cultures are placed in a GasPak jar or other gas-tight container. A GasPak Disposable Hydrogen + Carbon Dioxide Generator Envelope with palladium-coated alumina pellet catalyst, and an anaerobic indicator are also set inside the jar. Water is added to the envelope and the container sealed. The hydrogen gas combines with oxygen to form water and provide anaerobic conditions. Some CO_2 is also generated and is beneficial, and sometimes necessary for the growth of certain organisms. Large volumes can be made anaerobic by using more than one envelope. In the GasPak Disposable Pouch™ system, a variation is used to produce the anaerobic atmosphere. Here iron powder and carbonate, along with an anaerobic indicator, are contained within a plastic bag. After specimens, plates, etc. are placed inside the bag citric acid solution is added. Contact of this with iron powder leads to iron oxidation and hydrogen production, both leading to reduction of oxygen levels to less than 1%. The chemical reaction of citric acid with carbonate generates a small amount of CO_2 (15). While convenient, transportable, and yielding good anaerobic conditions within the bag, it has only limited space to contain materials. Other similar systems are also available, such as the Pouch System and Bio-Bag™ (Photo 16-2).

3. Prereduced media:

Prereduced anaerobically sterilized (PRAS) media have become commonly used for the culture of anaerobic bacteria. They are prepared so as to achieve highly reduced media. This is done by mixing constituents, boiling to drive off dissolved oxygen, filling the void space with oxygen-free gas, and adding a reducing agent to the medium. The containers are then tightly sealed and autoclaved. For inoculation, methods must be used that will exclude air from the container (13, 22). PRAS media can, without proper equipment, be a challenge to prepare, however, it can be obtained commercially.

4. Gas-exchange methods:

An anaerobic atmosphere can be obtained by merely replacing air with the desired O_2-free gas. These usually include mixtures of CO_2 and/or H_2 in N_2, and some CO_2, which, again, is helpful in the isolation of some organisms. H_2 aids in decreasing the Eh since it can combine with any O_2 to form water (in the presence of catalyst), and must be present (5). Gas exchange procedures may be done in anaerobic jars that are evacuated and refilled with the needed gas mixture containing CO_2 and H_2. It is recommended that the jar be evacuated to a level of 50 mm of mercury, then

refilled with gas, repeating this cycle 3 times. Other containers also may be employed for anaerobic incubation. Anaerobic incubators or chambers (Photo 16-3) may be desirable for large-volume laboratories. These use a continuous flow of O_2-free gas to maintain anaerobic conditions. All such containers must have palladium catalyst to allow removal of any traces of residual oxygen in the gas (5, 22).

Plating Media (7, 22)

Both isolation and identifying media have been developed for the anaerobic bacteria. (A discussion concerning identifying media will be covered later in Exercises 16 and 17.) Isolation plating media are enriched to enable the most fastidious organisms to grow. Thus, 5% laked sheep blood agar using *Brucella* agar base, and containing hemin and vitamin K_1 (K_1BA) is used as a non-selective medium. Hemin encourages the growth of pigmented *Bacteroides*; vitamin K_1 the *B. fragilis* group. However, because anaerobic infections are usually polymicrobic, selective agents are frequently used. Laked sheep blood agar supplemented with kanamycin, vancomycin, hemin, and vitamin K_1 (KVBA) is such a medium inhibiting most organisms except *Bacteroides*. Furthermore, the lysing of red cells encourages earlier coloration of pigmented forms. *Bacteroides* bile esculin (BBE) medium containing bile, esculin, and gentamicin also encourages growth of the *B. fragilis* group. Finally, phenylethanol agar (PEA) with blood allows the growth of most anaerobes, but inhibits facultative Gram-negative bacteria, as enterics, that may be troublesome contaminants. Unlike PRAS broths, isolation plates are not prepared in a prereduced form, therefore, they should be placed in an anaerobic atmosphere 24-48 hours before use to allow reduction to occur.

Identification Methods

Specific identification methods for anaerobic bacteria will be described in Exercises 16 and 17. However, some general comments will be useful.

Approaches taken in identification are generally outlined in Figure 16-1. They commonly use microscopic examination and other methods of direct sample examination discussed earlier. Catalase production, determination of motility, capacity to grow in the presence of 20% bile, pigment formation, and/or physiological patterns as assessed by carbohydrate fermentations, en-

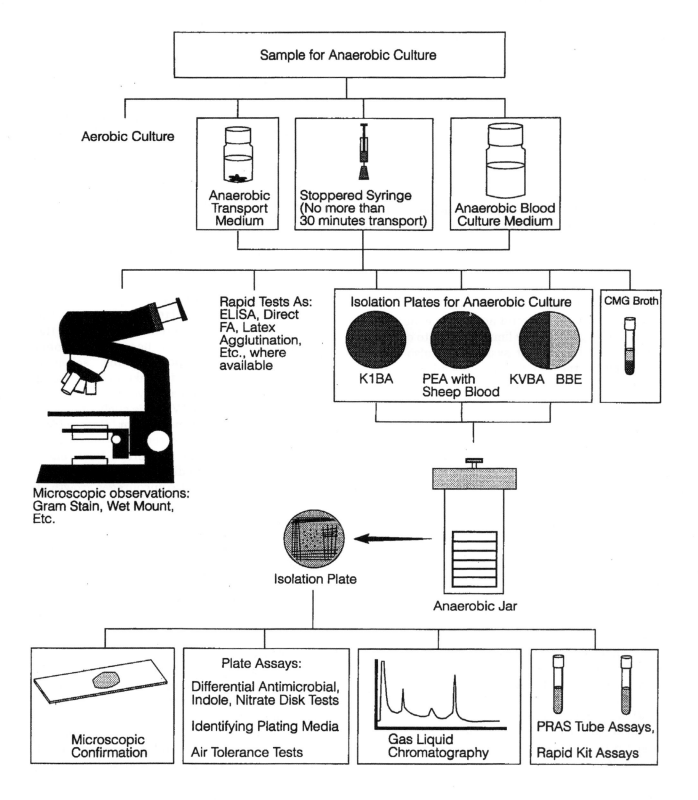

Figure 16-1: Schematic diagram for identification of anaerobes.. See text for details of procedure and full names of media.

zymes produced, etc. may be used. Of course, the ability to grow in the presence of oxygen is also an important criterion. Sensitivity to antimicrobial differentiation disks also provides valuable information, along with identification of kinds and patterns of fatty acids produced as determined by gas liquid chromatography (GLC). For physiological patterns, standard tube-type assays employing PRAS media can be used. However several miniaturized and rapid tests are commercially available, a few of which are discussed below.

Several rapid test systems similar to those originally designed for non-anaerobic bacteria are used for anaerobic bacteria (e.g. API20A®, and BBL® Minitek™ Anaerobe Set II). These require the growth of organisms in inoculated wells or cupules, each containing a separate substrate, including several carbohydrates. After incubation for 24 to 48 hours, reactions are read, and probable identifications made from appropriate manufacturer's data base references. Although such assays perform well for strongly saccharolytic organisms, those that are non-saccharolytic or are weakly so may not give clear reactions (13).

More recently, rapid assays have been developed that do not require microbial growth directly in the assay kit itself. Rather, only the presence of sufficient organisms to provide enzymes to produce a reaction is needed. Many of these are now available, including An-Ident®, RapID™ ANA II System, and the ANI Anaerobe Card with the Vitek System (see Exercise 1, page 6 for a description of this system). Several advantages make such kits attractive, besides their miniaturized form. They do not require anaerobic incubation (at least for the test itself), can ordinarily be read within two to four hours, and can provide a broader range of substrates than is commonly used in the PRAS tube system. Because of this, they have the potential for identifying a broader range of anaerobic bacteria. However, accuracy at the species level varies quite widely, especially for bacteria that are less commonly encountered (13, 14). Therefore, at this point, it is recommended that supplementary methods are included to verify identification. However, as more experience is gained with these and specific data bases become enlarged, it appears likely that these kinds of kits will displace the now standard tube tests (13).

QUESTIONS

1. Categorize bacterial genera or families in Exercise 1-15 into one of the following groups:
   a. Strict aerobe
   b. Facultatively anaerobic
   c. Microaerophilic
   d. Anaerobic
2. Exposure of strict anaerobes to excessive levels of oxygen (more than 0.5%) causes them to die. This does not occur with moderate anaerobes. What is the probable explanation for this?
3. Most anaerobic infections are due to organisms that are indigenous to us as part of our normal flora. Obviously, in most cases, they are harmless and of low pathogenic potential. Yet, under the proper circumstances they cause infection. They are, therefore, types of opportunistic organisms. Using B. fragilis as an example, speculate on the reason for this. What types of "opportunities" are needed to allow it to produce infection? Why doesn't it induce infection under usual circumstances as part of the normal flora? And, what factors does it produce that allows it to be opportunistic?

REFERENCES

1. Ali, M. S., D. Y. C. Fung, and C. L. Kastner. 1991. Comparison of rapid methods for isolation and enumeration of Clostridium perfringens in meat. J. Food Sci. 56:367-370.
2. Balows, A., W. J. Hausler, Jr., K. L. Herrmann, H. D. Isenberg, and H. J. Shadomy (ed.). 1991. Manual of clinical microbiology, 5th ed. American Society for Microbiology, Washington, D. C. p. 488-553.
3. Bartlett, J. G. 1990. Anaerobic bacteria: general concepts, p. 1828-1842. In G. L. Mandell, R. G. Douglas, Jr., and J. E. Bennett (ed.), Principles and practices of infectious diseases, 3rd ed. Churchill Livingstone, New York.
4. Bartlett, J. G., N. Sullivan-Sigler, T. J. Louie, and S. L. Gorbach. 1976. Anaerobes survive in clinical specimens despite delayed processing. J. Clin. Microbiol. 3:133-136.
5. Costilow, R. N. 1981. Biophysical factors in growth, p. 66-78. In P. Gerhardt, R. G. E. Murray, R. N. Costilow, E. W. Nester, W. A. Wood, N. R. Krieg, and G. B. Phillips (ed.), Manual of methods for general bacteriology. American Society for Microbiology, Washington, D. C.
6. Crow, W. D., R. Machanoff, and H. I. Adler. 1985. Isolation of anaerobes using oxygen reducing membrane fraction: experiments with acetone butanol producing organisms. J. Microbiol. Meth. 4:133-139.
7. Edelstein, M. A. C. 1989. Laboratory diagnosis of anaerobic infections in humans, p. 111-135. In S. M. Finegold, and W. L. George (ed.), Anaerobic infections in humans. Academic Press, Inc., San Diego, CA.
8. Finegold, S. M. 1989. Classification and taxonomy of anaerobes, p. 23-36. In S. M. Finegold, and W. L. George (ed.), Anaerobic infections in humans. Academic Press, Inc., San Diego, CA.

9. Finegold, S. M. 1990. Anaerobes: problems and controversies in bacteriology, infections, and susceptibility testing. Rev. Infect. Dis. **12**(Suppl. 2):S223-S230.

10. Finegold, S. M., E. J. Baron, and H. M. Wexler. 1992. A clinical guide to anaerobic infections. Star Publishing Co., Belmont, CA. p. 3-13, 95-110.

11. Krieg, N. R., and J. G. Holt (ed.). 1984. Bergey's manual of systematic bacteriology, Vol. 1. Williams & Wilkins, Baltimore. p. 602-662, 680-685.

12. Loesche, W. J. 1969. Oxygen sensitivity of various anaerobic bacteria. Appl. Microbiol. **18**:723-727.

13. Murray, P. R., and D. M. Citron. 1991. General processing of specimens for anaerobic bacteria, p. 488-504. *In* A. Balows, W. J. Hausler, Jr., K. L. Herrmann, H. D. Isenberg, and H. J. Shadomy (ed.), Manual of clinical microbiology, 5th ed. American Society for Microbiology, Washington, D. C.

14. Phillips, I. 1990. New methods for identification of obligate anaerobes. Rev. Infect. Dis. **1**(Suppl. 2):S127-S132.

15. Power, D. A., and P. J. McCuen (ed.). 1988. Manual of BBL products and laboratory procedures, 6th ed. Becton Dickinson Microbiology Systems, Cockeysville, MD. p. 311-316.

16. Rodloff, A. C., P. C. Appelbaum, and R. J. Zabransky. 1991. Practical anaerobic bacteriology. Cumitech 5A, Coord. ed. A. C. Rodloff, American Society for Microbiology, Washington, DC. 17p.

17. Shah, H. N., and D. M. Collins. 1990. *Prevotella*, a new genus to include *Bacteroides melaninogenicus* and related species formerly classified in the genus *Bacteroides*. Int. J. Syst. Bacteriol. **40**:205-208.

18. Shah, H. N., and M. D. Collins. 1988. Proposal for reclassification of *Bacteroides asaccharolyticus, Bacteroides gingivalis,* and *Bacteroides endodontalis* in a new genus, *Porphyomonas*. Int. J. Syst. Bacterol. **38**:128-131.

19. Shah, H. N., and M. D. Collins. 1989. Proposal to restrict the genus *Bacteroides* (Castellani and Chalmers) to *Bacteroides fragilis* and closely related species. Int. J.Syst. Bacteriol. **39**:85-87.

20. Sneath, P. H. A., N. S. Mair, M. E. Sharpe, and J. G. Holt (ed.). 1986. Bergey's manual of systematic bacteriology, Vol. 2. Williams & Wilkins, Baltimore. p. 1043-1434.

21. Sondag, J. E., M. Ali, and P. R. Murray. 1980. Rapid presumptive identification of anaerobes in blood cultures by gas liquid chromatography. J. Clin. Microbiol. **11**:274-277.

22. Summanen, P., E. J. Baron, D. M. Citron, C. A. Strong, H. M. Wexler, and S. M. Finegold. 1993. Wadsworth anaerobic bacteriology manual, 5th ed. Star Publishing Co., Belmont, CA. p. 1-93; 129-159; 189-204.

23. Summanen, P., E. J. Baron, D. M. Citron, C. A. Strong, H. M. Wexler, and S. M. Finegold. 1993. Wadsworth anaerobic bacteriology manual, 5th ed. Star Publishing Co., Belmont, CA. 230p.

24. Tally, F. P., P. R. Stewart, V. L. Sutter, and J. E. Rosenblatt. 1975. Oxygen tolerance of fresh clinical anaerobic bacteria. J. Clin. Microbiol. **1**:161-164.

25. Walden, W. C., and D. I. Hentges. 1975. Differential effects of oxygen and oxidation-reduction potential on the multiplication of three species of anaerobic intestinal bacteria. Appl. Microbiol. **30**:781-785.

26. Willis, A. T. 1989. History, p. 1-22. *In* S. M. Finegold, and W. L. George (ed.), Anaerobic infections in humans. Academic Press, Inc., San Diego, CA.

27. Wilson, G. S., and A. A. Miles. 1964. Topley and Wilson's principles of bacteriology and immunity, 5th ed., Vol. 1. Williams & Wilkins Co., Baltimore. p. 1046-1092.

28. Yotis, W., C. Gopalsami, K. Hoerman, J. Keene, and L. Simonson. 1990. Substitution of the anaerobic chamber with Oxyrase for the growth of *Treponema denticola*. Ann. Meet. Am. Soc. Microbiol. Abst., p. 213.

EXERCISE 16
The Nonsporeforming Anaerobic Bacteria

I. Gram-negative Anaerobic Bacteria

The Gram-negative nonsporulating rods are the most commonly isolated anaerobic bacteria from clinical material. They are found in more than 50% of specimens cultured for these organisms (13). Of these *Bacteroides fragilis* (Photo 16-4, 16-5, 16-6) and *B. thetaiotaomicron* are among the most frequently encountered species, along with the pigmented species *Prevotella melaninogenica*, and other *Prevotella* and *Bacteroides* spp. The *B. fragilis* group is commonly isolated from perirectal abscesses, intrabdominal infections, ulcers of the decubitus type and of the foot, and soft tissue infection below the waist. In contrast, the pigmented types of *Prevotella* and other *Bacteroides* spp. are more frequently isolated from infection of neck and head, oral infections, and those from human and animal bites, etc. (10).

Members of the *Fusobacterium* are also isolated. Of these, *F. nucleatum* (Photo 16-7, 16-8) is isolated most often from infection. Among those most frequently involved are central nervous system, soft tissue, and bite infections (10). *F. necrophorum*, a potentially highly virulent organism, produces infections of the oral cavity (13), especially Vincent's angina (10).

A new Gram-negative species, *Bilophila wadsworthia*, was identified in 1989 (4), and is being shown to be both a normal flora bacterium, as well as associated with disease (3). In the latter case, most isolates have been derived as part of a mixed flora from cases of appendicitis, although it has also been present in a variety of other infections. This organism can be isolated on *Bacteroides* bile esculin agar and is strongly catalase positive, a feature that led to its original recognition.

Veillonella is one of three genera of the Gram-negative cocci family *Veillonellaceae* (22). This genus, especially *V. parvula* (Photo 16-9), is found in clinical material, although its relative frequency is low (1), and all are essentially considered nonpathogens. Nevertheless, their presence in a specimen cannot be disregarded. Therefore, characteristics of *Veillonella parvula* are shown, along with *Bacteroides, Prevotella, Phorphyromonas assacharolytic* and *Fusobacterium* in Table 16-3.

Table 16-3 gives similarities and differential characteristics of a few of the Gram-negative anaerobes. There are, however, some general characteristics that will aid in the early separation of these and other organisms. Gram stain morphology has already been mentioned as important in the introduction to this exercise. *F. nucleatum* especially shows a unique microscopic morphology (Photo 16-7), having an arrangement and appearance of thrown straw. Also, their colonies have a flecked surface visible by reflected light (Photo 16-8) (18). Several *Prevotella* spp. (e.g. *P. melaninogenica*) and all *Porphyromonas* spp. form heavily pigmented colonies, and produce a brick-red fluorescence when exposed to UV light. *Veillonella* produce a red fluorescence, and, of course, are cocci.

II. Gram-positive Nonsporeforming Anaerobic Bacteria

Among the most important and frequently encountered nonsporeforming anaerobes that are Gram-positive are members of the genus *Propionibacterium*, *Eubacterium*, and *Peptostreptococcus*. Of the first of these, *Propionibacterium acnes* (Photo 16-10, 16-11) predominate among Gram-positive anaerobes. They primarily reside on the skin, although found in other areas of the body as well (see Table 16-2). While it is the most common isolate, it is not a potent pathogen. Although sometimes involved in infection as acnes (5), central nervous system and animal bite, and other infections (10), it is usually present as a contaminant. This is commonly ascribed to its being present as normal flora in large numbers on the skin, and inadequate sampling procedures (5). In one medical center study of almost 4,000 samples analyzed for anaerobes, for example, 20.5% (816 samples) contained *Propionibacterium* (of which, incidentally, 88.8% were *P. acnes*). However, only 11.5% of these (94 isolates) could be identified as the cause of infection (6).

Eubacterium spp., another rod form, are infrequently isolated (11), and rare agents of disease (9). When present, they are usually found in mixed abscess and wound infections (11). These organisms are widely distributed in humans, especially in the feces. The genus consists of 34 recognized species (17), of which *E. lentum* is most commonly observed (11).

Table 16-3
Characteristics of Selected Species of Gram-Negative and Gram-positive Non-sporeforming Anaerobic Bacteria

Genus-species	Colony Hemolysis[b]	Colony Pigment	Colony Fluorescent	Catalase	Disk Sensitivity[c] Kana	Vanco	Colis	Growth in 20% Bile	Esculin Hydrol.	Gelatin Liquif.	NO₃ Red.	Indole	Lipase	Ferm. Arab	Cello	Gluc	Mal	Treh	Xyl	Major Fermentation Products from PYG[e]
I. GRAM-NEGATIVE ANAEROBIC BACTERIA (1, 2, 13, 14, 21, 23)																				
Rod Forms:																				
Bacteroides fragilis	–	–[a]	–	+	R	R	R	+[f]	+	–	–	–	–	–[d]	–	+	+	–	+	S, A, p, pa
B. thetaiotaomicron	–	–	–	+	R	R	R	+	+	–	–	+	–	+	+	+	+	+	+	S, A, p, pa
Prevotella melaninogenica		+	Brick red	–	R	R	R	–	–	+	–	–	–	+	–	+	+	–	–	S, A
Porphyromonas asacharolytica	+	+	Brick red	–	R[c]	S	R	–	–	–	–	+	–	–	–	–	–	–	–	S, A, B, IV, ib, p
Fusobacterium																				
F. necrophorum	–	–		–	S	R	S	–	–	+	–	+	+	–	–	–	–	–	–	B[e], a, p
F. nucleatum		Green		–	S	R	S	–	–	–	–	+	–	–	–	–	–	–	–	B, a, p
Cocci:																				
Veillonella parvula	–		red	V	S	R	S	–	–	–	+	–	–	–	–	–	–	–	–	A, p
II. GRAM-POSITIVE ANAEROBIC BACTERIA (2, 7, 11, 14, 21)																				
Rods:																				
Propionibacterium acnes				+	S	S	R	–	–	+	+	+	–	–	–	+	–	–	–	A, P
Eubacterium lentum				–	S	S	R	–	–	–	+	–	–	–	–	–	–	–	–	A
Cocci:																				
Peptostreptococcus																				
P. anaerobius				–	R	S	R	–	–	–	–	–	–	–	–	+	–	–	–	A, IC, b, ib, iv
P. asaccharolyticus				V	S	S	R	–	–	–	–	+	–	–	–	–	–	–	–	A, B
P. magnus				–	S	S	R	–	–	V	–	–	–	–	–	–	–	–	–	A

a += usually positive; – = usually negative; V = variable (except see footnote[d] below).

b Hemolysis on sheep blood agar (14).

c Kana = kanamycin at 1000 µg; Vanco = vancomycin at 5 µg; and Colis = colistin at 10 µg. Zone diameter of <10 mm are resistant. R = resistant; S = sensitive; V = variable.

d Arab = arabinose; Glu = glucose; Cello = cellobiose; Malt = maltose; Treh = trehalose; and Xyl = xylose. Carbohydrate reactions only: + = pH<5.5; – = pH>5.7.

e A and a = acetic acid; B = butyric acid; IB = isobutyric acid; IV = isovaleric acid; P and p = propionic acid; S = succinic acid; pa = phenylacetic acid. Capital letters = major product; lower case letters = minor product. Only acids consistently produced are shown.

f Bile enhances the growth of *B. fragilis*.

Several anaerobic Gram-positive cocci are also found in clinical samples. Up to the early 1980's most of these were considered to be in the genera *Peptococcus* and *Peptostreptococcus*, names reflecting their microscopic arrangement. Thus, the latter resembled the streptococci and the former that of staphylococci. However, a taxonomic reorganization of this group occurred, primarily based on mol % G + C relationships. Several species of *Peptococcus* were transferred to *Peptostreptococcus* leaving only *Peptococcus niger* in the former group (11, 19, 20). As one might expect, this has practical implications. Several frequently encountered anaerobic, Gram-positive cocci formerly addressed as *Peptococcus* are now *Peptostreptococcus*, no matter their microscopic arrangement. These include *P. magnus* and *P. asacharolyticus* (8). Although older nomenclature continues to be used in many cases, this manual will apply the updated taxonomy.

Peptostreptococcus are normal flora of the intestinal tract, oral cavity, skin, upper respiratory tract, and external genitalia (Table 16-2). As disease agents, they are more important than either of the two Gram-positive rod forms discussed above. They are isolated from a variety of infections including periodontitis, ulcers, osteomyelitis, brain abscesses, endometritis, bacteremia and others (10, 11, 15). Those members that are most commonly isolated include *P. anaerobius, P. magnus, P. asaccharolyticus,* and *P. prevotii* (9).

Selected characteristics that are useful in the identification of *Propionibacterium, Eubacterium lentum,* and the more common *Peptostreptococcus* spp. are shown in Table 16-3. This exercise will exemplify several of these characteristics. For the Gram-negative anaerobes, *B. fragilis* and *F. nucleatum* will be used; for the Gram-positive bacteria, the rod form *P. acnes* and the coccus *P. anaerobius* will be studied.

MATERIALS

Part 1

Per pair of students

1 culture each of *Bacteroides fragilis, Fusobacterium nucleatum, Propionibacterium acnes* and *Peptostreptococcus anaerobius* in enriched thioglycollate broth.

5 plates of prereduced 5% sheep blood agar supplemented with hemin and vitamin K₁ (K₁BA)

1 plate of reduced *Bacteroides* bile esculin agar (BBE)

4 tubes 20% bile in prereduce anaerobically sterilized (PRAS) peptone yeast glucose (PYG) broth

4 tubes PRAS PYG broth (without bile)

4 each of the following antimicrobial disks:
 Kanamycin, 1 mg
 Colistin, 10 μg
 Vancomycin, 5 μg

4 Nitrate reductase disks

Per Bench

1 Anaerobic jar with supplies to produce an anaerobic atmosphere and an anaerobiosis dye indicator strip

1 Anaerobic inoculating device

Part 2

Per Pair of students:

5 filter paper disks for indole test
 Empty petri dish

For each bench, 1 set of each of the following:

1 50 ml beaker
 Nitrate reductase test reagents
 1% *p*-dimethylaminocinnamaldehyde in a dropper bottle
 pH meter
 pH standard buffers

LABORATORY PROCEDURES

Part 1

Each pair of students will be provided with stock cultures of *Bacteroides fragilis, Fusobacterium nucleatum, Propionibacterium acnes,* and *Peptostreptococcus anaerobius* in enriched thioglycollate broth. With these carry out the following:

A. Prepare a Gram stain and microscopically observe.

B. Inoculate each species into the following using reduced or prereduced media:

1. One hemin and vitamin K₁-supplemented sheep blood agar plate (K₁BA). Streak for isolation, but cover about half the plate in the first direction with heavy culture inoculum. After this, do the remainder of the streak directions as usual.

2. Heavily inoculate each of the four organisms onto one quadrant of the following reduced agar plates:
 a. A K₁BA plate
 b. A BBE plate

3. Inoculate each species into the following PRAS tubes. You must maintain anaerobic conditions within these tubes. Do so by using an anaerobic culturing device, such as that described by Holdeman, Cato, and Moore (12) (available from Bellco Glass Co., Inc.).
   a. 1 tube PRAS PYG broth containing 20% bile.
   b. 1 tube PRAS PYG broth that does not contain bile.

C. To the heavily inoculated section of your four K_1BA isolation plates, each containing a separate species, aseptically place the following disks, locating them as far apart from each other as possible:
   1. Kanamycin, 1 mg
   2. Vancomycin, 5 μg
   3. Colistin, 10μg
   4. Nitrate reductase

D. Place the four K_1BA isolation and four BBE plate cultures under anaerobic conditions as directed by instructor. The remaining K_1BA plate is to be incubated in a candle jar. (Why a candle jar, rather than full aerobic conditions?) The PRAS tubes are to be incubated under normal conditions on the open shelf. Maintain at 37°C for 48 hours. Do not open anaerobic containers before this time.

Part 2

A. Observe cultures inoculated previously:
   1. Describe the colony characteristics of each organism on K_1BA. Is hemolysis present? Note presence of blackening of BBE agar indicating growth and esculin hydrolysis. Recall that this medium is somewhat selective for the *Bacteroides fragilis* group and *Biophila wadsworthia*. (What gives this medium its selective character?)
   2. Measure inhibition zones about each kanamycin, vancomycin, and colistin disk. Record a zone diameter of less than 10 mm as R (resistant), 10 mm or more as S (sensitive). These sensitivity characteristics can be very useful in the early grouping of both Gram-negative and Gram-positive anaerobes. For example, organisms resistant to kanomycin and vancomycin include the *Bacteroides fragilis* group and *Prevotella*. Conversely, *Fusobacterium* spp. and *Veillonella* spp. are susceptible to kanamycin. The patterns shown for the selected

representative organisms in Table 16-3, therefore, generally apply for the broader groups in sensitivity characteristics.

3. Compare the amount of growth in the PYG broth containing bile to that without bile. Is it comparable? Increased? Inhibited? *B. fragilis* is usually stimulated by the presence of bile.

4. Test for indole production (16). Do so by placing a filter paper disk atop an area of heavy growth on the anaerobically incubated K_1BA plate with *B. fragilis*. Be sure the disk makes good contact with the microbial growth. After 5 minutes, transfer the disk to an empty petri dish. Add a drop of 1% *p*-dimethylaminocinnamaldehyde solution to it. A positive reaction is visible as a blue color within one minute. Repeat this test with *F. nucleatum*, *P. acnes*, and *P. anaerobius* cultures. Also, carry out a control test using a disk without organisms. (Note: For this test to succeed, the growth medium must contain tryptophan. Why?)

5. Carry out the test to detect nitrate reductase using the disk test (25). Do so by placing a drop of **disk test reagents** A and B on the nitrate reductase disks contained in each culture. A pink to red color is observed in a positive test. If none develops within 5 minutes, add a small amount of zinc dust to the disk. [(If nitrate is present, what reaction would you expect? If absent, what should happen? (See Exercise 1, *Part 2* A-5, page 11.)]

6. Determine glucose fermentation by measuring the pH. Decant a small amount of culture into a beaker to do the measurement, putting the contents back in the original tube after the measurement. A pH of <5.5 is acid, 5.6-5.8 weak acid, and >5.9 or more is negative (23). Use the same beaker for all measurements, then use for containing washes of electrodes. Dispose of beaker and its contents in the proper area for subsequent autoclaving.

Record all results and discuss them. Do characteristics of your cultures correspond to that given in Table 16-3?

B. Demonstration of analysis of PYG culture by gas liquid chromatography (GLC).

Identification of anaerobic bacteria is aided by gas liquid chromatography. The most common application of this procedure

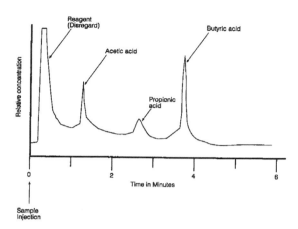

Figure 16-2: Typical gas liquid chromatography for a *Fuso-bacterium* sp. grown in PYG broth. Types of acids are characteristic for this genus, which consistently demonstrate large amounts of butyric acid.

for anaerobes is the detection of end products of glucose fermentation. The presence of volatile fatty acids (i. e. formic, acetic, propionic, isobutyric, butyric, isovaleric, valeric, isocaproic, caproic, and heptanoic acids), alcohols (ethanol, propanol, isobutanol, butanol, isopentanol, and pentanol), and non-volatile fatty acids (pyruvic, lactic, oxalacetic, oxalic, malonic, fumaric, and succinic acids) can be determined. The presence of one or more of those products following growth of the culture is frequently characteristic of the genus or species (see Table 16-3). For example, *Bacteroides* produces a variety of these, but butyric acid is usually not a major product. When it is, isobutyric and isovaleric acids are also produced. Conversely, *Fuso-bacterium* produces butyric acid as a major product, either without or with minor amounts of isobutyric and isovaleric acids (14). *P. acnes* differs from these by having large amounts of propionic acid, while *P. anaerobius* gives isocaproic acid as a major product. Thus, these four species could be distinguished based on Gram stains and GLC alone. Refinement of this kind of data also can be used as an aid in separating other species. The *V. P. I. Anaerobe Manual* provides gas chromatographic patterns that can be expected from many species of anaerobic bacteria (12). The *Wadsworth Anaerobic Bacteriology Manual*

also summarizes the major end products expected from commonly isolated anaerobic genera (23).

Another approach to microbial identification using GLC is by analysis of cellular fatty acids rather than end products of metabolism. It has the potential for being highly discriminating in identification. In this procedure, whole cell fatty acids are extracted from harvested cells, methylated, and analyzed. The fatty acids here range in length from 9 to 20 carbons. Unique profiles are generated reflecting the microbial species. Although sample preparation is the major impediment to routine diagnostic use at this time, many studies have been done using medically-important organisms. These are reviewed by Welch (24).

In principle, identification of fatty acids by GLC is similar to other types of chromatography, but in practice it is quite different. Here, sample compounds volatilize on entering a heated (up to 375°C) column with flowing inert gasses to carry the sample. The column itself is a tube containing an inert matrix (as fused silica) coated with a polar or non-polar substance that is liquid at operating temperature. A sample compound is carried through the column at a rate dependent on its solubility in the liquid phase. Partitioning from other components of the sample therefore occurs as it progresses through the column with those of lower solubility moving more rapidly than those of higher solubility. When the several components move out of the column, therefore, they do so in concentrated bands. As each exits the column, their presence and relative concentration is detected, usually by flame ionization or thermal conductivity types of detectors. In either case, an electrical current generated is proportional to the concentration of the compound detected, and from this, a chart recording is produced (26). An idealized example of such a result for *Fusobacterium* is shown in Figure 16-2. The identity of each peak is determined from control GLC patterns generated from pure known compounds (12, 23).

An automated GLC system (MIDI Microbial Identification System) is available where, following pure culture growth and extraction of samples, the methylated fatty acids are introduced into the gas chromatograph. The remainder of the process is automated and occurs in less than 30 minutes. Analysis of fatty acid content is done, and a pattern produced. This is compared to existing microbial libraries by computer and from this a report generated that, among other information, provides a probable identification. Many species are included in the microbial libraries, including anaerobic, as well as aerobic bacteria.

Although the following will be done as a demonstration, the procedures are included should you wish to test your samples from *Part 1* of this exercise. Also, it will allow a better understanding of how GLC is accomplished.

1. For volatile fatty acids (21, 23):
   a. Grow cultures of *B. fragilis* and *P. anaerobius* in PYG as described in *Part 1* B-3. (If available, PYG cultures from *Part 2* A-6 can be used here. Supernatant liquid from cooked meat glucose (CMG) also may be used.)
   b. Remove 5 ml from each culture tube, and place into separate, clean tubes. Acidify this by adding 2 drops of 50% H_2SO_4 to each, then centrifuge at 2,000 rpm for 5 minutes.
   c. Place the clear supernate into clean tubes.
   d. Inject 1.0 μl of supernatant liquid from each tube into the flame ionization chamber. Observe and interpret results, comparing to patterns given by standard compounds.
2. For non-volatile fatty acids (21, 23):
   a. Transfer 1 ml of supernate from step B1-c immediately above to a clean glass tube.
   b. Methylate samples by adding 2 ml methyl alcohol and 0.4 ml 50% H_2SO_4 to each. Stopper tube and vigorously agitate, Place these into a 60°C water bath for 30 minutes, then hold overnight at room temperature.
   c. Extract the non-volatile fatty acids by adding 1 ml water and 0.5 ml chloroform. Mix well with a vortex mixer, and centrifuge at 1000-2000 rpm for 2 minutes.
   d. Remove up to 14 μl of sample from the chloroform layer at the bottom of the tube and inject into the detector.

   e. Repeat Steps 2a-d using a mixture of known standard non-volatile fatty acids.
   f. Observe and record the results that were given by the gas chromatograph.
3. Compare results between the GLC traces obtained from the samples and the known standards in this demonstration. Also, prepare an analysis of your samples compared with the results provided in the *V. P. I. Anaerobe Laboratory Manual* (12). Are they similar? If not, explain the reason for the differences.

REFERENCES

1. Appelbaum, P. C. 1987. Anaerobic infections: nonsporeformers, p. 45-109. *In* B. B. Wentworth (ed.), Diagnostic procedures for bacterial infections, 7th ed. American Public Health Association, Inc., Washington, D. C.
2. Baron, E. J., L. R. Peterson, and S. M. Finegold. 1994. Bailey & Scott's diagnostic microbiology, 9th ed. Mosby-Year Book, Inc., St. Louis. p. 504-550.
3. Baron, E. J., M. Curren, G. Henderson, J. Jousimies-Somer, K. Lee. L. Lechowtiz, C. A. Strong, P. Summanen, K. Tunér, and S. M. Finegold. 1992. *Bilophila wadsworthia* isolates from clinical specimens. J. Clin. Microbiol. **30**:1882-1884.
4. Baron, E. J., P. Summanen, J. Downes, M. C. Roberts, H. Wexler, and S. M. Finegold. 1989. *Biophila wadsworthia*, gen. nov. and sp. nov., a unique gram-negative anaerobic rod recovered from appendicitis specimens and human faeces. J. Gen. Microbiol **135**:3405-3411.
5. Bartlett, J. G. 1990. Anaerobic Gram-positive nonsporulating bacilli, p. 1869-1870. *In* G. L. Mandell, R. G. Douglas, Jr., and J. E. Bennett (ed.), Principles and practices of infectious diseases, 3rd ed. Churchill Livingstone, New York.
6. Brook, I., and E. H. Frazier. 1991. Infections caused by *Propionibacterium* species. Rev. Infect. Dis. **13**:819-822.
7. Edelstein, M. A. C. 1989. Laboratory diagnosis of anaerobic infections in humans, p. 111-135. *In* S. M. Finegold, and W. L. George (ed.), Anaerobic infections in humans. Academic Press, Inc., San Diego, CA.
8. Ezaki, T., N. Yamamoto, K. Ninomiya, S. Suzuki, and E. Yabuuchi. 1983. Transfer of *Peptococcus indolicus, Peptococcus assacharolyticus, Peptococcus prevotii,* and *Peptococcus magnus* to the genus *Peptostreptococcus* and proposal of *Peptostreptococcus tetradius* sp. nov. Int. J. Syst. Bacteriol **33**:683-689.
9. Finegold, S. M. 1989. General aspects of anaerobic infection, p. 137-153. *In* S. M. Finegold, and W. L. George (ed.), Anaerobic infections in humans. Academic Press, Inc., San Diego, CA.
10. Finegold, S. M., E. J. Baron, and H. M. Wexler. 1992. A clinical guide to anaerobic infections. Star Publishing Co., Belmont, CA. p. 3-13.
11. Hillier, S., and B. J. Moncla. 1991. Anaerobic Gram-positive nonsporforming bacilli and cocci, p. 522-537. *In* A. Balows, W. J. Hausler, Jr., K. L. Herrmann, H. D. Isenberg, and H. J. Shadomy (ed.), Manual of clinical microbiology, 5th ed. American Society for Microbiology, Washington, D. C.
12. Holdeman, L. V., E. P. Cato, and W. E. C. Moore (ed.). 1977. Anaerobe laboratory manual, 4th ed. V. P. I. Anaerobe Laboratory, Virginia Polytechnic Institute and State University, Blacksburg, VA. p. 117-136.
13. Jousimies-Somer, H. R., and S. M. Finegold. 1991. Anaerobic Gram-negative bacilli and cocci, p. 538-553. *In* A. Balows, W. J. Hausler, Jr., K. L. Herrmann, H. D. Isenberg, and H. J. Shadomy

(ed.), Manual of clinical microbiology, 5th ed. American Society for Microbiology, Washington, D. C.

14. Koneman, E. W., S. D. Allen, W. M. Janda, P. C. Schreckenberger, and W. C. Winn, Jr. 1992. Color atlas and textbook of diagnostic microbiology, 4th ed. J. B. Lippincott Co., Philadelphia. p. 519-607.

15. Krepel, C. J., C. M. Gohr, A. P. Walker, S. G. Farmer, and C. E. Edmiston. 1992. Enzymatically active *Peptostreptococcus magnus*: association with site of infection. J. Clin. Microbiol. **30**:2330-2334.

16. Lombard, G. L., and V. R. Dowell, Jr. 1983. Comparison of three reagents for detecting indole production by anaerobic bacteria in microtest systems. J. Clin. Microb. **18**:609-613.

17. Moore, W. E. C., and L. V. H. Moore. 1986. Genus *Eubacterium* Prévot 1938, p. 1353-1373. In P. H. A. Sneath, N. S. Mair, M. E. Sharpe, and J. G. Holt (ed.), Bergey's manual of systematic bacteriology, Vol. 2. Williams & Wilkins, Baltimore.

18. Moore, W. E. C., L. V. Holdeman, and R. W. Kelley. 1984. *Fusobacterium* Knorr 1922, p. 631-637. *In* N. R. Krieg, and J. G. Holt (ed.), Bergey's manual of systematic bacteriology, Vol. 1. Williams & Wilkins, Baltimore.

19. Moore, L. V. H., J. L. Johnson, and W. E. C. Moore. 1986. Genus *Peptococcus* Kluyver and van Niel 1936, p. 1082-1083. *In* P. H. A. Sneath, N. S. Mair, M. E. Sharpe, and J. G. Holt (ed.), Bergey's manual of systematic bacteriology, Vol 2. Williams & Wilkins, Baltimore.

20. Moore, L. V. H., J. L. Johnson, and W. E. C. Moore. 1986. Genus *Peptostreptococcus* Kluyver and van Niel 1936, p. 1083-1092. *In* P. H. A. Sneath, N. S. Mair, M. E. Sharpe, and J. G. Holt (ed.), Bergey's manual of systematic bacteriology, Vol. 2. Williams & Wilkins, Baltimore.

21. Murray, P. R., and D. M. Citron. 1991. General processing of specimens for anaerobic bacteria, p. 488-504. *In* A. Balows, W. J. Hausler, Jr., K. L. Herrmann, H. D. Isenberg, and H. J. Shadomy (ed.), Manual of clinical microbiology, 5th ed. American Society for Microbiology, Washington, D. C.

22. Rogosa, M. 1984. *Veillonellaceae* Rogosa 1971, p. 680-681. *In* N. R. Krieg, and J. G. Holt (ed.), Bergey's manual of systematic bacteriology, Vol. 1. Williams & Wilkins, Baltimore.

23. Summanen, P., E. J. Baron, D. M. Citron, C. A. Strong, H. M. Wexler, and S. M. Finegold. 1993. Wadsworth anaerobic bacteriology manual, 5th ed. Star Publishing Co., Belmont, CA. p. 49-93; 103-110; 147-159; 189-204.

24. Welch, D. F. 1991. Applications of cellular fatty acid analysis. Clin. Microbiol. Rev. **4**:422-438.

25. Wideman, P. A., D. M. Citronbaum, and V. L. Sutter. 1977. Simple disk technique for detection of nitrate reduction by anaerobic bacteria. J. Clin. Microbiol. **5**:315-319.

26. Wood, W. A. 1981. Physical methods, p. 286-327. *In* P. Gerhardt, R. G. E. Murray, R. N. Costilow, E. W. Nester, W. A. Wood, N. R. Krieg, and G. B. Phillips (ed.), Manual of methods for general bacteriology. American Society for Microbiology, Washington, D. C.

Exercise 16
Data Table 1: Non-sporeforming Anaerobic Bacteria Results

		Culture	B. fragilis		F. nucleatum		P. acnes		P. anaerobius	
		Age	K$_1$BA	Other	K$_1$BA	Other	K$_1$BA	Other	K$_1$BA	Other
Colony size and Colony Form	mm									
	Punctiform									
	Irregular									
	Circular									
	Rhizoid									
	Filamentous									
	Other									
Colony Surface	Flat									
	Raised									
	Convex									
	Pulvinate									
	Other									
Colony Margin	Entire									
	Undulate									
	Lobate									
	Erose									
	Other									
Colony Consistency	Butyrous									
	Viscid									
	Membranous									
	Brittle									
	Other									
Colony Optical Character	Opaque									
	Translucent									
	Dull									
	Glistening									
	Other									
Colony Surface	Smooth									
	Rough									
	Other									
Colony color										
Hemolysis	Type									
Other										

Exercise 16
Data Table 2: Non-Sporeforming Anaerobic Bacteria Results

		Culture Age	B. fragilis	F. nucleatum	P. acnes	P. anaerobius
Catalase test	Culture source:					
Gram stain	Culture source:					
	Reaction					
	Morphology					
	Arrangement					
Aerobic Growth						
BBE agar	Growth					
	Esculin hydrolysis					
Sensitivity Assays[a]	Kanamycin, 1 mg					
	Vancomycin, 5 μg					
	Colistin, 10 μg					
Indole Nitrate Nitrite						
	Reduced					
	Reduced					
PYG-20% bile	Enhanced growth					
	Normal growth					
PYG	pH 5.9 or more (-)					
	pH 5.6 - 5.8 (wk. acid)					
	pH <5.5 (Acid)					
GLC Demo.: Fatty Acids Present[b]	Volatile					
	Non-volatile					
Other						

[a] S = sensitive with inhibition zone of >10 mm; R = resistant with zone of 10 mm or less.
[b] Designate fatty acids by initials given in Table 16-3.

Exercise 16: Non-sporeforming Anaerobic Bacteria Results
Laboratory Notes

EXERCISE 17
Clostridium, The Sporeforming Anaerobic Rod

The genus *Clostridium* is an anaerobic, sporeforming group of organisms consisting of over 100 species, though only 14 are potentially or clearly pathogenic (8). It is included in the family *Bacillaceae,* along with the genus *Bacillus,* their aerobic and facultatively anaerobic sporeforming counterparts that we will study in Exercise 18. Most clostridia are widely distributed in our environment (1). Within humans, those that are carried as normal flora organisms are mostly found in the colon (14).

When the clostridia produce infections, they, like other anaerobes, are found with a mixture of other organisms. However, some, as *C. botulinum,* are usually not invasive, producing symptoms through toxins that are formed before entry into the body. All of the clostridia that cause diseases do so by synthesis of one or more toxins that contribute to clinical symptoms as neurotoxins, hemolysins, enterotoxins, phospholipases, etc. (8). The organisms can be separated into five major categories based upon the type of symptoms they produce. They include: (i) those causing gas gangrene (or myonecrosis) and other histotoxic damage due to *C. perfringens, C. novyi* and others; (ii) the tetanus group caused by *C. tetani*; (iii) those producing botulism, the *C. botulinum* group; (iv) the pseudomembranous enterocolitis agents, mostly *C. difficile*; and (v) a miscellaneous group that includes agents producing diseases other than those in groups (i) through (iv). Such diseases as food poisoning, septicemia, etc. are placed in this category (1, 2).

The major virulence factors responsible for the clinical symptoms within the categories are well studied. With *C. perfringens,* the most common agent of the gas gangrene group, for example, at least 12 are produced, though not necessarily all at once. Of these, lecithinase (or α toxin) is thought to be most significant, with others contributing to a lesser amount. Five of these 12 toxins are lethal for mice and are antigenically distinct as determined through mouse protection studies. This has therefore allowed for the separation of this species into serologic types A through E, with type A most

commonly causing disease in humans. Type C is responsible for enteritis necroticans (gangrenous necrosis and hemorrhaging in the small bowel) in humans and lower animals (1, 3), while Types B, D, and E affect lower animals, especially sheep, goats, and calves (15).

C. tetani and *C. botulinum* are potent toxin-producing bacteria. In these the toxins have an affinity for nerve tissue, causing paralysis. However, the syndromes of tetanus and botulism are very distinct because the toxic effect on target tissue differs. In any case, while *C. tetani* produces a single antigenic types of toxin, this is not so of *C. botulinum.* The latter, therefore, has been placed into distinct serological groups A-G (Type C consists of C_α and C_β subtypes, and the organism producing Type G has been renamed *C. argentinense* (13)) to reflect these differences in toxin. Human botulism is most often caused by Types A, B, and E, while C and D occur in lower animals (1). Each type of toxin can be neutralized only by its own specific antitoxin.

C. difficile causes diarrhea and pseudomembranous enterocolitis precipitated by using antimicrobial agents. Symptoms are ascribed to at least 3 toxins of which Toxin A (enterotoxin) and B (cytotoxin) are considered most important in giving clinical symptoms. There is only a single serologic type of this organism.

It should be apparent that toxins are the cause of symptoms, and their action in some clostridial syndromes can progress very quickly and be irreversible once they appear. Therefore, clinical diagnosis may not await laboratory diagnosis (3, 5, 12) as described below.

Laboratory diagnosis of clostridial infections follows the general procedures given in the introduction to anaerobic bacteria (Pages 236 to 241). There are, however, clues that suggest their presence in a specimen. For most, a helpful early sign is the observation of Gram-positive bacilli with endospores that usually cause the vegetative cell to become distended. If the spores are located terminally, they have been likened to "racket" and "drumstick" shapes (Photo 17-1, 17-2); if subterminal, "club-shaped" (Photo 17-3); or centrally, then "spindle-shaped." However, caution must be noted since spore location is not constant, and for some, as *C. perfringens*, it is very difficult to observe the presence of spores (Photo 17-4). With *C. perfringens*, though, their presence is signaled by a "double zone" of hemolysis on sheep blood agar (6), and "stormy fermentation" in tubed milk medium (14). The former of these is seen as a clear inner zone of lysis around the colony surrounded by a partially lysed turbid outer zone. With the latter, a shredding of the milk clot and spattering of particles of the clot about the tube due to vigorous gas production is evident.

Selective media are also available in the isolation of clostridia. Phenylethanol agar with sheep blood, as previously discussed (page 239), can be useful to inhibit selectively facultative anaerobes. Commercially prepared plating agars have also been developed for the selective isolation of *C. perfringens* and *C. difficile*. An example of the latter is CCFA that is made selective by addition of the antimicrobials cycloserine and cefitoxin, with fructose used for the carbohydrate source. *C. difficile* forms large yellow colonies on this medium (14). Sulfadiazine, oleandomycin phosphate, and polymyxin are the selecting antimicrobial compounds in OPSP agar for *C. perfringens*, which form black colonies on this medium. As with the nonsporeforming anaerobes, physiological characterization, including gas liquid chromatography, can be used to identify the clostridia. Table 17-1 provides data for many of those most commonly encountered.

Besides the rapid assays discussed in the introductory section on anaerobes, that are designed to identify anaerobes primarily through physiological and enzymatic patterns, additional methods are available for clostridia. For *C. botulinum* toxin, detection and typing are done using specific anti-Type A, B, and E antiserum. A mouse toxicity test is used to confirm diagnosis of botulism, and a passive protection assay in mice for the toxin type (12). This information is useful in therapy, since antitoxin treatment is the only method of directly neutralizing toxin formed *in vivo*. However, once symptoms of toxicity occur, the toxin combined to tissue cannot be reversed with antitoxin. Therefore, since almost all cases of botulism are due to Types A, B or E, polyvalent antiserum containing antibodies against these may be administered without waiting for the results of laboratory typing (12). But, knowing the toxin serological type can obviously have confirmatory importance, as well as epidemiologic significance in detecting the probable food source responsible for the outbreak (1).

Tetanus is also treated with antitoxin therapy, however, there is little need for laboratory diagnosis since determination of its presence is fully based upon clinical findings (1, 5). Furthermore, because there is only a single antigenic type of toxin, there is no possibility, of course, of administering the wrong type of antitoxin as could occur in botulism.

For the gas gangrene group, antisera are needed to learn the serological type of *C. perfringens* (Types A-E) and *C. novyi* (Types A-C) (6). However, since antitoxin therapy is not employed for the disease caused by these organisms typing of these is primarily for laboratory and epidemiological purposes. *C. perfringens* also causes food poisoning due to its ability to produce an enterotoxin that forms *in vivo* during sporulation. Indeed, it is the most common agent of this following that due to *Salmonella* and *Staphylococcus* (9, 11). As with myonecrosis, the common *C. perfringens* involved is Type A. Beyond this, however, added steps are necessary to establish its etiologic role, especially since this organism is part of our normal flora. Thus, plate counts establishing $>10^5$ organisms/g of suspected food and $>10^6$ spores/g of stool sample collected within 24 hours of onset of symptoms are helpful indicators (1, 11). Serotyping of both should be done to assure matching antigens. Finally, enterotoxin production can be demonstrated by use of reverse passive latex agglutination (RPLA) test (9). This assay works like a standard latex agglutination test (see Exercise 2, Section 4, page 47). The "reverse" aspect of the test merely shows that specific antibody instead of antigen is attached to the latex bead. In one limited study, this assay positively selected all patients with symptoms of enteritis in an outbreak (4).

For *C. difficile* toxin, the most widely accepted assay is that based on detection of its cytotoxicity on cells in human fibroblast culture (1). Although this test is commercially available, up to 48 hours are required to obtain results. Several rapid assays which use antibodies have become available. These include those that are based on latex agglutination (as the Culturette Brand CDT® test and Meritec™-*C. difficile*), and enzyme-linked

Table 17-1
Characteristics of Selected Clostridial Species (1, 6)

Clostridium species	Spore Position[b]	Motility	Esculin Hydrolysis	Gelatin Liquifaction	Indole	Lecithinase[c]	Lipase[c]	Meat Digest[d]	Milk Clot	Milk Digestion	Hemolysis	Fermentation[e] Cello	Glu	Lac	Malt	Treh	Major PYG Fermentation Products[f]
Tetanus Group																	
C. tetani	T	V−	−[a]	+	V	−	−	V−		V+	+	−	−	−	−	−	A, B, p
Histotoxic Group																	
C. perfringens	S	−	V	+	−	+	−	V+	+[g]	+	+[g]	V−	+	+	+	V	A, B, L
C. novyi[h]	S	V	−	V+	V	V+	V−	V+	V	V	+	−	+	−	V	−	A, B, P
C. septicum	S	V+	+	+	−	−	−	−	+	+	+	+	+	+	+	+	A, B
C. histolyticum	S	V+	−	+	−	−	−	+		+	+	−	−	−	−	−	A
C. bifermentans	S	+	V+	+	+	+	−	+		+	+	−	+	−	−	−	A, F
Botulism Group																	
C. botulinum[h]	S	V+	V−	+	−	−	+	V	V	V	+	−	+	−	V	V	A, B
Toxic Colitis Group																	
C. difficile	S	V+	+	+	−	−	−	−	−	−	−	+	+	−	−	−	A, B, ib, ic, iv
Miscellaneous																	
C. ramosum	T	−	+	−	−	−	−	+	−	−		+	+	+	+	+	A, F, I
C. sporogenes	S	V+	+	+	−	−	+	+		+	+	−	+	−	−	−	A, B, ib, iv

[a] + = >90% positive; − = <10% positive; V+ = most strains positive; V− = most strains negative.
[b] T = terminal location; S = subterminal position in sporangium. For *C. perfringens* and *C. ramosum*, spores frequently difficult to show.
[c] Reactions on egg yolk agar. [d] Digestion of cooked meat.
[e] Cello = cellobiose; Glu = glucose; Lac = lactose; Malt = maltose; treh = trehalose.
[f] A = acetic acid; B = butyric acid; F = formic acid; L = lactic acid; P = propionic acid; ib = isobutyric acid; ic = isocaproic acid; iv = isovaleric acid. Capital letters indicate 1 meq or more/100 ml; lower case letters indicates <1 meq/100 ml. Only those acids produced consistently are shown.
[g] *C. perfringens* shreds clot in milk due to gas production ("stormy fermentation"), and produces a "double zone" of hemolysis.
[h] Specific antitoxin required for definitive identification of type. *C. botulinum* consists of 6 types, A-F; *C. novyi* has 3 types, A-C.

immunoassays (EIA) (including Cytoclone™ A+B EIA, *C. diff*-CUBE™, Premier *C. difficile* Toxin A, and CDA® *Clostridium difficile* Toxin A assay kit). The basis for all these is detection of toxin in stool extracts, eliminating the need for *C. difficile* culture and cytotoxic cell culture assays. Conversely, potential cross reactions with other clostridia in the latex-type assays require confirmation by other methods (1). EIA methods need further comparative evaluation, but, in at least one study the Premier kit yielded an accuracy comparable to cytotoxic assays (7).

As in many other cases, alternative technology is being applied to *C. difficile* also. For example, PCR reaction to detect this organism through its Toxin A gene appears promising (10) being highly specific for it, as well as for only those that are toxin-producers. Similarly, hybridization with a DNA probe for the toxin A gene shows efficiency in its detection (16). However, neither of these types of assays are yet available for the routine detection of this organism.

MATERIALS

Part 1

Per pair of students:

1 culture each of *Clostridium tetani*, *C. botulinum*, *C. perfringens* and *C. difficile* in cooked meat medium.

4 Hemin-Vitamin K_1-sheep blood agar (K_1BA) plates

1 Egg yolk agar (EYA) plate
4 tubes each of:
  Prereduced anaerobically sterilized (PRAS)
    peptone yeast glucose (PYG) broth
  PRAS peptone yeast lactose (PYL) broth
2 tubes skimmed milk
Per bench:
  1 tube cooked meat medium
  1 anaerobic container and supplies for generating anaerobic atmosphere.
  Spore stain reagents

Part 2

pH meter and pH standard
50 ml beaker

LABORATORY PROCEDURE

Part 1

A. Known cultures: Each pair of students do the following with stock cultures of *C. perfringens*, *C. tetani*, *C. botulinum*, and *C. difficile* in cooked meat medium.

  1. Gram stain and spore stain by the Wirtz-Conklin procedure each organism. The latter is done by the following steps:

    a. Prepare smears and heat-fix in usual manner.

    b. Place slide over a boiling water bath and flood surface with malachite green.

    c. Steam slide with stain for 5 minutes.

    d. Remove stain by gently rinsing in tap water.

    e. Counterstain with safranine for 30 seconds, wash and dry.

    f. Observe smear. Spores stain green, cells red.

  Especially note the general position of the spores and morphology of the organisms on microscopic examination. Describe. Because the usual laboratory procedure is to examine smears after Gram-staining, you should especially observe the appearance of spore-forming organisms after this procedure. (Note: Slides containing pathogenic sporeforming-bacteria should not be hand-cleaned unless first autoclaved.)

  2. Observe your stock cooked meat cultures for the relative degree of digestion of meat and of gas production. Compare to the uninoculated control tube made available for this purpose. Digestion is noted by the breakdown of the larger meat particles into finely divided sediment. Gas production can be observed by the displacement of intact meat particles upwards in the tube. Also, note the odor. After using these for stock cultures purposes below, incubate and reexamine after 7 days.

  3. Streak each organism for isolation on ½ of each of two different K₁BA plates (therefore a total of four plates for all four species). After inoculation, incubate one set containing all four species anaerobically, and the other aerobically (in a candle jar) for 48 hours at 37°C.

  4. Inoculate organisms for the lecithinase and lipase tests. To do this, streak each species in a single straight line with a loop parallel to each other, but as far apart as possible, such that they cross the egg yolk agar (EYA) plate. Incubate anaerobically in an anaerobic jar, preferably separate from that containing the K₁BA plates, for up to 7 days at 37°C.

  5. Inoculate each species into the following PRAS media:
    a. PYG
    b. PYL

  6. Inoculate *C. perfringens* and *C. difficile* only into skimmed milk tubes.

  7. Incubate all plates as described above. Tube cultures, including your stock cooked meat and the uninoculated control tube, should be incubated at 37°C for 48 hours and examined, then reincubated if necessary.

Part 2

A. Known cultures:

  1. K₁BA plates: Describe colonies that developed under anaerobic conditions. Give the type of hemolysis. Does any species show a "double zone" of red cell lysis? Does any species demonstrate spreading across the plate surface due to motility? Did the clostridia grow aerobically?

  2. Observe the lecithinase and lipase action on EYA. The former is seen as an opaque zone along the streak of organisms. Lipase is noted by a zone of iridescence (as the appearance of an oil drop on water) seen by reflected light on the surface of growth, especially along the margins. It may be necessary to reincubate this plate since the lipase test sometimes does not become positive for one week.

3. Determine acid production due to fermentation of sugars using a pH meter as described in Exercise 16, *Part 2* A-6.

4. Examine *C. perfringens* and *C. difficile* in skimmed milk for clot formation, digestion, or gas production. Especially observe for "stormy fermentation."

5. Again observe cooked meat cultures for digestion and gas production.

6. Tabulate results and discuss.

Part 3

A. *C. difficile* on a selective medium:

Observe the demonstration CCFA plate that has been inoculated on one side with *C. difficile* and on the other with *C. perfringens*, then incubated anaerobically at 37°C. Describe the relative amounts of growth of the two organisms, and other characteristics requested in Data Table 1. Be sure to record the culture age at the time of your observations.

B. Demonstration of tetanus in the mouse: One-tenth milliliter of an aged culture of *C. tetani* heated at 90°C for 15 minutes and suspended 1:2 in 10% lactic acid, will be injected intramuscularly (IM) into a mouse. (What is the function of the lactic acid?) Another animal will be similarly injected with the organism suspended in saline. Observe these animals daily for one week and describe and explain your observations. What are the symptoms of tetanus in the mouse?

QUESTIONS

1. What is the Nagler reaction and what is its usefulness?

2. Give the major source of *Clostridium tetani* in our environment?

REFERENCES

1. Allen, S. D., and E. J. Baron. 1991. *Clostridium*, p. 505-521. *In* A. Balows, W. J. Hausler, Jr., K. L. Herrmann, H. D. Isenberg, and H. J. Shadomy (ed.), Manual of clinical microbiology, 5th ed. American Society for Microbiology, Washington, D. C.

2. Baron, E. J., L.R. Peterson and S. M. Finegold. 1994. Bailey & Scott's diagnostic microbiology, 9th ed. Mosby-Year Book, Inc., St. Louis. p. 504-523.

3. Bartlett, J. G. 1990. Gas gangrene (other clostridium-associated diseases), p. 1850-1860. *In* G. L. Mandell, R. G. Douglas, Jr., and J. E. Bennett (ed.), Principles and practices of infectious diseases, 3rd ed. Churchill Livingstone, New York.

4. Birkhead, G., R. L. Vogt, E. M. Heun, J. T. Snyder, and B. A. McClane. 1988. Characterization of an outbreak of *Clostridium perfringens* food poisoning by quantitative fecal culture and fecal enterotoxin measurement. J. Clin. Microbiol. **26**:471-474.

5. Care, T. R. 1990. Clostridium tetani (tetanus), p. 1842-1846. *In* G. L. Mandell, R. G. Douglas, Jr., and J. E. Bennett (ed.), Principles and practices of infectious diseases, 3rd ed. Churchill Livingstone, New York.

6. Cato, E. P., W. L. George, and S. M. Finegold. 1986. Genus *Clostridium* Prazmowski 1880, p. 1141-1200. *In* P. H. A. Sneath, N. S. Mair, M. E. Sharpe, and J. G. Holt (ed.). Bergey's manual of systematic bacteriology, Vol. 2. Williams & Wilkins, Baltimore.

7. Di Girolami, P. C., P. A. Hanff, K. Eichelberger, L. Longhi, H. Teresa, J. Pratt, A. Cheng, J. M. Letourneau, and G. M. Thorne. 1992. Multicenter evaluation of a new enzyme immunoassay for detection of *Clostridium difficile* enterotoxin A. J. Clin. Microbiol. **30**:1085-1088.

8. Hatheway, C. L. 1990. Toxigenic clostridia. Clin. Microbiol. Rev. **3**:66-98.

9. Johnson, C. C. 1989. *Clostridium perfringens* food poisoning, p. 629-638. *In* S. M. Finegold, and W. L. George (ed.), Anaerobic infections in humans. Academic Press, San Diego, CA.

10. Kato, N., C.-Y. Ou, H. Kato, S. L. Bartley, V. K. Brown, V. R. Dowell, Jr., and K. Ueno. 1991. Identification of toxigenic *Clostridium difficile* by the polymerase chain reaction. J. Clin. Microbiol. **29**:33-37.

11. Koneman, E. W., S. D. Allen, W. M. Janda, P. C. Schreckenberger, and W. C. Winn, Jr. 1992. Color atlas and textbook of diagnostic microbiology, 4th ed. J. B. Lippincott Co., Philadelphia. p. 588-607.

12. Schaffner, W. 1990. Clostridum botulinum (botulism), p. 1847-1850. *In* G. L. Mandell, R. G. Douglas, Jr., and J. E. Bennett (ed.), Principles and practices of infectious diseases, 3rd ed. Churchill Livingstone, New York.

13. Suen, J. C., C. L. Hatheway, A. G. Steigerwalt, and D. J. Brenner. 1988. *Clostridum argentinense*, sp. nov.: a genetically homologous group composed of all strains of *Clostridium botulinum* toxin type G and some nontoxigenic strains previously identified as *Clostridium subterminale* or *Clostridium hastiforme*. Int. J. Syst. Bacteriol. **38**:375-381.

14. Summanen, P., E. J. Baron, D. M. Citron, C. A. Strong, H. M. Wexler, and S. M. Finegold. 1993. Wadsworth anaerobic bacteriology manual, 5th ed. Star Publishing Co., Belmont, CA. p. 1-20; 129-159; 189-204.

15. Timoney, J. F. J. H. Gillespie, F. W. Scott, and J. E. Barlough. 1988. Hagan and Bruner's microbiology and infectious diseases of domestic animals, 8th ed. Comstock Publishing Associates, Ithica, NY. p.223-240.

16. Wren, B. W., C. L. Clayton, N. B. Castledine, and S. Tabaqchali. 1990. Identification of toxigenic *Clostridium difficile* strains by using a toxin A gene-specific probe. J. Clin. Microbiol. **28**:1808-1812.

Exercise 17
Data Table 1: *Clostridium*

		Culture	C. perfringens		C. tetani		C. botulinum		C. difficile	
		Age	K₁BAᵃ	CCFAᵇ	K₁BA	Other	K₁BA	Other	K₁BA	CCFAᵇ
Colony size and Colony Form	mm									
	Punctiform									
	Irregular									
	Circular									
	Rhizoid									
	Filamentous									
	Other									
Colony Surface	Flat									
	Raised									
	Convex									
	Pulvinate									
	Other									
Colony Margin	Entire									
	Undulate									
	Lobate									
	Erose									
	Other									
Colony Consistency	Butyrous			■						■
	Viscid			■						■
	Membranous			■						■
	Brittle			■						■
	Other			■						■
Colony Optical Character	Opaque									
	Translucent									
	Dull									
	Glistening									
	Other									
Colony Surface	Smooth									
	Rough									
	Other									
Colony color										
Hemolysis	Type			■						■
	Double zone			■						■
				■						■
Other	Surface spreading			■						■
	Aerobic growth			■						■

ᵃ K₁BA = Hemin-Vitamin K₁ - supplemented sheep blood agar.
ᵇ CCFA = cycloserine, cefoxitin, and fructose-containing agar.

Exercise 17
Data Table 2: *Clostridium*

		Culture Age	C. perfringens		C. tetani		C. botulinum		C. difficile	
			K₁BA	Other	K₁BA	Other	K₁BA	Other	K₁BA	Other
Gram stain	Culture source:									
	Reaction									
	Morphology									
	Arrangement									
Spore stain	Culture source:									
	Spore Density[a]									
Egg yolk agar	Lecithinase									
	Lipase									
Skimmed milk	Coagulation									
	Digestion									
	Gas									
	Stormy fermenter									
Cooked meat	Digestion									
	Gas									
	Odor									
Fermentation[b]	PYG									
	PYL									
Other										

[a] Record relative density or numbers at +1 to +4, or −.
[b] PYG, and PYL = peptone yeast broth with glucose or lactose, respectively. Acid = pH <5.5; weak acid = 5.6-5.8, and negative = 5.9 or more.

Exercise 17
Data Table 3: *Clostridium*

Tetanus Demonstration Results

Postinoculation		Observations
Date	Day	
	1	
	2	
	3	
	4	
	5	

Other Laboratory Notes:

EXERCISE 18
Bacillus, the Aerobic and Facultatively Anaerobic Sporeforming Rods

The genus *Bacillus* is the aerobic and facultatively anaerobic sporeforming member of the *Bacillaceae* that contains species pathogenic for humans and lower animals. However, because their incidence in disease, at least in the United States, is low, they hold relatively less importance in medical microbiology. The two most significant species in humans are *B. anthracis* (Photo 18-1, 18-2), the agent of anthrax, and *B. cereus* (Photo 18-3, 18-4), most commonly involved in food poisoning, both of the emetic and diarrheal types. However, only 16 outbreaks (1.8% of total) of this latter disease have been reported to the Centers for Disease Control from 1983-1987 (3). For anthrax, only 9 cases have been reported in the 10 years ending 1988 (4).

This is not to say, however, that *B. anthracis* and *B. cereus* are not important. Anthrax, for example, is endemic in many countries, and enzootic and epizootic in some (8, 15). Herbivores are those primarily infected with this organism, and then it is transmitted to humans and other animals, either directly or indirectly. Because the spores are highly resistant, soils contaminated from infected animals can be a source of further infection for many years. *B. cereus,* while incapable of causing anthrax, has been, besides food poisoning, associated with pneumonia, eye infections, bacteremia, and other conditions in humans (14), and bovine mastitis, and bovine abortions (15).

B. anthracis and *B. cereus* are genetically very similar organisms. Their 16S rRNA, for instance, shows high sequence similarity (99.9-100%) (1), and they also have many phenotypic similarities, some of which are shown in Table 18-1. Morphologically, they cannot be differentiated by Gram stain, although a capsule is formed only by *B. anthracis.* Virulence has, though, always been an outstanding difference. Only *B. anthracis* can cause anthrax, a fact diagnostically demonstrated in the laboratory using mice. This is because it contains two plasmids, pX01 and pX02 (12). The first of these codes for "anthrax toxin," an exotoxin that actually consists of three com-

ponents; the second is responsible for the poly-d-glutamic acid capsule (8). An interesting taxonomic puzzle that has yet to be resolved is whether *B. anthracis* that lacks its plasmids, and therefore avirulent, represents a strain of *B. cereus.* At the practical level, though, there are fortunately other laboratory methods of differentiation between these two organisms. These include that motility, hemolysis, and growth on phenylethanol agar are positive for *B. cereus* and not *B. anthracis.* Conversely, lysis by gamma phage and susceptibility to penicillin are positive for *B. anthracis,* but not *B. cereus* (7, 15).

Unfortunately, the problem of identification is more complex than just the separation of *B. anthracis* and *B. cereus.* The genus contains at least 34 species (5). These, like *B. cereus,* are widely distributed, especially in soil, and therefore can be found as contaminants in clinical samples. The presence of *B. cereus,* for example, may therefore represent such a contaminant, while others commonly present, as *B. subtilus* (Photo 18-5) and *B. circulans,* have been rarely isolated as agents of human infection (15), thus cannot be completely disregarded as contaminants when present. However, one needs to consider also "pseudoepidemics." This phenomenon can occur through persisting isolation of an organism as *B. cereus* above baseline levels (11), when in fact its isolation is unrelated to any clinical condition, but due to contamination.

Commercial assays are available for identification of members of *Bacillus.* API® Rapid CH and Rapid CHB and the Biolog System are two examples. Both are based on physiological patterns for identification. Antibody-based, nucleic acid-based, or other types of identification systems are not available for routine laboratory use (15). The problem does not lie in the lack of effort to develop such assays, but more in the similarities between species. For example, no differences can be found in whole cell fatty acid analysis by gas chromatography if *B. cereus* and *B. anthracis* are grown in a complex medium. However, useful differences are found if these

Table 18-1
Differential Characteristics of Some *Bacillus* spp. (2, 5, 7, 13)

Bacillus species	Catalase	Hemolytic	Penicillin Sensitive[b]	Voges-Proskauer Test	Nitrate Reduced	Starch Hydrolysis	Litmus Milk Reactions Coagulation	Digestion	Motility	Anaerobic Growth	Fermentation of:[c] Arab	Glucose	Maltose	Mannitol	Sal	Xyl
B. anthracis[d]	+	−[a]	+	+	+	+	+	+	−	+	−	+	+	−	−	−
B. cereus	+	+	−	+	+	+	V	+	+	+	−	+	+	−	+	−
B. circulans	+	−	−	−	V	+	+		+	V	+	+	+	+	+	+
B. licheniformis	+	+	+	+	+	+			V	+	+	+	+	+		+
B. megaterium	+	−	·	−	V	+	+		V	−	V	+	V	V	V	V[a]
B. pumilus	+	V	+	+	−	−	V	+	+	−	+	+	−	+	+	+
B. sphaericus	+	−	−	−	−	−	−	+	−	−	−	−	−	−	−	−
B. subtilus	+	V	+	+	+	+	+		V	−	+	+	V	+		+

[a] + = 90% or more positive reactions; − = 10% or less negative; V = 11-89% positive.
[b] Penicillin disk of 10µg concentration.
[c] Abbreviations: Arab = arabinose; Sal = salicin, and Xyl = xylose.
[d] Gamma phage specifically identifies.

were grown in a synthetic medium (9), although such differences are not great. In another study, monoclonal antibodies against *B. anthracis* could not distinguish between *B. anthracis* and all strains of *B. cereus* (6).

The following exercise will demonstrate some of the more prominent characteristics of *B. anthracis*, *B. cereus*, and *B. subtilus*. The latter is a rare opportunist, but a common contaminant. Although *B. anthracis* can be studied under Biosafety Level 2 containment conditions (16), it can cause infection through inhalation, of which most documented cases have been fatal (8). If a potential for aerosol production exists, Biosafety Level 3 containment is recommended (16). Also, residual spores are difficult to eliminate should culture spillage occur. For these reasons, cultures of this organism will be made available only through demonstration.

MATERIALS

Part 1
Per pair of students:
- 1 culture each of *B. cereus* and *B. subtilus*
- 2 plates sheep blood agar (SBA)
- 1 plate phenylethanol agar (PEA)
- 2 tubes litmus milk
- 2 Penicillin disks, 10µg/disk

Per bench:
- 1 tube litmus milk
  Spore stain reagents
  Apparatus for anaerobic incubation

Part 2
Catalase reagent

LABORATORY PROCEDURES

Part 1
Known cultures: Each pair of students will be given stock cultures of *B. cereus* and *B. subtilus*. With these carry out the following.

1. Gram stain and spore stain (Photo 18-5) by the Wirtz-Conklin method. Observe your preparations for the presence of spores. Do spores cause the sporangium to swell? After observations have been completed, do not attempt to recycle these slides. Discard.

2. Streak each organism for isolation on ½ of two sheep blood agar plates. Place a disk containing 10µg penicillin per disk on the heavily inoculated segments of each species of one of the plates. Incubate this plate containing the penicillin sensitivity disk *aerobically*. Incubate the second plate anaerobically as specified by the instructor.

3. Inoculate each organism onto ½ of a PEA plate in approximately equal concentrations and streaking pattern (so that a comparison of growth can be made later). Incubate aerobically.

4. Inoculate each organism into litmus milk. An uninoculated control tube will be provided per bench. One pair of students should incubate this with their cultures for the entire bench. This is then to be made available for comparative purposes.

5. Incubate all cultures for 24-48 hours at 35°C.

Part 2

1. Describe colony characteristics on SBA plates incubated aerobically and anaerobically. Use a magnifying lens or a dissecting microscope to observe the surface texture of isolated *Bacillus* colonies of the aerobic plate. Are they rough? Dull or glistening? Can the appearance of either be likened to the appearance of "ground glass?" Also, are the margins entire? Or irregular? *B. cereus,* like *B. anthracis,* may form "Medusa head" colonies, so called because of their surface texture and stringy extensions radiating out from the colony margin (Photo 18-2, 18-4).

If growth has not occurred on the anaerobic plate (should there be growth?) incubate an additional 24 hours at 35°C aerobically and reexamine. Compare the anaerobic growth of the *Bacillus* spp. with each other. Are colonies similar in size?

2. Find the sensitivity of the two species to 10μg penicillin by measuring the zone of inhibition, if any.

3. Test for catalase production by each species using proper methods.

4. Examine the growth on PEA. Is that of either species inhibited?

5. Read litmus milk cultures and describe. Do they change litmus milk? Several reactions are observable in this medium. Acid production causes litmus to change to a pink color, the presence of alkali causes it to turn purple, while reducing conditions make it become colorless. Also, curd may form due to acid or enzyme (usually rennin) under alkaline conditions, and digestion of casein can occur. Finally, gas production

can be observed by shredding or breaking of an acid curd. If severe, the term "stormy fermentation" is sometimes applied (10).

6. Can *B. cereus* and *B. subtilus* be distinguished based upon the minimal tests employed here? How? If not, give one or more tests from Table 18-1 that should be done to differentiate these species.

Part 3:
Demonstration of *Bacillus anthracis.*

A. Observe the demonstration slide of the *B. anthracis.* Carefully note the arrangement of cells and their morphology within chains that are present. Do they have ends that appear "flattened?" A "bamboo rod" appearance has been used to describe the appearance of chains of these organisms. Compare these with your preparations of *B. cereus* and *B. subtilus.* Are those of *B. anthracis* comparable to that seen with either of these species?

B. Sheep blood agar and PEA plate, each inoculated with *B. anthracis*: A disk containing 10μg penicillin was placed on the heavily inoculated area of the SBA plate. With these plates, do the following, but **DO NOT OPEN**:

1. Measure the zone of inhibition around the penicillin disk, if any.

2. Determine colony characteristics of each species on SBA, as specified on Data Table 1 at the end of this exercise. Again, do not open these plates to make any observation.

3. Record the relative amount of growth on PEA. Use the scale described in Data Table 1.

C. Discuss your data. Especially note differential characteristics between *B. anthracis* as shown in this demonstration and *B. cereus* you cultivated above.

QUESTIONS

1. What is Ascoli's test? How is it done?

2. Of organisms studied in Exercises 1 through 17, give an example of one that causes an emetic type and one that causes a diarrheal type of food poisoning. Of all those that can cause food poisoning, are there others besides *B. cereus* that can cause both types? If so, give the name of one.

3. Give characteristics that will distinguish members of the genus *Bacillus* from those of *Clostridium* early in the sequence of identification.

REFERENCES

1. Ash, C., J. A. E. Farrow, M. Dorsch, E. Stackebrandt, and M. D. Collins. 1991. Comparative analysis of *Bacillus anthracis, Bacillus cereus,* and related species on the basis of reverse transcriptase sequencing of 16S rRNA. Int. J. Syst. Bacteriol. **41**:343-346.

2. Baron, E. J., L. R. Peterson, and S. M. Finegold. 1994. Bailey & Scott's diagnostic microbiology, 9th ed. Mosby-Year Book, Inc., St. Louis. p. 451-456.

3. California Dept. of Health Services, Infectious Disease Branch. 1991. Three outbreaks of *Bacillus cereus* food poisoning. Calif. Morbid. **39/40** (Oct. 4.)

4. Centers for Disease Control. 1988. Human cutaneous anthrax - North Carolina, 1987. MMWR **37**:413-414.

5. Claus, D., and R. C. W. Berkeley. 1986. Genus *Bacillus* Cohn 1872, p. 1105-1139. *In* P. H. A. Sneath, N. S. Mair, M. E. Sharpe, and J. G. Holt (ed.), Bergey's manual of systematic bacteriology, Vol. 2. Williams & Wilkins, Baltimore.

6. Ezzell, J. W., Jr., T. G. Abshire, S. F. Little, B. C. Lindgerding, and C. Brown. 1990. Identification of *Bacillus anthracis* by using monoclonal antibody to cell wall galactose-N-acetylglucosamine polysaccharide. J. Clin. Microbiol. **28**:223-231.

7. Koneman, E. W., S. D. Allen, W. M. Janda, P. C. Schreckenberger, and W. C. Winn, Jr. 1992. Color atlas and textbook of diagnostic microbiology, 4th ed. J. B. Lippincott Co., Philadelphia. p. 468-475.

8. LaForce, F. M. 1990. Bacillus anthracis (anthrax), p. 1593-1595. *In* G. L. Mandell, R. G. Douglas, Jr., and J. E. Bennett (ed.), Principles and practices of infectious diseases, 3rd ed. Churchill Livingstone, New York.

9. Lawrence, D., S. Heitefuss, and H. S. H. Seifert. 1991. Differentiation of *Bacillus anthracis* from *Bacillus cereus* by gas chromatographic whole-cell fatty acid analysis. J. Clin. Microbiol. **29**:1508-1512.

10. MacFaddin, J. F. 1980. Biochemical tests for identification of medical bacteria, 2nd ed. Williams & Wilkins, Baltimore. p. 194-200.

11. Morrell, R. M., Jr., and B. L. Wasilauskas. 1992. Tracking laboratory contamination by using *Bacillus cereus* pseudo-epidemic as an example. J. Clin. Microbiol. **30**:1469-1473.

12. Robertson, D. L., T. S. Bragg, S. Simpson, R. Kaspar, W. Xie, amd M. T. Tippetts. 1990. Mapping and characterization of the *Bacillus antracis* plasmids pX01 and pX02, p. 55-58. *In* P. C. B. Turnbull (ed.), Proceedings of the international workshop on antrax. Salisbury Medical Bull., No. 68, Special Supplement. (Original not seen. Cited from P. C. B. Turnbull, R. A. Hutson, M. J. Ward, M. N. Jones, C. P. Quinn, N. J. Finnie, C. J. Duggleby, J. M. Kramer, and J. Melling. 1992. *Bacillus antracis* but not always anthrax. J. Appl. Bacteriol **72**:21-28)

13. Smith, N. R., and R. Gordon. 1957. Genus I. *Bacillus* Cohn, 1872, p. 613-634, *In* R. S. Breed, E. G. D. Murray, and N. R. Smith (ed.), Bergey's manual of determinative bacteriology, 7th ed., William & Wilkins, Baltimore.

14. Tuazon, C. U. 1990. Other Bacillus species, p. 1595-1598. *In* G. L. Mandell, R. G. Douglas, Jr., and J. E. Bennett (ed.), Principles and practices of infectious diseases, 3rd ed. Churchill Livingstone, New York.

15. Turnbull, P. C. B., and J. M. Kramer. 1991. *Bacillus,* p. 296-303. *In* A. Balows, W. J. Hausler, Jr., K. L. Herrmann, H. D. Isenberg, and H. J. Shadomy (ed.), Manual of clinical microbiology, 5th ed. American Society for Microbiology, Washington, D. C.

16. U. S. Public Health Service, Centers for Disease Control and National Institutes of Health. 1988. Biosafety in microbiological and biomedical laboratories, 2nd ed. Publication No. (NIH 88-8395). U. S. Dept. of Health and Human Services, Washington, D. C. p. 55-56.

Exercise 18
Data Table 1: *Bacillus* Results

		Culture	B. cereus			B. subtilus			B. anthracis		
		Age	SBA[a]	PEA	Other	SBA	PEA	Other	SBA	PEA	Other
Colony size and Colony Form	mm										
	Punctiform										
	Irregular										
	Circular										
	Rhizoid										
	Filamentous										
	Other										
Colony Surface	Flat										
	Raised										
	Convex										
	Pulvinate										
	Other										
Colony Margin	Entire										
	Undulate										
	Lobate										
	Erose										
	Other										
Colony Consistency	Butyrous								■	■	■
	Viscid								■	■	■
	Membranous								■	■	■
	Brittle								■	■	■
	Other								■	■	■
Colony Optical Character	Opaque										
	Translucent										
	Dull										
	Glistening										
	Other										
Colony Surface	Smooth										
	Rough										
	Other										
Colony color											
Hemolysis	Type			■			■			■	
Relative Growth[b]			■		■	■		■	■		■
			■		■	■		■	■		■
Other											

[a] Abbreviations: SBA = sheep blood agar; PEA = Phenylethanol agar.
[b] Relative growth: +4 = maximum growth to 1+ = minimum growth; − = no growth.

Exercise 18
Data Table 2: *Bacillus* Results

		Culture	B. cereus			B. subtilus			B. anthracis		
		Age	SBA[a]	PEA	Other	SBA	PEA	Other	SBA	PEA	Other
Catalase test											
Culture source:											
Gram stain	Reaction										
Culture source:	Morphology										
	Arrangement										
Spore stain											
Anaerobic	Anaerobic										
Plate Growth	Aerobic										
Litmus milk	Reduced										
	Acid										
	Alkaline										
	Gas										
	Digestion										
Penicillin	Zone size										
Sensitivity	mm										
Other											

[a] Abbreviations: SBA = sheep blood agar; PEA = phenylethanol agar.

LABORATORY NOTES

EXERCISE 19
Listeria and *Erysipelothrix*

I. *Listeria*

The genus *Listeria* is composed of six species (5, 21) of which *L. monocytogenes* is the most significant pathogen, causing listeriosis in both humans and lower animals. The disease is most frequently seen as stillbirths, meningoencephalitis, and septicemia in both (1, 29). The only other member of this genus that rarely causes disease in humans, but is common in lower animals is *L. ivanovii*. Listeriosis is actually considered a zoonosis, with transmission to humans by using animals or their products as food, leading to epidemics as well as localized outbreaks of this disease. Focal infections, as skin and ocular disease, also may occur through direct contact with infected animals, or with the organism in laboratory employees (1, 23). In a study by CDC during 1988-1990 (9), an annual incidence of 7.4 cases/million population occurred, making it an infrequent disease, but with a mortality of 23%. Also, it was found that 33% of the 301 cases that were identified in this study were among pregnant women or their newly born offspring. Nearly all that contracted listeriosis had at least one type of immunocompromising circumstance, as use of corticosteroids, cancer, or AIDS, an observation made in other studies (1). Data also suggested that a major source of the infecting organisms was food, as soft cheeses and undercooked chicken (9).

Listeria monocytogenes (and other species of this group) are widely distributed in our environment. At least 1% of normal humans are fecal excreters (1), and it is contained in large numbers in the feces of ruminants (29). The latter is a result of consumption of foliage containing these organisms.

Listeria are Gram-positive, nonsporeforming short rods (Photo 19-1). At room temperature they are motile, showing a "tumbling" motility by their one to five peritrichous flagella. At 37°C, these flagella may fail to develop, therefore, most appear non-motile. They also are aerobic to facultatively anaerobic, produce catalase, but not oxidase. Other characteristics are shown in Table 19-1.

The approach to isolation of *Listeria* may be determined by the type of specimen presented. If it is a food, for example, enrichment is usually required. Because *L. monocytogenes* can grow at refrigeration temperatures, cold enrichment has been employed to encourage its selective growth over contaminating organisms. Unfortunately, this may require weeks to months (1). Therefore, selective broths that can be incubated at higher temperatures have been developed for this purpose (various formulations available commercially). Following this, the enriched sample is plated on selective agar. LPM agar containing lithium chloride, phenylethanol, and moxalactam (17) is highly selective, but not differential. PALCAM (containing polymyxin, acriflavin, lithium chloride, ceftazidime, esculin, and mannitol) (30), Oxford medium (10) and modified Oxford agars have both properties. It should be noted that LPM, however, is a transparent medium that allows visualization of the typical blue-green colony sheen of *L. monocytogenes* when observed with oblique lighting (the Henry effect (12)). This property is not visible on differential agars (5, 23). Clinical specimens suspected of containing *L. monocytogenes*, as amniotic fluid, cerebrospinal fluid, or blood generally do not require enrichment. Furthermore, unless heavily contaminated, selective agars are not needed, though they may be helpful in allowing preliminary identification. It does grow satisfactorily on nonselective agars, as blood, brain heart infusion, and similar media. The Henry effect can be seen on clear media, and hemolysis on sheep blood agar. *L. monocytogenes* produces a narrow zone of lysis (Photo 19-2), which may not be visible unless the colony is scraped aside. *L. ivanovii* and *L. seeligeri* are also hemolytic, but the former causes broad double or triple zones; that of the latter is a weak beta lysis (25). Other differential and identifying characteristics are presented in Table 19-1.

Not shown in Table 19-1 is that systems of bacteriophage and antigenic typing are available for *Listeria*, especially *L. monocytogenes*. While the phage set has been useful for epidemiological purposes, many *L. monocytogenes* cannot be

Table 19-1
Identifying Characteristics of *Listeria*[a] and *Erysipelothrix rhusiopathiae* (5, 14, 23, 25)

Genus-species	Catalase Reaction	Hemolysis on SBA[b,c]	CAMP Test with:		Motility at 25°C	Esculin Hydrolysis	V-P[c] Reaction	H$_2$S on TSI	Fermentation of:			
			S. aureus	R. equi					Lac	Mann	L-Rham	Xyl
Listeria												
L. grayi	+[d]	−	−	−	+	+	+	−	+	+		−
L. innocua	+	−	−	−	+	+	+	−	+	−	V	−
L. ivanovii	+	β	−	+	+	+	+	−	+	−	−	+
L. monocytogenes	+	β	+	+ or −[e]	+	+	+	−	V	−	+	−
L. seeliger	+	β(w)	+	−	+	+	+	−	−	−	V	+
L. welshimeri	+	−	−	−	+	+	+	−	−	V		+
Erysipelothrix												
E. rhusiopathiae	−	α			−	−	−	+	+(w)	−	−	−

[a] *L. denitrificans* has been reclassified as *Jonesia denitrificans* (22); *L. grayi* and *L. murrayi* are now a single species, *L. grayi* (21); and *L. ivanovii* consists of two subspecies, *L. ivanovii* subsp. *ivanovii* and *L. ivanovii* subsp. *londoniensis* (8).

[b] Hemolytic characteristics of *L. monocytogenes* = narrow zone; of *L. ivanovii* = broad zone.

[c] Abbreviations: SBA = sheep blood agar; V-P = Voges Proskauer; Lac = lactose; Mann = mannitol; L-Rham = L-rhamnose; and Xyl = xylose.

[d] + = 90% or more positive; − = 10% or less positive; V = 11-89% positive; (w) = weak reaction.

[e] Different reactions reported by different investigators (24).

typed. The use of antibody typing is based on the organism's content of somatic and flagellar antigens giving eleven serotypes, of which most cases of human listeriosis are caused by types 1/2a 1/2b, and 4c (23). Antibody also can be detected in infected patients.

Unfortunately, both antibody-based methods for typing and for antibody detection are of limited value. In the latter case, *Staphylococcus aureus* and *Enterococcus faecalis* induce antibodies that can cross-react with *L. monocytogenes* giving the potential for false-positive reactions. In typing, because a limited number of serotypes are associated with human disease, its application to epidemiological studies is also limited. Finally, because serotypes are not species specific, serotyping cannot be used for identification without other assays (5, 23). However, genus-specific assays based on the use of antibodies are commercially available (11), especially for use in food samples.

Non-traditional methods of identification are also being applied to the *Listeria*. A non-commercial miniaturized assay has been used by Kämpfer, et al. (15) to characterize phenotypically

and successfully identify them. API® 50CH, though successful in identification of *L. monocytogenes*, uses more substrate tests than needed, and is relatively expensive (16). An evaluation of the API® 20 STREP system showed it to be useful in discriminating at the genus level, but deficient in identification at the species level (18). This is improved by the use of API® *Listeria* system (6) and the MICRO-ID LISTERIA system (2), where 85% and 98.8% of listerial species were correctly identified, respectively. The latter, however, also contained several unneeded assays, and required the use of the CAMP test (see *Part 3*, below) to achieve best accuracy. Fatty acid profiles are also available for all species in the MIDI identification system, but listerial fatty acid composition can be similar to several other Gram-positive rods requiring auxiliary methods for identification (3, 31). Finally, an Accuprobe™ kit is available for detection of *L. monocytogenes*.

Experimental studies are exploring methods to improve identification of *Listeria*. PCR, for example, is capable of identifying listerial meningitis directly from samples of cerebrospinal fluid (13). While considered useful in diagnosis, variations in comparison to culture were found with occurrence of some false positive and negative reactions. Multilocus enzyme electrophoresis is also being applied to identify strains and species of this organism with some success. This procedure analyzes genetic variation of organisms through their content of enzyme polymorphism as shown by electrophoresis (26). Its application is proving useful both in epidemiology of listeriosis (4, 7), and its taxonomy (8, 21).

II. *Erysipelothrix rhusiopathiae*

E. rhusiopathiae is the single species of this genus (14). Like *Listeria,* it is an oxidase-negative, facultatively anaerobic, Gram-positive rod. Morphologically, it is similar to them as well. Table 9-1 gives important distinguishing characteristics to separate it from the latter, however. In contrast to *Listeria* for example, *E. rhusiopathiae* is catalase negative, non-motile, negative in the Voges-Proskauer test, and produces H_2S when grown in a TSI agar slant. Also, not shown in Table 19-1, is that this organism produces clotting of citrated bovine and rabbit plasma, a characteristic not seen in listerial species. However, unlike *S. aureus,* this property does not correlate with virulence of *E. rhusiopathiae* (28). The mechanism of clotting also appears to be different, being due to depletion of calcium ions by the latter, rather than by enzyme factors directly activating the clotting mechanism, as staphcoagulase does (27).

Erysipeloid is the condition produced in humans by *E. rhusiopathiae.* This infrequent disease usually occurs as cutaneous invasion through an abrasion of the hand or other site from a source containing the bacteria, as raw fish and meat (19). Septicemia, arthritis, and endocarditis also may occur. It is, however, more common as a zoonotic pathogen causing, for example, swine erysipelas, polyarthritis in lambs and calves, and septicemia in ducks and turkeys (29).

MATERIALS

Part 1

Per pair of students:
  1 culture each of *L. monocytogenes* and *E. rhusiopathiae*
  1 Sheep blood agar (SBA) plate
  1 Brain heart infusion (BHI) agar plate
  2 tubes 0.1% dextrose semisolid (DSA) agar
  2 tubes nutrient gelatin (NG)

  2 tubes triple sugar iron agar

Part 2

Per Bench
  1 bottle catalase test reagent

LABORATORY PROCEDURES

Part 1

Known culture: Each pair of students will be provided with a culture of *L. monocytogenes* and *E. rhusiopathiae.* Transfer these organisms to the following:

1. Sheep blood agar, streaking each organism for isolation on one-half of a plate.
2. BHI agar, again streaking each organism for isolation on one-half of a plate.
3. Stab-inoculate two tubes of 0.1% dextrose semisolid agar (DSA) with *L. monocytogenes.* Repeat this procedure by inoculating *E. rhusiopathiae* into each of two tubes of nutrient gelatin (NG). Be sure to use a straight inoculating needle for these.
4. TSI agar using the usual streak and stab technique. Incubate all of the above cultures at 35°C for 48 hours, except one DSA and one NG tube of each species, which should be incubated at room temperature for the same period.
5. Gram-stain organisms from your stock cultures. Observe and describe. Especially note their relative sizes and arrangement. Compare to that of *Bacillus* studied in Exercise 18.

Part 2

Known cultures:

1. Observe the SBA plate for colony characteristics and hemolysis. If hemolysis is not visible, move one or more colonies aside with a loop so that observations can be made directly under its location.
2. Observe the color of colonies using a method modified from that of Henry (20). Do so by placing the BHI plate on the glass plate stage of a dissecting microscope. Shine a light at the culture plate at a 45° angle onto a mirror positioned to strike the underside of colonies to be observed (see Figure 19-1, which also contains additional information). Observe colonies for a blue-green sheen.

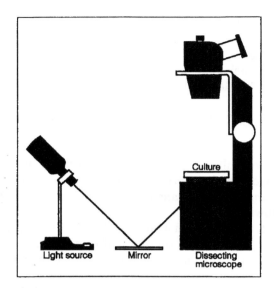

Figure 19-1: Dissecting microscope and lighting arrangement for observation of listerial colonies by oblique illumination as described by McLain and Lee (20). They also recommend an AO635 variable focus light source. Either a concave or a flat surface mirror to reflect light at the required 45° angle is satisfactory.

3. Examine the two tubes of DSA and two tubes of NG. Describe the pattern of growth occurring in each type of medium when incubated at room temperature and at 35°C. Motile *L. monocytogenes* produce a growth that has been likened to an umbrella. *E. rhusiopathiae*, in contrast, forms a "pipe cleaner" or "test tube brush" appearance in nutrient gelatin at room temperature (14). Now, remove some growth from each tube and prepare wet mounts. Make a comparison of motility by phase-contrast microscope observation and describe.

4. Is H$_2$S produced in either tube of TSI? From Table 19-1, *E. rhusiopathiae* only should be positive.

5. Do a catalase test directly on colonies contained in the BHI plate, doing so within a biohazard hood. Is either organism catalase positive? Record and discuss your data.

Part 3

1. Observe the plate of Oxford agar that has been streaked with *L. monocytogenes*, *L. ivanovii*, and *E. rhusiopathiae*. These organisms were each streaked for isolation on one-third of this plate and subsequently incubated at 35°C for 48 hours.

   Describe the appearance of each species as designated in Data Table 1. Does this medium inhibit the growth of one or more of them? Is it differential for *Listeria* at the genus level? At the species level?

2. A CAMP test is also available for observation. This plate has been streaked with *S. aureus* and *Rhodococcus equi* across the plate in single parallel lines next to each other near the center. *L. monocytogenes*, *L. ivanovii*, and *E. rhusiopathiae* were then streaked in a single line perpendicular to (but not across) the previously streaked *S. aureus* and *R. equi* (see Figure 19-2). This plate was then incubated at 35°C for 48 hours. Is a CAMP reaction produced by the *Listeria* spp. or *E. rhusiopathiae*? Can one or more be differentiated by this assay? Record your results and discuss them.

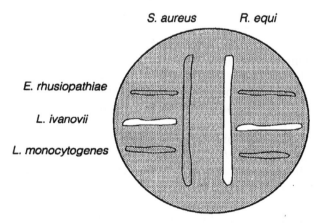

Figure 19-2: CAMP test for differentiation of listerial species. *Staphylococcus aureus* and *Rhodococcus equi* serve as the source of hemolysin for the CAMP reaciton by *Listeria monocytogenes* and *L. ivanovii*.

QUESTIONS

1. Give the reason that Oxford (also modified Oxford and PALCAM agars) is differential for *Listeria*. (Hint: Note the ingredients of Oxford agar shown in Appendix 4.) What is the compound responsible for the formation of the dark halo appearing around the listerial colonies?

2. What is the purpose of the Anton test? How is it done?
3. A virulence test is available for both *L. monocytogenes* and for *E. rhusiopathiae*. Describe it.

1. Armstrong, D. 1990. Listeria monocytogenes, p. 1587-1593. *In* G. L. Mandell, R. G. Douglas, Jr., and J. E. Bennett (ed.), Principles and practices of infectious diseases, 3rd ed. Churchill Livingstone, New York.
2. Bannerman, E., M.-N. Yersin, and J. Bille. 1992. Evaluation of the Organon-Teknika MICRO-ID LISTERIA system. Appl. Environ. Microbiol. **58**:2011-2015.
3. Bernard, K. A., M. Bellefeuille, and E. P. Ewan. 1991. Cellular fatty acid composition as an adjunct to the identification of asporogenous, aerobic Gram-positive rods. J. Clin, Microbiol. **29**:83-89.
4. Bibb, W. F., B. G. Gellin, R. Weaver, B. Schwartz, B. D. Plikaytis, M. W. Reeves, R. W. Pinner, and C. V. Broome. 1990. Analysis of clinical and food-borne isolates of *Listeria monocytogenes* in the United States by multilocus enzyme electrophoresis and application of the method to epidemiological investigations. Appl. Environ. Microbiol **56**:2133-2141.
5. Bille, J., and M. P. Doyle 1991. *Listeria* and *Erysipelothrix*, p. 287-295. *In* A. Balows, W. J. Hausler, Jr., K. L. Herrmann, H. D. Isenberg, and H. J. Shadomy (ed.), Manual of clinical microbiology, 5th ed. American Society for Microbiology, Washington, D. C.
6. Bille, J., B. Catimel, E. Bannerman, C. Jacquet, M.-N. Yersin, J. Caniaux, D. Monget, and J. Rocourt. 1992. API *Listeria*, a new and promising one-day system to identify *Listeria* isolates. Appl. Environ. Microbiol. **58**:1857-1860.
7. Boerlin, P., and J.-C. Piffaretti. 1991. Typing of human, animal, food, and environmental isolates of *Listeria monocytogenes* by multilocus enzyme electrophoresis. Appl. Environ. Microbiol. **57**:1624-1629.
8. Boerlin, P., J. Rocourt, F. Grimont, P. A. D. Grimont, C. Jaquet, and J.-C. Piffaretti. 1992. *Listeria ivanovii* subsp. *londoniensis* subsp. nov. Int. J. Syst. Bacteriol. **42**:69-73.
9. Centers for Disease Control. 1992. Update: Foodborne listeriosis-United States, 1988-1990. MMWR **41**:251, 257-258.
10. Curtis, G. D. W., R. G. Mitchell, A. F. King, and E. J. Griffin. 1989. A selective differential medium for the isolation of *Listeria monocytogenes*. Lett. Appl. Microbiol. **8**:95-98.
11. Farber, J. M., and P. I. Peterkin. 1991. *Listeria monocytogenes*, a food-borne pathogen. Microbiol. Rev. **55**:476-511.
12. Henry, B. S. 1933. Dissociation in the genus Brucella. J. Infect. Dis. **52**:374-402.
13. Jaton, K., R. Sahli, and J. Bille. 1992. Development of polymerase chain reaction assays for detection of *Listeria monocytogenes* in clinical cerebrospinal fluid samples. J. Clin. Microbiol **30**:1931-1936.
14. Jones, D. 1986. Genus *Erysipelothrix* Rosenbach 1909, p. 1245-1249. *In* P. H. A. Sneath, N. S. Mair, M. E. Sharpe, and J. G. Holt (ed.). Bergey's manual of systematic bacteriology, Vol. 2. Williams & Wilkins, Baltimore.
15. Kämpfer, P., S. Böttcher, W. Dott, and H. Rüden. 1991. Physiological characterization and identification of Listeria species. Zbl. Bakt. **275**:432-435.
16. Kerr, K. G., N. A. Rotowa, P. M. Hawkey, and R. W. Lacey. 1990. Evaluation of the Mast ID and API CH systems for identification of *Listeria* spp. Appl. Environ. Microbiol. **56**:657-660.
17. Lee, W. H., and D. McLain. 1986. Improved *Listeria monocytogenes* selective agar. Appl. Environ. Microbiol. **52**: 1215-1217.
18. MacGowen, A. P., R. J. Marshall, and D. S. Reeves. 1989. Evaluation of API 20 STREP system for identifying *Listeria* species. J. Clin. Pathol. **42**:548-550.
19. McLain, J. B. 1990. Erysipelothrix rhusiopathiae, p. 1599-1600. *In* G. L. Mandell, R. G. Douglas, Jr., and J. E. Bennett (ed.), Principles and practices of infectious diseases, 3rd ed. Churchill Livingstone, New York.
20. McLain, D., and W. H. Lee. 1988. Development of USDA-FSIS method for isolation of *Listeria monocytogenes* from raw meat and poultry. J. Assoc. Off. Anal. Chem. **71**:660-664.
21. Rocourt, J., P. Boerlin, F. Grimont, C. Jacquet, and J.-C. Piffaretti. 1992. Assignment of *Listeria grayi* and *Listeria murrayi* to a single species, *Listeria grayi*, with a revised description to *Listeria grayi*. Int. J. System. Bacteriol. **42**:171-174.
22. Rocourt, J., U. Wehmeyer, and E. Stackebrandt. 1987. Transfer of *Listeria denitrificans* to a new genus *Jonesia* gen. nov. as *Jonesia denitrificans* comb. nov. Int. J. Syst. Bacteriol. **37**:266-270.
23. Schuchat, A., B. Swaiminathan, and C. V. Broome. 1991. Epidemiology of human listeriosis. Clin. Microbiol. Rev. **4**:169-183.
24. Schuchat, A., B. Swaminathan, and C. V. Broome. 1991. Letter to the editor. *Listeria monocytogenes* CAMP reaction. Clin. Microbiol. Rev. **4**:396.
25. Seeliger, H. P. R., and D. Jones. 1986. Genus *Listeria* Pirie 1940, p. 1235-1245. *In* P. H. A. Sneath, N. S. Mair, M. E. Sharpe, and J. G. Holt (ed.). Bergey's manual of systematic bacteriology, Vol. 2. Williams & Wilkins, Baltimore.
26. Selander, R. K., D. A. Caugant, H. Ochman, J. M. Musser, M. N. Gilmour, and T. S. Whittan. 1986. Methods of multilocus enzyme electrophoresis for bacterial population genetics and systematics. Appl. Environ. Microbiol. **51**: 873-884.
27. Takahashi, T., I. Takahashi, Y. Tamura, T. Sawada, T. Yoshida, S. Suzuki, and M. Muramatsu. 1990. Mechanism of plasma clotting by *Erysipelothrix rhusiopathiae*. J. Clin. Microbiol. **28**:2161-2164.
28. Tesh, M. J., and R. L. Wood. 1988. Detection of coagulase activity in *Erysipelothrix rhusiopathiae*. J. Clin. Microbiol. **26**:1058-1060.
29. Timoney, J. F., J. H. Gillespie, F. W. Scott, and J. E. Barlough. 1988. Hagan and Bruner's microbiology and infectious diseases of domestic animals, 8th ed. Comstock Publishing Associates, Ithica, NY. p.197-205; 241-246.
30. van Netten, P., I. Perales, A. van de Moosdijk, G. D. W. Curtis, and D. A. A. Mossel. 1989. Liquid and solid selective differential media for the detection and enumeration of *Listeria monocytogenes* and other *Listeria* spp. Int. J. Food Microbiol. **8**:299-316.
31. Von Graevenitz, A., G. Osterhout, and J. Dick. 1991. Grouping of some clinically relevant Gram-positive rods by automated fatty acid analysis. APMIS **99**:147-154.

Exercise 19
Data Table 1: *Listeria* and *Erysipelothrix*

		Culture Age	L. monocytogenes		L. ivanovii		E. rhusiopathiae	
			Sheep Blood	Oxford agar	Oxford agar	Other	Sheep Blood	Oxford agar
Colony size and Colony Form	mm							
	Punctiform							
	Irregular							
	Circular							
	Rhizoid							
	Filamentous							
	Other							
Colony Surface	Flat							
	Raised							
	Convex							
	Pulvinate							
	Other							
Colony Margin	Entire							
	Undulate							
	Lobate							
	Erose							
	Other							
Colony Consistency	Butyrous							
	Viscid							
	Membranous							
	Brittle							
	Other							
Colony Optical Character	Opaque							
	Translucent							
	Dull							
	Glistening							
	Other							
Colony Surface	Smooth							
	Rough							
	Other							
Colony color								
Hemolysis	Type							
	Zone size (mm)							
Other								

Exercise 19
Data Table 2: *Listeria* and *Erysipelothrix*

Assay		Culture Age	L. monocytogenes	L. ivanovii	E. rhusiopathiae
Catalase test	BHI plate				
Gram stain	Reaction				
Culture source:	Morphology				
	Arrangement				
Motility:					
Macroscopic	DSA*a* at 35°C				
	DSA at RT				
	NG at 35°C				
	NG at RT				
Microscopic	DSA*a* at 35°C				
	DSA at RT				
	NG at 35°C				
	NG at RT				
TSI	Growth				
	H₂S produced				
CAMP Reaction	S. aureus				
	R. equi				
Other					

a Abbreviations: DSA = Dextrose semisolid agar; NG = nutrient gelatin; TSI = triple sugar iron agar; RT = room temperature.

Other Data:

Colony color of growth on BHI agar using oblique lighting (*Part 2-2*):

Culture Age: _____   Date: _____

L. monocytogenes: _____

L. ivanovii: _____

OTHER LABORATORY NOTES

EXERCISE 20
Corynebacterium

The genus *Corynebacterium* is within a group of organisms known as "coryneforms" or "diphtheroids" typifying the morphology of this broader group. *Bergey's Manual of Systematic Bacteriology* lists 16 that fit within the generic definition being developed for *Corynebacterium*. These criteria include a cell wall that contains meso-diaminopimelic (DAP) acid and arabinogalactan, presence of mycolic acid of 22-36 carbons, 8 to 9 isoprene units on dihydrogenated menaquinones, fatty acids that are primarily straight chains, and a G + C content of 51-63 mol% (4). Several others continue to be listed as species of *Corynebacterium*, including seven plant pathogenic species; however, these do not belong to this genus in the strict sense. Also, other bacteria that either appear to be corynebacteria or are closely related to this group continue to arise. The Centers for Disease Control's Special Bacteriology Reference Laboratory in Atlanta, GA has had an especially important role in this respect. As examples, their designated Groups D2 and JK are diphtheroids received by them for identification over many years. Most of these are from urinary tract infections and endocarditis, respectively, particularly from immunocompromised patients. D2 and JK, along with *C. diphtheriae* are now considered major pathogens within the coryneforms (1). Subsequent study of these CDC groups has confirmed that these organisms are indeed *Corynebacterium*, and they have been formally added to the genus. D2 is now *C. urealyticum* (15), and JK is *C. jeikeium* (10). There are several other CDC Groups that have not yet been given formal names, many of which are listed by Coyle and Lipsky (5). Conversely, *C. ulcerans*, an organism similar to *C. diphtheriae* and associated with human pharyngitis, as well as diseases of lower animals, is unrecognized on a formal basis, neither appearing in *Bergey's Manual* (4), nor in the approved *List of Bacterial Names* (16). However, the name continues to be used on a practical level.

The corynebacteria are found in water, air, and soil, and as plant and animal pathogens. From a human disease standpoint, *C. diphtheriae* has

Table 20-1
Some Characteristics of *Corynebacterium* spp. of Medical Importance (1, 4, 5, 10, 15)

Corynebacterium species	Beta Hemolysis	Urease	Nitrate Reduced	Phosphatase Produced	Carbohydrate fermentations:				
					Glucose	Maltose	Sucrose	Starch	Trehalose
C. diphtheriae									
biotype *gravis*	V	−a	+	−	+	+	−	+	−
biotype *intermedius*	−	−	+	−	+	+	−	−	−
biotype *mitis*	+(w)	−	+	−	+	+	−	−	−
C. jeikeium (CDC Group JK)	−	−	−	−	+	V	−	−	−
C. matruchotii	−	−	+	−	+	+	+	−	−
C. minutissimum	−	−	−	+	+	+	+	−	−
C. pseudodiphtheriticum	−	+	+	−	−	−	−	−	−
C. pseudotuberculosis	−	+	V	−	+	+	−	−	−
C. striatum	−	−	+	+	+	−	+	+	V
*C. ulcerans*b	+	+	−	+	+	+	−	+	+
C. urealyticum (CDC Group D2)	−	+(s)	−		−	−	−	−	−
C. xerosis	−	−	+	−	+	V	+	−	−

a + = 90% or more positive; − = 90% or less positive; V = 11-89% positive; (w) = weak reaction; (s) = strong reaction.
b Informal name.

historically been most important due to its property of exotoxin production leading to diphtheria. Fortunately, today its incidence in the U. S. and Europe is low, although it remains endemic in areas of Third World countries (12). Other species, such as some strains of *C. ulcerans* and *C. pseudotuberculosis*, may produce an antigenically identical toxin (11). However, though the former can cause a diphtheria-like infection (3), the latter has not been identified as such a cause, although it can opportunistically cause endocarditis (13). Others uncommonly implicated in human infection besides those mentioned above, include *C. minutissimum, C. xerosis*, and *C. striatum, C. pseudodiphtheriticum*, as well as CDC Groups, some of which eventually may be included as *Corynebacterium*. It also should be recognized that *C. xerosis, C. striatum*, and *C. pseudodiphtheriticum*, along with *C. matruchotii* are most commonly isolated as normal flora bacteria. (3, 5). Some corynebacterial species are also important in infection of lower animals. *C. renale, C. cystidis*, and *C. pilosum*, also known as the *C. renale* group, primarily cause urinary tract infection in cattle (18).

Corynebacterium spp. are Gram-positive, straight to curving nonsporeforming rods (Photo 20-1). They are nonmotile and usually show characteristic metachromatic granules (Photo 20-2), "palisade" and "Chinese letter" cell arrangement, and pleomorphic morphology. All give a negative cytochrome oxidase reaction, but are catalase positive. Further identifying and differential characteristics of medically important species are shown in Table 20-1.

Although there is only a single species of *C. diphtheriae*, three biotypes are usually recognized: *gravis, intermedius*, and *mitis*. Differential characteristics for these are included in Table 20-1. Furthermore, they have differing colony characteristics when grown on blood and tellurite-containing agar. *C. diphtheriae* biotype *gravis* usually exhibits large, gray colonies with radial striations and variable hemolysis. Biotype *intermedius*, in contrast, yields small, gray to black non-hemolytic forms (Photo 20-3). Finally, Biotype *mitis* colonies are intermediate in size, and shiny, black in color and weakly hemolytic (4, 11). While these characteristics along with others in Table 20-1 will aid in their differentiation, speciation is most significant. All three produce the same toxin and have the same clinical effect. In fact, the

disease should be treated as soon as it is suspected, even without cultural confirmation since the therapeutic outcome is greatly influenced by early treatment (12).

Sampling methods and transport of specimens containing corynebacteria are similar to those described for other organisms. Should diphtheria be suspected, a throat swab is taken, and immediately streaked onto sheep blood agar and a tellurite-containing medium, as cystine-tellurite agar. If transport is required, Stuart or Amies are suggested (See Figure 20-1). *Corynebacterium* form gray to black colonies on tellurite media. This character is very helpful in differentiation, although some *Staphylococcus* and *Streptococcus* species also present colored colonies. Thus, correctly establishing morphology is important. The typical form of corynebacteria is best viewed by culture material taken from media as Pai or Loeffler's slants and stained with Loeffler's methylene blue stain (11). (It is possible that metachromatic granules contained by these rod forms can be mistaken for chains of cocci, especially when using the Gram stain.) Once having established the presence of a coryneform, bacterial identification can now be accomplished by carrying out assays shown in Table 20-1.

Since diphtheria is due to a toxin, its presence must be verified. This can be done *in vivo* or *in vitro* (Figure 20-2). The *in vivo* assay is usually done in guinea pigs by inoculating two animals, one unprotected and the other protected with 500 to 1000 International Units of diphtheria antitoxin, with an isolate of suspected toxigenic *C. diphtheriae*. If the organism produces toxin, the unprotected animal will die within the four days. The protected animal, on the other hand, will show little or no reaction because of neutralization of toxin by the antitoxin (11).

The more commonly done *in vitro* assay establishes the presence of toxin production through use of the precipitin test in a gel as devised by Elek (7). Since this test is done below (*Part 3*B), it will be described in detail there.

Alternate assays are available for identification of corynebacterial species. Coyle and Lipsky (5) summarize evaluations of many of these, both non-commercial and commercially available types. Among the latter, the Minitek System was found to identify correctly all species of 50 corynebacterial stock cultures in 12-18 hours (17). Furthermore, the API® Coryne gave a 96.7%

correspondence to conventional techniques with 240 clinical isolates (8). Other studies using physiological methods, as that using the Rapid Identification Method (9), are primarily directed toward identification of *C. jeikeium* and *C. urealyticum*. In terms of cellular fatty acid analysis, similar discrimination levels have been encountered as discussed for *Listeria* (2, 19). Speciation of corynebacteria using this method frequently requires supplementary assays.

The PCR (polymerase chain reaction) has also been studied to aid in identification of *Corynebacterium diphtheriae*, especially for detection of toxin-bearing strains. In at least one investigation (14), it was found to be able to identify the presence of the toxin gene, whether in a mixture of organisms or in pure culture. Furthermore, the test was rapidly done, giving same day results. There is one disadvantage, however, this being the assay could potentially identify an inactive gene, leading to a false-positive result.

The following exercise will demonstrate many methods used in identifying *Corynebacterium* species by standard methods.

MATERIALS

Part 1

A. Per pair of students:
  1 culture each of *C. diphtheriae* biotype *gravis* (or other biotype), *C. jeikeium*, and *C. pseudodiphtheriticum* on Loeffler's slants
  1 "Y" plate each of cystine-tellurite (C-T) and sheep blood agar (SBA)
  3 tubes glucose fermentation broth
  3 tubes nitrate broth
  Catalase reagent
  Loeffler's methylene blue and Gram stain reagents
Per student:
  1 sterile swab
  1 tube containing 2 ml trypticase soy broth
  1 tube Loeffler's medium

Part 2

B. Per student:
  1 plate cystine-tellurite (C-T) agar
  1 plate sheep blood agar (SBA)

Part 3

A. Per student
  1 tube containing 0.5 ml trypticase soy broth

  1 tube each of glucose, sucrose, and nitrate broths
  1 tube Christensen urea agar
  Catalase reagent
  Loeffler's methylene blue and Gram stain reagents
B. Per pair of students:
  1 KL antitoxin-impregnated filter paper strip
  1 sterile petri dish
  10 ml KL-virulence test medium
  1 pair forceps
  1 bottle of 95% ethanol

LABORATORY PROCEDURES

Part 1

A. Known cultures: Each pair of students will be provided with *Corynebacterium diphtheriae* of known biotype, *C. jeikeium*, and *C. pseudodiphtheriticum* on Loeffler's serum medium. Carry out the following with these:
  1. Observe the appearance of each species on Loeffler's serum slants. Prepare two smears of each organism. Stain one with Gram stain and the other with Loeffler's methylene blue. The latter is simply done by applying stain to a heat-fixed smear of microorganisms for one minute. After this, the stain is washed away with tap water, blotted dry, and observed. Organisms are blue.

     Record your observations. Are metachromatic granules present? How does the morphology of these organisms compare to that of *Listeria* (Exercise 19)? To *Bacillus* (Exercise 18)? To *Propionibacterium* (Exercise 16)?
  2. Streak for isolation on a "Y" plate of cystine-tellurite (C-T) agar and an SBA plate, placing one species on each segment.
  3. Place each organism into glucose and nitrate broths.
  4. Incubate all cultures at 35°C for 24-48 hours.
  5. Carry out a catalase test on each stock culture.
B. Isolation of *Corynebacterium* species (1, 11): Each student accomplish the following in an attempt to isolate a corynebacteria (see also Figure 20-1):
  1. Using a swab wet in sterile trypticase soy broth, have your partner swab your throat.

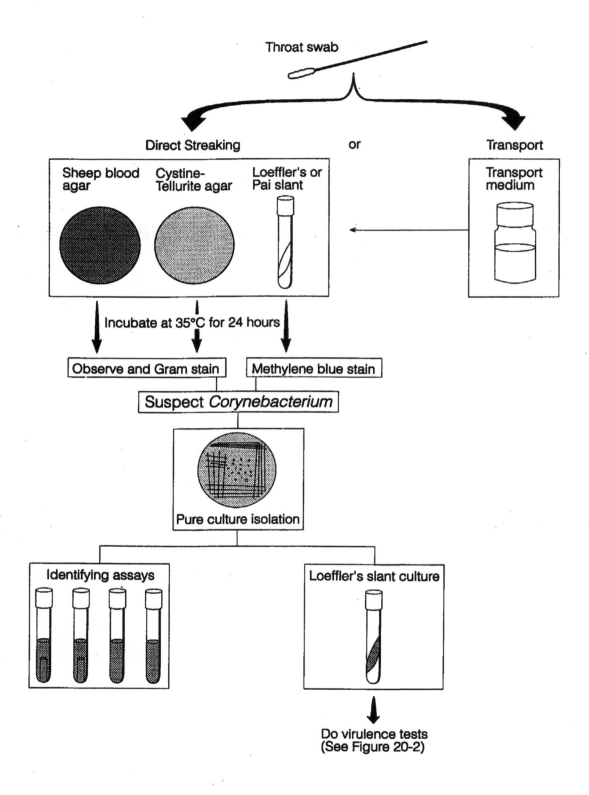

Figure 20-1: Cultural examination of corynebacterial isolate starting with throat swab. If isolate is suspected to be a toxin-producing strain, then virulence tests should be done by a procedure such as shown in Figure 20-2.

2. Inoculate the surface of a Loeffler's slant with the swab. Incubate for 18 to 24 hours at 35°C. When low concentrations are anticipated, as is true here, inoculation of this medium as a first step then subculturing to agar plates is recommended (1).

Part 2

A. Known cultures:

1. Examine colonies on cystine-tellurite (Photo 20-3) and sheep blood agar plates (Photo 20-4). Especially note the differences in morphology, color, and size of colonies between the three species on C-T agar, and the presence of hemolysis on SBA. (Note: Hold C-T plate at 4°C for use in *Part 3*.)

   Potassium tellurite in C-T agar and other types of tellurite-containing media serves two purposes. It makes these media somewhat selective, inhibiting most normal throat flora organisms. Also, it is taken up by corynebacteria to give black to gray colonies. These colony characteristics should always be considered in early identification, along with microscopic findings obtained from culture on Loeffler's medium, and the organism's hemolytic characteristics on SBA. Blood agar also serves to allow growth of some strains that may be inhibited by tellurite in C-T agar.

   It should be mentioned that another medium, Tinsdale agar, is available, and recommended as a differential aid following isolation of corynebacteria (11). It contains tellurite, serum, thiosulfate, and cystine. *C. diphtheriae* produces gray to black convex colonies surrounded by a brown halo, the intensity of which increases with continued incubation. While other organisms will grow on this medium, no halo is produced (6). Evidence of the presence of *C. diphtheriae* also may be obtained from stabbed areas of Tinsdale agar. This is seen by browning around the stab within 10-12 hours, thus aiding in early diagnosis. Unfortunately, this medium reportedly has a short shelf life of 4 days.

2. Is acid formed from glucose? Nitrate reduced to nitrite or beyond?

B. Throat isolates:

1. Prepare smears of colony material from the Loeffler's slant. Stain by Gram and methylene blue methods.

2. Streak suspected corynebacteria for isolation onto C-T medium and SBA. One plate of each will be available per individual. Incubate for 24 and 48 hours at 35°C, examining plates at each period.

Part 3

A. Throat isolates:

1. Observe C-T medium and SBA plates for presence of typical corynebacteria. Select potential *Corynebacterium* colonies, prepare Gram and methylene blue stains, and observe.

2. Using one colony that you think is a diphtheroid, carry out the following:

   a. Suspend in 0.5 ml trypticase soy broth (TSB).

   b. Inoculate from TSB to glucose, sucrose and nitrate broths, and incubate cultures at 35°C for 24-48 hours.

   c. Streak the surface of a Christensen urea agar slant.

3. Use your isolate for the *in vitro* virulence test, given in *Part 3*B. A pure culture on Loeffler's medium is recommended for this purpose; however, because of time constraints, other sources of inoculum will be employed here.

4. Determine whether your isolate produces catalase.

B. The *in vitro* virulence test (7): Since diphtheria is a toxicosis due to the elaboration of exotoxin, it is important that the presence of that toxin is shown from the isolate suspected to be the cause of infection. The following will show a procedure to detect such toxins (also see Figure 20-2).

   Each pair of students is to carry out the following using known and unknown throat isolate cultures:

1. Aseptically pour 10 ml KL-virulence medium cooled to 45-50°C into a sterile petri dish.

2. *Before* the agar hardens, gently (and aseptically) place a KL antitoxin-containing strip of filter paper on the surface. Push the strip so it will lie just below the surface. (See Figure 20-2).

3. Allow the agar to harden and to dry. This latter is important to obtain discrete streaks of growth. It can be done by gently heating the entire bottom of the plate until warm, then inverting on the bench top for about 10 minutes. Remove the lid and shake excess

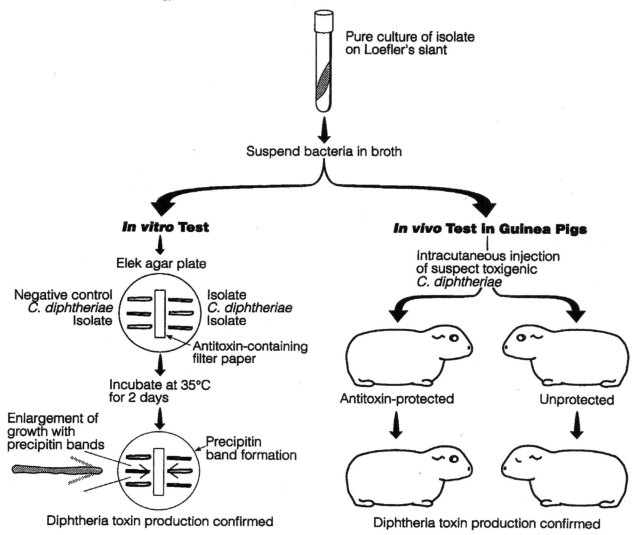

Figure 20-2: The *in vitro* and *in vivo* virulence tests for the detection of diphtheria toxin producing *C. diphtheriae.*

moisture from it. Examine the surface of the agar. If moisture is still present repeat the procedure. Alternately, if time permits, drying may be accomplished by leaving the lid of the dish slightly ajar for 1 to 2 hours.

4. After the surface of the agar has been "dried," heavily streak, in a single line with a loop, the known *C. diphtheriae* and *C. pseudodiphtheriticum* perpendicular to the antitoxin strip and parallel to one another approximately 1.5 cm (or more if space permits) apart. With your partners and your own isolate, carry out the same procedure on the same plate parallel to the known organisms and at least 1.5 cm from them.

5. Incubate at 35°C for 48 hours. If reactions do not appear by this time, continue incubation in your drawer at room temperature.

Part 4

A. *Corynebacterium* isolates:
  1. Describe reactions obtained in glucose, sucrose, nitrate and urea media.
  2. Tabulate results obtained from the culture of your isolate. Attempt to identify the organism based upon these results.

B. *In vitro* virulence test:
  Observe your test for the presence of precipitin bands as diagrammed in Figure 20-2. The interpretation of such bands is as follows: The organisms producing

toxin elaborate this substance into the medium. The antitoxin contained in the filter paper strip also diffuses into the medium. When the antitoxin and toxin in the medium meet in concentrations approximating their equivalence zone, a visible antigen-antibody reaction occurs. In this case it will be manifest as a line of precipitate that is observable in the agar. Thus, if toxin is produced, a band will be seen extending out from the line of growth of the organism. If toxin is not elaborated, no such band will result (7).

QUESTIONS

1. In the clinical testing of colonies for toxigenic *C. diphtheriae*, it is recommended that testing is done on several colonies. This is because some may test negative, while others are positive, although they all come from the same individual (11). How is this possible? What is responsible for the ability of positive strains to produce toxin?

2. Diphtheria toxin is measured in terms of a guinea pig minimum lethal dose (MLD). Antitoxin is also measured in units. For example, strips used in the *in vitro* virulence test are prepared by dipping into antiserum containing 500-1000 International Units (IU)/ml (11). In therapy, 20,000 to 100,000 units are recommended for human treatment, depending on the severity of disease (12). Is there a relationship in the guinea pig MLD and the antitoxic unit? What is a guinea pig MLD and how is it determined? What are other standards of measurement of diphtheria toxin?

3. Describe the Schick test. What is its purpose?

REFERENCES

1. Baron, E. J., L. R. Peterson, and S. M. Finegold. 1994. Bailey & Scott's diagnostic microbiology, 9th ed. Mosby-Year Book, Inc., St. Louis. p. 462-467.

2. Bernard, K. A., M. Bellefeuille, and E. P. Ewan. 1991. Cellular fatty acid composition as an adjunct to the identification of asporogenous, aerobic Gram-positive rods. J. Clin. Microbiol. **29**:83-89.

3. Brown, A. E. 1990. Other corynebacteria, p. 1581-1587. *In* G. L. Mandell, R. G. Douglas, Jr., and J. E. Bennett (ed.), Principles and practices of infectious diseases, 3rd ed. Churchill Livingstone, New York.

4. Collins, M. D., and C. S. Cummins. 1986. Genus *Corynebacterium* Lehmann and Newmann 1896, p. 1266-1283. *In* P. H. A. Sneath, N. S. Mair, M. E. Sharpe, and J. G. Holt (ed.). Bergey's manual of systematic bacteriology, Vol. 2. Williams & Wilkins, Baltimore.

5. Coyle, M. B., and B. A. Lipsky. 1990. Coryneform bacteria in infectious diseases: clinical and laboratory aspects. Clin. Microbiol. Rev. **3**:227-246.

6. Difco Laboratories. 1984. Difco manual, 10th ed. Difco Laboratories, Inc., Detroit, MI. p. 965-967.

7. Elek, S. D. 1948. The recognition of toxogenic bacterial strains *in vitro*. Brit. Med. J. **1**:493-496.

8. Freney, J., M. T. Duperron, C. Courtier, W. Hasen, F. Allard, J. M. Boeufgras, D. Monget, and J. Fleurette. 1991. Evaluation of API Coryne in comparison with conventional methods for identifying coryneform bacteria. J. Clin. Microb. **29**:38-41.

9. Grasmick, A. E., and D. A. Bruckner. 1987. Comparison of rapid identification method and conventional substrates for identification of *Corynebacterium* Group JK isolates. J. Clin. Microbiol. **25**:1111-1112.

10. Jackman, P. J. H., D. G. Pitcher, S. Pelczynska, and P. Borman. 1987. Classification of corynebacteria associated with endocarditis (Group JK) as *Corynebacterium jeikeium* sp. nov. Syst. Appl. Microbiol. **9**:83-90.

11. Kretch, T., and D. G. Hollis. 1991. *Corynebacterium* and related organisms, p. 777-286. *In* A. Balows, W. J. Hausler, Jr., K. L. Herrmann, H. D. Isenberg, and H. J. Shadomy (ed.), Manual of clinical microbiology, 5th ed. American Society for Microbiology, Washington, D. C.

12. MacGregor, R. R. 1990. Corynebacterium diptheriae, p. 1574-1581. *In* G. L. Mandell, R. G. Douglas, Jr., and J. E. Bennett (ed.), Principles and practices of infectious diseases, 3rd ed. Churchill Livingstone, New York.

13. Morris, A., and I. Guild. 1991. Endocarditis due to *Corynebacterium pseudodiphtheriticum*: five case reports, review, and antibiotic susceptibilities of nine strains. Rev. Infect. Dis. **13**:887-892.

14. Pallen, M. J. 1991. Rapid screening for toxigenic Corynebacterium diphtheriae by the polymerase chain reaction. J. Clin. Pathol. **44**:1025-1026.

15. Pitcher, D., A. Soto, F. Soriano, and P. Valero-Guillén. 1992. Classification of coryneform bacteria associated with urinary tract infection (Group D2) as *Corynebacterium urealyticum* sp. nov. Int. J. Syst. Bacteriol. **42**:178-181.

16. Skerman, V. B. D., V. McGowan, and P. H. A. Sneath (ed.). 1989. Approved lists of bacterial names. American Society for Microbiology, Washington, DC. 188p.

17. Slifkin, M., G. M. Gil, and C. Engwall. 1986. Rapid identification of group JK and other corynebacteria with the Mintek system. J. Clin. Microbiol. **24**:177-180.

18. Timoney, J. F., J. H. Gillespie, F. W. Scott, and J. E. Barlough. 1988. Hagan and Bruner's microbiology and infectious diseases of domestic animals, 8th ed. Comstock Publishing Associates, Ithica, NY. p. 247-253.

19. Von Graevenitz, A., G. Osterhout, and J. Dick. 1991. Grouping of some clinically relevant Gram-positive rods by automated fatty acid analysis. APMIS **99**:147-154.

Exercise 20
Data Table 1: *Corynebacterium* Results

		Culture	*C. diphtheriae* biotype ____			*C. jeikeium*			*C. pseudodiphtheriticum*		
		Age	C-T[a]	SBA	Other	C-T	SBA	Other	C-T	SBA	Other
Colony size and Colony Form	mm										
	Punctiform										
	Irregular										
	Circular										
	Rhizoid										
	Filamentous										
	Other										
Colony Elevation	Flat										
	Raised										
	Convex										
	Pulvinate										
	Other										
Colony Margin	Entire										
	Undulate										
	Lobate										
	Erose										
	Other										
Colony Consistency	Butyrous										
	Viscid										
	Membranous										
	Brittle										
	Other										
Colony Optical Character	Opaque										
	Translucent										
	Dull										
	Glistening										
	Other										
Colony Surface	Smooth										
	Rough										
	Other										
Colony	color										
	Hemolysis		▓		▓	▓		▓	▓		▓
Loeffler's Slant	Culture Color		▓		▓	▓			▓		
Other											

[a] C-T = cystine-tellurite agar; SBA = sheep blood agar.

Exercise 20
Data Table 2: *Corynebacterium* Results

		Culture	C. diphtheriae biotype _____			C. jeikeium			C. pseudodiphtheriticum		
		Age	C-T[a]	SBA	Other	C-T	SBA	Other	C-T	SBA	Other
Catalase test											
Gram stain	Reaction										
(1000X)	Morphology										
	Arrangement										
	Branching										
Methylene	Description										
blue stain	Metachromatic										
(X)	granules										
Source:											
Loeffler's											
Glucose	Fermented										
Nitrate	Reduction										
Other											

[a] C-T = cystine-tellurite agar; SBA = sheep blood agar

Other Laboratory Notes

Exercise 20
Data Table 3: Coryneform Isolate Results

		Culture Age	Throat Coryneform Isolate No.								
			1			2			3		
			C-T[a]	SBA	Other	C-T	SBA	Other	C-T	SBA	Other
Colony size and Colony Form	mm										
	Punctiform										
	Irregular										
	Circular										
	Rhizoid										
	Filamentous										
	Other										
Colony Elevation	Flat										
	Raised										
	Convex										
	Pulvinate										
	Other										
Colony Margin	Entire										
	Undulate										
	Lobate										
	Erose										
	Other										
Colony Consistency	Butyrous										
	Viscid										
	Membranous										
	Brittle										
	Other										
Colony Optical Character	Opaque										
	Translucent										
	Dull										
	Glistening										
	Other										
Colony Surface	Smooth										
	Rough										
	Other										
Colony	Color										
	Hemolysis		■		■		■		■		■
Loeffler's Slant	Culture Color		■			■			■		
Other											

[a] C-T = cystine-tellurite agar; SBA = sheep blood agar.

Exercise 20
Data Table 4: Coryneform Isolate Results

		Culture	Throat Coryneform Isolate No.								
			1			2			3		
		Age	C-Tᵃ	SBA	Other	C-T	SBA	Other	C-T	SBA	Other
Catalase test											
Gram stain	Reaction										
(1000X)	Morphology										
	Arrangement										
	Branching										
Methylene	Description										
blue stain	Metachromatic										
(X)	granules										
Source:											
Loeffler's											
Glucose	Fermented										
Nitrate	Reduction										
Other											

ᵃ C-T = cystine-tellurite agar; SBA = sheep blood agar

Part 3B: *In vitro* Virulence Test Results

Incubation Starting Date: _____

Incubation Time (days): _____

Incubation Temperature: _____

Description (Include diagram):

Other Laboratory Notes

EXERCISE 21
Mycobacterium

The genus *Mycobacterium*, the only member of the family *Mycobacteriaceae*, includes at least 53 accepted species (53). Many of these, as seen in Table 21-1, are associated with humans, either as disease agents or as saprophytic organisms. Species are also found in lower animals and in the environment. Of course, those associated with humans are of most interest here.

1. Clinical Groups

The mycobacterioses consist of two general groups of human disease: tuberculosis and nontuberculosis. The former is caused by *M. tuberculosis*, *M. bovis* (Photo 21-1), and *M. africanum*. *M. tuberculosis* continues to be the most frequent and important in the group causing pulmonary infection, though *M. bovis* and *M. africanum* (which is only found in Africa) also produce this disease. All other species infecting humans therefore cause nontuberculosis disease. For example, *M. avium-M. intracellulare* (the most common of opportunistic mycobacteria, and frequently called a complex because of their similarities), *M. kansasii*, *M. xenopi* and *M. fortuitum* also produce pulmonary tuberculosis-like disease. All, like those of the tuberculosis group, may disseminate to other areas of the body. Conversely, *M. marinum*, *M. ulcerans*, and *M. haemophilum* do not primarily target the lung, preferring the skin or subcutaneous tissue. Also, *M. scrofulaceum* is a nonpulmonary agent producing cervical lymphadenitis (Table 21-1). All these organisms and others of the genus except *M. leprae* (Photo 21-2), the etiologic agent of leprosy (Hansen's disease), may be cultured *in vitro*. Saprophytic mycobacteria, as *M. phlei*, *M. smegmatis*, or *M. gordonae* also can appear in clinical samples.

2. Epidemiology

The non-tuberculous group of agents and their opportunistic nature became prominently evident with the AIDS epidemic. Furthermore, unlike tuberculosis-causing agents, they can be found in dust, soil and water of the environment, and are less contagious (54). *M. leprae*, though included in this group, is an exception because it is contagious and not found free-living in our environment (7).

Epidemiologic data leaves little doubt as to the importance of the mycobacterial induced diseases. Worldwide it is estimated by the World Health Organization (WHO) that there are 10-12 million cases of leprosy, with over 570,000 new cases occurring in 12 months during 1989-1990 (32). For tuberculosis, over 1700 million people, or one-third of the world population were estimated to be infected, and that between 2.6 and 2.9 million died of this disease in 1990 (41). Africa and South East Asia, with an estimated 220,000 cases/100,000 population and 194 cases/100,000, respectively, represent those areas with the highest rates. In contrast, the U. S. rate for the same year was 10.33 cases/100,000, and the total was 25,701 cases (11). Although this is of relatively low incidence, it unfortunately has been increasing since 1988 when 9.13 cases/100,000 was achieved. This rise is attributed to a variety of factors, including economic, immigration, and social factors, and human immunodeficiency virus (HIV) infection (10). In the latter, the virus targets the $CD4^+$ and $CD8^+$ T-lymphocyte function (e.g. 30) important in immunity against mycobacteria. Thus, rates of tuberculosis and nontuberculosis disease have increased remarkably in these highly susceptible, immune-impaired individuals. For example, in the 14-49 year-old group in Africa for 1990, an estimated increase of 20% of cases of tuberculosis occurred because of HIV infection (41). The trend in the U. S. will present a challenge to achieve the national goal of eliminating tuberculosis in this country by the year 2010 (9).

3. Classification and informal grouping of mycobacteria

The classification and categorization of mycobacteria have been approached in many ways. Of course, formal classification based on genetic and phenotypic characteristics serve as our basic method of reference. They all are Gram-positive, though they stain poorly by this procedure. Furthermore, they are acid-fast, have an aerobic metabolism, and may show branching. It has also been proposed that the mycolic acid content (which, incidentally, gives their acid fast character) be of C_{22} to C_{26} fatty acid methyl esters chain length following pyrolysis, and G + C content of

Table 21-1
Agents of Human Mycobacterioses (34, 54, 56)

Groups	Species of *Mycobacterium*	Most Common Form or Site of Disease and Comments
Disease agents:		
M. tuberculosis complex	*M. tuberculosis*	Pulmonary (common isolate)
	M. bovis	Pulmonary
	M. africanum	Pulmonary; only in Africa
M. avium complex (MAC) or *M. avium*	*M. avium*	Pulmonary; tb-like; common in HIV-infected patients; present in environment.
M. intracellulare (MAI) complex	*M. intracellulare*	Similar to *M. avium*
M. fortuitum complex	*M. fortuitum*	Skeletal and soft tissue
	M. chelonae	Skeletal and soft tissue
Others	*M. asiaticum*	Pulmonary (rare isolate)
	M. haemophilum	Subcutaneous forming nodules and ulcers
	M. kansasii	Pulmonary; tb-like disease
	M. leprae	Skin and nervous tissue
	M. malmoense	Pulmonary
	M. marinum	Cutaneous (following abrasion)
	M. scrofulaceum	Lymphadenitis (usually children)
	M. shimoidei	Pulmonary (rare isolate)
	M. simiae	Pulmonary (rare isolate)
	M. szulgai	Pulmonary
	M. ulcerans	Subcutaneous (after trauma)
	M. xenopi	Pulmonary
Rarely Pathogenic Saprophytes *M. terrae* complex	*M. gordonae*	*Common environmental organism*
	M. smegmatis	
	M. terrae	
	M. chromogenicum	
	M. triviale	

new species fall in the range of 61-71 mol% (51). Many other properties, of course, are used to speciate, some of which are shown in Table 21-2.

Beyond this, certain organisms have been grouped together because of their similarities. The *M. tuberculosis* complex, for example, encompasses *M. tuberculosis, M. bovis, M. africanum,* and *M. microti.* This clustering is primarily based on their similarities in DNA homology, antigens, and other phenotypic characteristics. Also, the clinical conditions that are produced are similar, excepting *M. microti,* which causes tuberculosis in voles, but not humans (17, 53). The term "tubercle bacillus" has a clinical connotation and overlaps with the *M. tuberculosis* complex, referring to either *M. tuberculosis* or *M. bovis* (17). In addition, there is the *M. avium complex* (MAC), also called

the *M. avium-M. intracellulare* (MAI) complex. Besides these two species, this group now includes the non-human pathogens *M. paratuberculosis* (agent of Johne's disease in cattle, sheep, goats, etc.), *M. lepraemurium* (infects rats, cats, and others) (43), and a probable new species, the wood pigeon bacillus (54). The members of the MAC are so similar in biochemical and growth characteristics that they are difficult to distinguish on these parameters alone, therefore they are usually referred to as a complex. However, *M. avium* and *M. intracellulare* do differ in the degree of nitrate reduction (53) and arylsulfatase activity (45), antigen content, and in DNA and RNA make-up (54). Finally, *M. fortuitum* and *M. chelonae* are sometimes referred to as the *M. fortuitum* complex, and *M. terrae, M. nonchromogenicum,* and *M.*

Table 21-2
Some Characteristics of Selected Mycobacterial Species (34, 36, 51, 53)

Mycobacterium species	Growth		Pigment[b] in		Catalase		Niacin	Susceptible to T2H[c], 10 µg/ml	NO$_3$ Reduced	Urease	5% NaCl Tolerance	Tween 80 hydrolysis (5 days)	Pyrazinamidase Activity (4 days)	Arylsufatase Activity (3 days)	Tellurite Reduction	MacConkey Agar Growth (5 days)
	Optimum °C	Rate	Light	Dark	>45mm column	Activity after 68°C										
M. tuberculosis	37	S[a]	−	−	−	−	+	−	+	+	−	V	+	−	V	−
M. bovis	37	S	−	−	−	−	−	+	−	+	−	−	−	−	−	−
M. avium and M. intracellulare	37	S	−	−	−	V	−	−	−	−	−	−	+	−	+	V
M. chelonae	37	R	−	−	+	V	V	−	−	+	V	V	+	+	+	+
M. fortuitum	37	R	−	−	+	+	V	−	+	+	+	V	+	+	+	+
M. haemophilum		S	−	−	−	−	−	−	−	−	−	−	+	−	−	−
M. kansasii	37	S	+	−	+	+	−	−	+	+	−	+	−	−	V	−
M. marinum	32	M	+	−	−	+	−	−	−	+	−	+	+	V	V	−
M. scrofulaceum	37	S	+	+	+	+	−	−	−	+	−	−	V	V	V	−
M. ulcerans	32	S	−	−	−	+	−	−	−	V	−	−	−	−		
M. gordonae	37	S	+	+	+	+	−	−	−	−	−	+	V	V	−	−
M. phlei		R	+	+	+	+			+		+	+	+	−	+	−
M. smegmatis	37	R	−	−	+	+			+		+	+			+	−

[a] + = >85% positive; − = <15% positive; V = 15-85% positive; S = slow; R = rapid; M = moderate growth rates.
[b] Pigment is yellow to orange color.
[c] T2H = thiophene-2-carboxylic acid hydrazide.

triviale as the *M. terrae* complex. This latter group includes species usually considered nonpathogens (54).

Another method of grouping of clinically important mycobacteria includes that based on (i) growth rates, and (ii) growth rate and pigment production, the Runyon groups (35). In the first instance, the organisms are either slow growers or rapid growers, depending on whether more than 6 days are required for growth to appear (54). As seen in Table 21-2, the former group includes *M. tuberculosis*, which may require four weeks before growth appears, and *M. bovis*, which can take up to 8 weeks. In contrast, *M. fortuitum*, *M. chelonae*, and *M. smegmatis*, among the rapid growers, require less than a week, and usually growth appears within 2-3 days, especially following primary isolation (36).

While Runyon's grouping also makes use of rapid growth as a defining characteristic, emphasis is placed on chromogenicity. Keep in mind that this method was originally published in the 1950's when the tubercle bacilli were dominant in mycobacteriology. To designate those bacteria that were not included in these "classical" forms, the terms "atypical" or "anonymous" was applied (44). These were then categorized into Groups. Group I is the photochromogens which are non-pigmented bacilli when grown in the absence of light, but become bright yellow to orange when exposed to light. This group includes, among others, *M. kansasii* and *M. marinum* (see Table 21-2). Group II, the scotochromogens, produces a reddish-orange pigment in the presence or absence of light, and contains *M. scrofulaceum* and *M. gordonae*. Group III organisms are the "non-photochromogens" and are non-pigmented. There are several species here, including *M. avium*, *M. intracellulare*, *M. ulcerans*, *M. xenopi*, and *M. haemophilus*. Finally, Group IV, the "rapid growers" encompass those mentioned above, *M. fortuitum*, *M. chelonae*, *M. phlei*, and *M. smegmatis*, as well as other species.

4. Laboratory Identification Procedures

Laboratory processing of specimens suspected of containing mycobacteria may take several routes (See Figure 21-1). Direct staining of the specimen by use of the acid fast stain or the fluorescent auramine O stain (with or without a

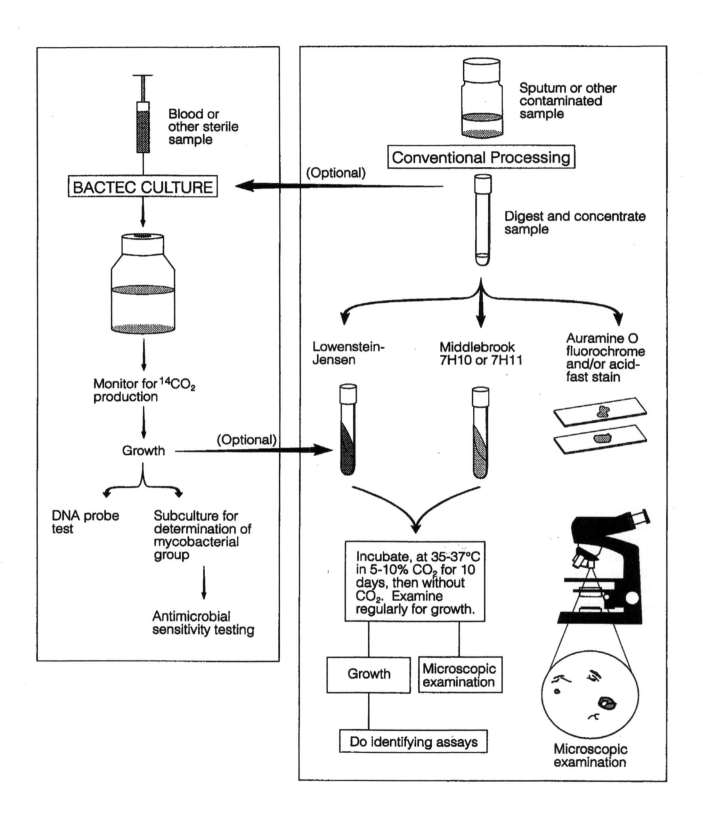

Figure 21-1: Outline of isolation and identification scheme for mycobacteria. See text for details of procedures.

rhodamine counterstain) is done on most samples other than blood. Depending on the specimen, smears may be prepared directly from it, as fecal material; or done following a concentration step, as urine; or after digestion and concentration steps, as with sputum (Photo 21-3), the most common type of sample. In any case, observation of acid fast bacilli (AFB), or fluorescing bacilli with the auramine O stain, should be reported immediately to the physician. Though not highly sensitive (perhaps 25-40% in the acid-fast stain), the specificity of the microscopic examination of stained smears is very good (up to 99%) (14). Along with clinical data, sufficient information may be provided for initiation of therapy without the delay of waiting for cultural confirmation. However, whether positive or negative information is revealed by staining, a cultural sequence as described below must be done.

The processing of a sputum specimen is a part of the work of this exercise, therefore its procedure will be described in detail later. In brief, it involves liquefaction of the sputum to release mycobacteria, followed by centrifugation to concentrate the microorganisms. The digesting solution contains a decontaminating component, as NaOH, oxalic acid, or Zephiran to reduce the microbial load from normal flora or other contaminating microorganisms. The digestant also may be the decontaminating NaOH, but trisodium phosphate, dithiothreitol, and N-acetyl-L-cysteine are also used (4, 34). Besides sputum, other contaminated specimens also can be subjected to decontamination. For example, if microscopic examination suggests the presence of mycobacteria in a stool specimen (which most commonly will represent the MAC from AIDS patients), the next step is to subject the sample to decontamination before culture (34). Always, but particularly with NaOH-containing digestants, care must be taken to follow published protocols, otherwise unwanted weakening or killing of the mycobacteria will occur yielding reduction in positive cultures. Sterile specimens do not require decontamination, but may need to be concentrated, either by centrifugation, or, especially in cerebral spinal fluid, by filtration. If the former case, leak-proof centrifuge containers should be used. Also, take care not to contaminate the lip of containers while transferring the specimen to it. Centrifuge speeds to achieve 2,000 to 4,000 x g for 20 to 30 minutes are satisfactory (4, 34), after which excess super-

natant fluid is discarded and smears and culture prepared from the sediment.

The standard culture steps involve inoculation of tube or bottled media followed by assay of growth from these. The primary culture media should include an agar-based medium (as Middlebrook 7H10 or 7H11), and an egg-based medium (as Lowenstein-Jensen or Petragnani), all of which are commercially available. Agar-based media have the advantage of being transparent allowing earlier detection, while egg-based media allows more organisms to grow and has a longer shelf life (34). Cultures are incubated in the presence of 5–10% CO_2 for up to 10 days, after which CO_2 is not required. Regular examination of cultures is done, perhaps 2–3 times per week. If mycobacterial growth is noted, smears are prepared, stained, and microscopically examined. Following adequate growth, identifying assays as seen in Table 21-2 are done.

It should be apparent that many of the most common species of mycobacteria associated with infection, as *M. tuberculosis*, the MAC, and *M. kansasii* may take weeks to identify. Many studies have therefore been done to find alternative methods to speed the identification process. One that has been successful and that is being used by many laboratories is the commercially-available BACTEC® TB System, especially in combination with a DNA probe, as that available from Gen-Probe. Briefly, BACTEC Middlebrook's 7H12 (BACTEC 12B medium) includes a ^{14}C-labeled substrate, growth factors, and antimicrobials to aid in selectivity. Samples processed as described above are injected into the vial and incubated. If $^{14}CO_2$ is produced, the presence of mycobacteria is suggested (34, 37). An acid fast or fluorochrome stain will confirm the presence of mycobacteria. Further differentiation is possible also by subculturing into BACTEC 12B containing p-nitro-α-acetyl-amino-β-hydroxypropriophenone (NAP). Only "mycobacteria other than tuberculosis" (MOTT) can grow in the presence of NAP, again measured by the release of $^{14}CO_2$. This system also can be used for susceptibility testing of mycobacteria by adding an antimicrobial to the 12B medium and then inoculating with the test organism. Each further antimicrobial to be tested requires a separate bottle of broth. Blood samples also can be cultured in the BACTEC system by adding blood from the patient directly into BACTEC 13A medium.

As a supplementary step, the Isolator™ Microbial Tube may be used for blood cultures. This contains an anticoagulant and saponin, a blood cell lysing agent. Centrifugation of the tube permits concentration of organisms prior to addition to BACTEC media or to standard plating media (34, 38, 57). Its use also has the advantage of inactivating HIV provided blood is held in the tube for at least 60 minutes (24). Isolator tubes are further useful to concentrate fungi in blood, as *Cryptococcus neoformans* (57) and *Candida* (42).

Detection of mycobacteria using the BACTEC system has reduced the time required for their detection as compared to standard culture. In one study of the BACTEC 12B system, about a 40% reduction for detection of the *M. tuberculosis* complex, and over 70% reduction for MOTT was reported (3). Other examples are reviewed in Reference 34.

Studies combining the BACTEC system with Gen-Probe radiolabeled DNA probes show that detection of mycobacteria can be hastened over that of BACTEC alone (12) since there is no need to subculture or do biochemical assays. This is because the *M. tuberculosis* complex and MAC are identified directly by the probe (20, 33). More recently, non-isotopically labeled Accuprobe™ has been used, but blood can cause false positive reactions, especially for the *M. tuberculosis* complex (21). This problem does not occur with culture-isolated bacteria where greater than 95% sensitivity can be achieved for it, MAC, and *M. gordonae*. The *M. kansasii* assay was, however, insensitive in limited testing (28). Recently a DNA probe that uses a non-radiolabeled alkaline phosphatase label (SNAP® Culture Identification Diagnostic Kit) has become available for the *M. tuberculosis* and *M. avium* complexes. The specificity and sensitivity of this system are 99% and 100%, respectively, when tested on L-J medium cultures (29). Such a system holds promise for other identification protocols.

A variety of other techniques has also been and are being investigated to achieve more rapid diagnosis of mycobacterial infections. Examples include the application of the PCR reaction (e.g. 13, 22, 39), which may be applicable to identification of an organism directly from sputum (19), even within one working day (50). Furthermore, it has promise for the identification of *M. leprae* for diagnosis of leprosy (23, 55). Gas chromatography (25), high performance gas liquid chromatography (8), electron capture GLC (6), and thin layer chromatography (5) have also been investigated. Furthermore, polyacrylamide gel electrophoresis of soluble protein patterns (15) and the use of monoclonal antibodies (48) are being examined.

Remembering that most cases of tuberculosis occur in underdeveloped nations, it is unfortunate that many techniques mentioned above are prohibitive because of cost and technical training required to do them. While stains and standard culture techniques are applicable and useful, development of inexpensive and technically simple rapid assays are needed.

Although not commonly done, typing of some mycobacteria also may be done for epidemiological purposes. *M. tuberculosis* can be placed in one of eight phage types (26, 40). Serological groupings have also been accomplished with *M. avium* and *M. intracellulare* (16, 46, 58).

The present exercise is designed to take you through some cultural methods of mycobacterial identification. However, you should be aware that the mycobacteria are a proven hazard to laboratory workers (47) and obviously can cause pulmonary infection. Therefore, beware of producing an aerosol from clinical and culture material. Always wear a laboratory gown or coat, and gloves when handling viable culture material. When working with open cultures (including smear preparations, transferring, testing cultures, etc.), do so within the confines of a biological safety hood. Remember to decontaminate your work area with ample amounts of disinfectant before and following your work.

MATERIALS

Part 1
For each pair of students:

1 Lowenstein-Jensen (L-J) culture each of *Mycobacterium tuberculosis* Strain H37Ra (ATCC No. 25177), *M. kansasii*, *M. avium*, and *M. phlei*

8 tubes Middlebrook 7H10 agar slants

2 tubes Tween 80 medium

2 tubes pyrazinamide test agar, 5 ml/tube

2 tubes mycobacterial nitrate broth, 2 ml/ tube

1 tube containing 5 ml distilled water

1 5 ml unplugged, unsterile pipette
5 pieces aluminum foil (to cover tubes)
For each bench:
Mycobacteria nitrate reduction reagents
(MNRR)-A, B, and C (Appendix 3)
1 set of color standards for nitrate test
Auramine O-rhodamine fluorochrome stain-
ing reagents (if fluorescent microscope avail-
able)
Ziehl-Neelsen acid-fast staining reagents
For Class:
5-10% CO_2 atmosphere incubator

Part 2

A. Per pair of students:
Sputum sample
1 50 ml leak proof centrifuge tube
1 pipette bulb,
1 10 ml pipette, unsterile
1 wide bore tip, unsterile 10 ml pipette,
cotton plugged
applicator sticks
10 cc digestant solution (Appendix 3)
45 ml M/15 phosphate buffer, pH 6.8
1 ml 0.2% bovine serum albumin solution
5 ml 5% phenol solution
cotton pledget
splash-proof discard container
2 tubes Lowenstein-Jensen slants
1 piece aluminum foil
Per Bench:
5-10% CO_2 atmosphere incubator
Ziehl-Neelsen acid-fast staining reagents
Vortex mixer
B. Per pair of students:
2 cotton plugged Pasteur pipettes
pipette bulb
2 12 X 75 mm unsterile tubes with stoppers
Niacin strips
Catalase reagent (with Tween 80)
Per bench:
1 dropper bottle containing 10% NaOH
1 dropper bottle with freshly-prepared 1%
ammonium ferroussulfate

Part 3

Catalase reagent (with Tween 80)
Ziehl-Neelsen acid-fast stain reagents

LABORATORY PROCEDURES

> **NOTE:** USE EXTREME CARE IN WORK-
> ING WITH ORGANISMS IN THIS EXER-
> CISE. Use a biohazard or other protective
> hood for work with the pathogenic myco-
> bacteria. Line the work area with absorbent
> paper and thoroughly wet (and keep wet) with
> disinfectant. Loops and needles are preferably
> sterilized within enclosed electrical heaters
> (e.g. Bacti-Cinerator® III or Steri-Loop®
> Bacteriology Incinerator). If suitable facilities
> are not available, it is recommended that
> culture procedures be restricted to those
> laboratories where the organisms can be
> properly and safely studied.
>
> Despite the use of organisms of relatively
> low virulence in this exercise, plan your work to
> be as efficient as possible. The fewer transfers
> made, the less opportunities for inadvertent
> contamination of the environment.

Part 1

Known cultures: Each pair of students will be
provided with cultures of *M. tuberculosis* H37Ra,
M. kansasii, *M. avium*, and *M. phlei* on
Lowenstein-Jensen slants. With these carry out
the following (4, 34, 49):

1. Examine each culture, describe, and record
your findings.
2. Carefully prepare smears of each culture
and stain by the Ziehl Neelsen acid-fast
procedure (Photo 21-4.) The procedure is
as follows: (i) Prepare smears and heat-fix
in the usual manner; (ii) stain smear 3-5
minutes with carbol fuchsin providing
sufficient heat to give gentle steaming, but
not active boiling; (iii) cool slide, briefly
rinse in water, then decolorize with acid-
alcohol until only a slight pink remains.
Wash in tap water; (iv) counterstain for
about 30 seconds with methylene blue and
again wash in tap water; and (v) allow smear
to dry, then examine. Acid-fast organisms
will appear red with blue granules, while
other organisms are blue.

Compare the morphology (relative length,
width, presence of granules, branching,
etc.) of the four species. Alternatively, if a
fluorescent microscope is available, first
carry out the auramine O-rhodamine fluorochrome stain (Appendix 2) and observe

each organism. The procedure for this is:

a. Fix smear at 65°C for at least 2 hours.

b. Stain smear at room temperature for 15 minutes.

c. Rinse slide with distilled water, then decolorize with acidified ethanol for two to three minutes, and again rinse well with distilled water.

d. Counterstain with permanganate solution for two to four minutes, then rinse with distilled water.

e. Microscopically examine with fluorescent microscope.

An advantage of the fluorochrome stain is that detection of organisms can be made more readily using a lower magnification. Thus, by this method, smears can be scanned with the 10X objective, and verification of morphology done with the 40-50X objective. If fluorescent-positive organisms are seen, these same smears are then restained by the acid-fast method and their acid fast character confirmed by conventional microscopy.

3. Transfer each organism to two slants of Middlebrook 7H10 agar. To test for photochromogenicity, shield one tube containing each species from light with aluminum foil; expose the other to light. Incubate in a 5-10% CO_2-air atmosphere, either within a CO_2 incubator or in a jar containing a CO_2-generating packet. Only after good growth (but still having individual colonies) is evident in the *uncovered* tube, examine the companion tube held in the dark as described in *Part 2B-2*.

Because of the differing growth rates of the stock culture bacteria, if a CO_2 jar is used, it will be necessary to open it to remove the rapid grower(s). If 10 days of incubation have not elapsed regenerate the CO_2 atmosphere for the remaining slower growers. However, after 10 days, all tubes are to be removed and incubated under normal atmospheric conditions. Examine at regular intervals to assess progress of growth.

4. Transfer a full loop of *M. avium* and *M. phlei* only to separate tubes of Tween 80 medium. Incubate for 5 days without added CO_2.

5. Inoculate full loops of *M. kansasii* and *M. avium* to separate tubes of pyrazinamide

agar. Incubate for 5 days without increased CO_2.

6. Incubate all cultures at 35-37°C. Do not over-tighten closures on tubes or growth of these aerobic organisms may be restricted. Examine cultures at times noted above.

7. Do the nitrate reduction test as follows:

a. In separate 16 X 125 mm tubes containing 2 ml $NaNO_3$ emulsify a loopful of culture from the stock cultures of *M. avium* and *M. phlei* only.

b. Gently shake tubes without tilting and incubate in a 37°C water bath for 2 hours.

c. Add to each tube 1 drop of mycobacterial nitrate reducing reagent (MNRR)-A (1:2 dilution HCl), and 2 drops each of MNRR-B (0.2% sulfanilamide), and MNRR-C (1% N-naphylethylenediamine) solutions.

d. Observe tubes for development of a red to pink color. If a color does not develop, add a small amount of zinc dust to confirm the negative test. The color reactions may be compared to color standards for further quantitation. (Method for the preparation of color standards is also given in Appendix 3).

8. For subsequent determination of niacin production by mycobacteria, carefully add 1.5 ml distilled water to each stock culture tube of *M. tuberculosis* and *M. avium* after all of the previous steps are completed. Clearly label these with your name, course number, then place in a container provided by the instructor. These will be autoclaved and returned for further analysis.

Part 2

A. Examination and culture of tubercle bacillus from sputum: The following procedure involves the use of sputum obtained from the clinical laboratory. Handle with care. Remember, tuberculosis is usually contracted by the respiratory route. Any procedure which leads to the formation of an aerosol could subsequently lead to infection. Continue to work in the biohazard hood. Line the work area with absorbent paper saturated with disinfectant.

1. Select one of the sputum samples provided (1 per pair of students).

2. Using a pipette with a large bore opening and a pipette bulb, *carefully* transfer 10 ml of sputum to a 50 ml leak proof centrifuge tube. Be sure the tube is not cracked or show signs of other damage. Use applicator sticks to aid in teasing the sputum apart at the tip of the pipette if necessary. (Don't forget to have appropriate containers for pipette and applicator stick disposal near your work area.)

3. Add an equal volume of digesting reagent (*N*-acetyl-L-cysteine/citrate/NaOH solution) to the tube.

4. Tightly close the centrifuge tube and mix on a vortex-type apparatus in the hood. Now, incubate for 15 minutes at room temperature with occasional gentle swirling.

5. Fill the tube to within ¾ inch of the top with M/15 phosphate buffer, pH 6.8. Again within the biohazard hood, centrifuge at 2000 x g for 15 minutes, then carefully decant supernatant liquid into the splash-proof liquid discard container provided. Wipe the lip of the tube with cotton soaked in 5% disinfectant solution.

6. With a loop that is 3 mm in diameter, prepare 2 smears of the sediment covering an area of about 2 mm x 3 mm, and stain by the acid-fast method. Observe both smear preparations at 1000X and report your results as follows (2):

Average No. Cells Observed	Report
0	Negative for AFB[a]
1-2 in 300 fields	±
1-9 in 100 fields	+1
1-9 in 10 fields	+2
1-9 in one field	+3
>9 in one field	+4

[a]AFB = acid fast bacilli

7. Add 1 ml of 0.2% solution of bovine serum albumin to the tube. Mix the sediment with a loop and transfer one loopful to each of two tubes of Lowenstein-Jensen medium. Wrap one tube in foil. Incubate at 35-37°C in a 5-10% atmosphere for at least the first

ten days. Observe at regular intervals. After growth expose contents of the wrapped tube to light. Report as with known cultures.

B. Known cultures:
1. On the fifth day examine only the unwrapped 7H10 cultures. Describe colony characteristics of *M. phlei*. Compare the relative amount of growth with that of *M. tuberculosis*, *M. avium*, and *M. kansasii*. Also, compare colony characteristics, including pigmentation, when good growth of the latter has been obtained.

2. When obvious visible growth (but culture is still actively growing, a requirement for the photochromogenic effect to occur) (35) is seen on each uncovered slant, unwrap its companion culture containing the same species. Note its color. Now, expose it to light from an incandescent lamp for not less than one hour. After further incubation at 35-37°C in the dark for 24 hours, compare the pigmentation of these to that of tubes that were not covered during the entire incubation period.

3. Observe whether Tween 80 has been hydrolyzed after 5 days of incubation. A positive test is seen by the pink to red color of the medium (not the cells). Discard positive cultures and reincubate negative cultures. Reexamine after 10-12 days of incubation then discard whether positive or negative. Record.

4. Complete the pyrazinamidase assay by adding 1 ml (20 drops) of freshly prepared ammonium ferrous sulfate to each tube of pyrazinamide agar containing *M. kansasii* and *M. avium*. Place in the refrigerator (to suppress growth of contaminants) until a pink band forms in the agar, or for up to four hours. Discard tubes after this. Does either organism produce pyrazinamidase? Does your data correspond to that of Table 21-2?

5. Complete the niacin test in the following manner:
a. Retrieve your autoclaved cultures of *M. tuberculosis* and *M. avium*.
b. Remove approximately 0.6 ml of liquid from each tube with a Pasteur pipette and deliver to separate 12 X 75 mm tubes.

c. With a pair of forceps, place a niacin strip into each tube with arrow at the bottom. Immediately stopper tube to avoid the escape of cyanogen bromide gas generated in subsequent chemical reactions.

d. Gently shake each tube without tilting. Shake again after 5 and 10 minutes. During this time acidified potassium thiocyanate and chloramine T, both contained in the strip, mix causing a release of cyanogen chloride. This reacts with niacin in the presence of p-amino-salicylic acid (also contained in the strip) to give a yellow color in the medium. A yellow color within 30 minutes is therefore a positive test (18). After tests are completed, add 1-2 drops of 10% NaOH to each tube to neutralize test reagents, then discard.

Is either *M. tuberculosis* or *M. avium* positive for niacin production? Examination of Table 21-2 will show that the former should be positive. Indeed, it alone of all mycobacterial species likely to be associated with humans regularly has this characteristic. Because of this tentative identification of *M. tuberculosis* can be made if such a result is obtained.

6. Test the 7H10 slant of each organism for the presence of catalase. This is done by placing a drop of catalase reagent (containing Tween 80) on the growth in one of each of the duplicate tube cultures, again within a biohazard hood. Observe for the evolution of gas. Discard this culture following the test. (Do not remove cultures from within the hood until reaction has stopped and cap tightened.)

7. Tabulate your results and discuss.

Part 3

Sputum cultures: Observe at regular intervals for growth up to 4 weeks. If growth occurs, describe. If none occurs, report as negative. Compare these results with that obtained by observing the acid fast stain of the original sputum concentrate (*Part* 2A-6). Does the amount of growth correspond to findings of the microscopic observation? Which is the more sensitive procedure? Why? Finally, if growth does occur, do an acid fast stain on it to confirm the presence of an acid fast bacillus. Apply catalase reagent as described in *Part* 2B-6. Is it catalase positive and acid fast positive?

Finally, remove the light shield from the companion tube, note the culture color, and compare this to the uncovered culture. Now, expose this formerly covered tube to light as described in *Part* 2B-2 and reincubate overnight.

Record and discuss all of your findings. Have you compiled sufficient information to speciate the known cultures? The sputum isolate (if any)? If not, give further assays required to name these organisms to species.

QUESTIONS

1. What importance does the tuberculin test have in the diagnosis of tuberculosis or tuberculosis-like infections?

2. Provide information concerning the following biochemical assays done in this exercise.

   a. Give the chemical name of Tween 80. What causes the appearance of a positive test, including the changing of the solution from colorless to pink? (Hint: See references 4, 27, and/or 31.)

   b. Describe the pyrazinamidase reaction, starting with the compound pyrazinamide shown below. (Hint: See references 1 and 52.)

Pyrazinamide

3. Among the battery of possible tests for mycobacterial separation and identification, some have more significance for a particular organism or group of organisms. The niacin test, as described in *Part* 2B-5, for example, is very useful for the identification of *M. tuberculosis*. For the following assays, give the organism(s) listed in Table 21-2 for which they are most useful in their separation from other species and identification.

   a. Pyrazinamidase test.
   b. Nitrate test.
   c. Arylsulfatase test.
   d. Thiophene-2-carboxylic acid hydrazide (T2H) test.

REFERENCES

1. Allen, W. S., S. M. Aronovic, L. M. Brancone, and J. H. Williams. 1953. Determination of the pyrazinamide content of blood and urine. Anal. Chem. **25**:895-897.

2. American Thoracic Society. 1981. Diagnostic standards and classification of tuberculosis and other mycobacterial diseases. Am. Rev. Respir. Dis. **123**:343-355.

3. Anargyros, P., D. S. J. Astill, and I. S. L. Lim. 1990. Comparison of improved BACTEC and Lowenstein-Jensen media for culture of mycobacteria from clinical specimens. J. Clin. Microbiol. **28**:1288-1291.

4. Baron, E. J., L. R. Peterson, and S. M. Finegold. 1994. Bailey & Scott's diagnostic microbiology, 9th ed. Mosby-Year Book, Inc., St. Louis. p. 590-633.

5. Bosne, S., and V. V.-Lévy-Frébault. 1992. Mycobactin analysis as an aid for the identification of *Mycobacterium fortuitum* and *Mycobacterium chelonae* subspecies. J. Clin. Microbiol. **30**: 1225-1231.

6. Brooks, J. B., M. I. Daneshvar, R. L. Haberberger, and I. A. Mikhail. 1990. Rapid diagnosis of tuberculous meningitis by frequency-pulsed electron-capture gas-liquid chromatography detection of carboxylic acids in cerebrospinal fluid. J. Clin. Microbiol. **28**:989-997.

7. Bullock, W. E. 1990. Mycobacterium leprae (leprosy), p. 1906-1914. In G. L. Mandell, R. G. Douglas, Jr., and J. E. Bennett (ed.), Principles and practices of infectious diseases, 3rd ed. Churchill Livingstone, New York.

8. Butler, W. R., and J. O. Kilburn. 1990. High performance liquid chromatography patterns of mycolic acid as criteria for identification of *Mycobacterium chelonae*, *Mycobacterium fortuitum*, and *Mycobacterium smegmatis*. J. Clin. Microbiol **28**:2094-2098.

9. Centers for Disease Control. 1989. A strategic plan for the elimination of tuberculosis in the United States. MMWR **38**(S-3): 1-25.

10. Centers for Disease Control. 1992. Prevention and control of tuberculosis in U. S. communities with at-risk minority populations and prevention and control of tuberculosis among homeless persons. MMWR **41**(RR-5):1-23.

11. Centers for Disease Control. 1991. Summary of notifiable diseases, United States 1990. MMWR **39**:1-61.

12. Colombrita, D., G. Ravizzola, G. Pinsi, R. Li Vigni, F. Pirali, and A. Turano. 1990. Rapid detection and identification of mycobacteria from blood of patients with acquired immune deficiency syndrome. J. Med. Microbiol. **32**:271-273.

13. Cousins, D. V., S. D. Wilton, B. R. Francis, and B. L. Gow. 1992. Use of polymerase chain reaction for rapid diagnosis of tuberculosis. J. Clin. Microbiol. **30**:255-258.

14. Daniel, T. M. 1990. The rapid diagnosis of tuberculosis. A selective review. J. Lab. Clin. Med. **116**:277-282.

15. De Jong, A., A. H. Hoetjen, and A. G. M. Van Der Zanden. 1991. A rapid method for identification of *Mycobacterium* species by polyacrylamide gel electrophoresis of soluble cell proteins. J. Med. Microbiol. **34**:1-5.

16. Denner, J. C., A. Y. Tsang, D. Chatterjee, and P. J. Brennan. 1992. Comprehensive approach to identification of serovars of *Mycobacterium avium* complex. J. Clin. Microbiol. **30**:473-478.

17. Des Prez, R. M., and C. R. Heim. 1990. Mycobacterium tuberculosis, p. 1877-1906. In G. L. Mandell, R. G. Douglas, Jr., and J. E. Bennett (ed.), Principles and practices of infectious diseases, 3rd ed. Churchill Livingstone, New York.

18. Difco Laboratories. 1984. Difco Manual, 10th ed. Difco Laboratories, Detroit, MI. p. 923-925.

19. Eisenach, K. D., M. D. Sifford, M. D. Cave, J. H. Bates, and J. T. Crawford. 1991. Detection of *Mycobacterium tuberculosis* in sputum samples using a polymerase chain reaction. Am. Rev. Respir. Dis. **144**:1160-1163.

20. Ellner, P. D., T. E. Kiehn, R. Cammarata, and M. Hosmer. 1988. Rapid detection and identification of pathogenic mycobacteria by combining radiometric and nucleic acid probe methods. J. Clin. Microbiol. **26**:1349-1352.

21. Evans, K. D., A. S. Nakasone, P. A. Sutherland, L. M. DE LA Maza, and E. M. Peterson. 1992. Identification of *Mycobacterium tuberculosis* and *Mycobacterium avium-M. intracellulare* directly from primary BACTEC cultures using acridinium-ester-labeled DNA probes. J. Clin. Microbiol. **30**:2427-2431.

22. Fries, J. W. U., R. J. Patel, W. F. Piessens, and D. F. Wirth. 1991. Detection of untreated mycobacteria by using polymerase chain reaction and specific DNA probes. J. Clin. Microbiol. **29**:1744-1747.

23. Hartskeerl, R. A., M. Y. L. De Wit, and P. R. Klatser. 1989. Polymerase chain reaction for detection of *Mycobacterium leprae*. J. Gen. Microbiol. **135**:2357-2364.

24. Hodinka, R. L., P. H. Gilligan, and L. Smiley. 1988. Survival of human immunodeficiency virus in blood culture systems. Arch. Pathol. Lab. Med. **112**:1251-1254.

25. Jantzen, E., T. Tangen, and J. Eng. 1989. Gas chromatography of mycobacterial fatty acids and alcohols: diagnostic applications. APMIS **97**:1037-1045.

26. Jones, W. D., Jr., R. C. Good, N. J. Thompson, and G. D. Kelly. 1982. Bacteriophage types of *Mycobacterium tuberculosis* in the United States. Am. Rev. Respir. Dis. **125**:640-643.

27. Koneman, E. W., S. D. Allen, W. M. Janda, P. C. Schreckenberger, and W. C. Winn, Jr. 1992. Color atlas and textbook of diagnostic microbiology, 4th ed. J. B. Lippincott Co., Philadelphia. p. 703-755.

28. Lebrun, L., F. Espinasse, J. D. Poveda, and V. Vincent-Lévy-Frébault. 1992. Evaluation of nonradioactive DNA probes for identification of mycobacteria. J. Clin. Microbiol. **30**:2476-2478.

29. Lim, S. D., J. Todd, J. Lopez, E. Ford, and J. M. Janda. 1991. Genotypic identification of pathogenic *Mycobacterium* species by using a nonradioactive oligonucleotide probe. J. Clin. Microbiol. **29**:1276-1278.

30. Meyaard, L., S. A. Otto, R. R. Jonker, M. J. Mijnster, R. P. M. Keet, and F. Miedema. 1992. Programmed death of T cells in HIV-1 infection. Science **257**:217-219.

31. Musial, C. E., and G. D. Roberts. 1987. Tuberculosis and other mycobacterioses, p. 539-580. In B. B. Wentworth (ed.), Diagnostic procedures for bacterial infections, 7th ed. American Public Health Association, Inc., Washington, D. C.

32. Noordeen, S. K., L. Lopez Bravo, and D. Daumerie. 1991. Global review of multidrug therapy (MDT) in leprosy. Wld. Hlth. Statist. Quart. **44**:2-15.

33. Peterson, E. M., R. Lu, C. Floyd, A. Nakasone, G. Friedly, and L. M. DE LA Maza. 1989. Direct identification of *Mycobacterium tuberculosis*, *Mycobacterium avium*, and *Mycobacterium intracellulare* from amplified primary cultures in BACTEC media using DNA probes. J. Clin. Microbiol. **27**:1543-1547.

34. Roberts, G. D., E. W. Koneman, and Y. K. Kim. 1991. *Mycobacterium*, p. 304-339. In A. Balows, W. J. Hausler, Jr., K. L. Herrmann, H. D. Isenberg, and H. J. Shadomy (ed.), Manual of clinical microbiology, 5th ed. American Society for Microbiology, Washington, D. C.

35. Runyon, E. H. 1959. Anonymous mycobacteria in pulmonary disease. Med. Clin. North Am. **43**:273-290.

36. Sanders, W. E., Jr., and E. A. Horowitz. 1990. Other mycobacterial species, p. 1914-1926. In G. L. Mandell, R. G. Douglas, Jr., and J. E. Bennett (ed.), Principles and practices of infectious diseases, 3rd ed. Churchill Livingstone, New York.

37. Schweinle, J. E. 1990. Evolving concepts of the epidemiology, diagnosis, and therapy of *Mycobacterium tuberculosis* infection. Yale J. Biol. Med. **63**:565-579.

38. Shanson, D. C., and M. S. Dryden. 1988. Comparison of methods for isolating *Mycobacterium avium-intracellulare* from blood of patients with AIDS. J. Clin. Pathol. **41**:687-690.

39. Sjöbring, U., M. Mecklenburg, Å. B. Andersen, and H. Miörner. 1990. Polymerase chain reaction for detection of *Mycobacterium tuberculosis*. J. Clin. Microbiol. **28**:2200-2204.

40. Snider, D. E., Jr., W. D. Jones, and R. C. Good. 1984. The usefulness of phage typing *Mycobacterium tuberculosis* isolates. Am. Rev. Respir. Dis. **130**:1095-1099.

41. Sudre, P., G. ten Dam, and A. Kochi. 1992. Tuberculosis: a global overview of the situation today. Bull. Wld. Hlth. Org. **70**:149-152.

42. Telenti, A., J. M. Steckelberg, L. Stockman, R. S. Edson, and G. D. Roberts. 1991. Quantitative blood cultures in candidemia. Mayo Clin. Proc. **66**:1120-1123.

43. Timoney, J. F., J. H. Gillespie, F. W. Scott, and J. E. Barlough. 1988. Hagan and Bruner's microbiology and infectious diseases of domestic animals, 8th ed. Comstock Publishing Associates, Ithica, NY. p. 270-289.

44. Timpe, A., and E. H. Runyon. 1954. The relationship of "atypical" acid-fast bacteria to human disease. A preliminary report. J. Lab. Clin. Med. **44**:202-209.

45. Tomioka, H., H. Saito, K. Sato, and D. J. Dawson. 1990. Arylsulfatase activity for differentiating *Mycobacterium avium* and *Mycobacterium intracellulare*. J. Clin. Microbiol. **28**:2104-2106.

46. Tsang, A. Y., J. C. Denner, P. J. Brennan, and J. K. McClatchy. 1992. Clinical and epidemiological importance of typing of *Mycobacterium avium* complex isolates. J. Clin. Microbiol. **30**:479-484.

47. U. S. Public Health Service, Centers for Disease Control and National Institutes of Health. 1988. Biosafety in microbiological and biomedical laboratories, 2nd ed. Publication No. (NIH) 88-8395. Dept. of Health and Human Services, Washington, DC., p. 45-92.

48. Verstijnen, C. P. H. J., H. M. Ly, K. Polman, C. Richter, S. P. Smits, S. Y. Maselle, P. Peerbooms, D. Rienthong, N. Montreewasuwat, S. Koanjanart, D. D. Trach, S. Kuijper, and A. H. J. Kolk. 1991. Enzyme-linked immunosorbent assay using monoclonal antibodies for identification of mycobacteria from early cultures. J. Clin. Microbiol. **29**:1372-1375.

49. Vestel, A. L. 1975. Procedures for the isolation and identification of mycobacteria. HEW Publication No. (CDC) 77-8230, U. S. Department of Health, Education, and Welfare, Center for Disease Control, Atlanta, GA., p. 33-39, 65-90, 125-126.

50. Victor, T., R. du Toit, and P. D. van Helden. 1992. Purification of sputum samples through sucrose improves detection of *Mycobacterium tuberculosis* by polymerase chain reaction. J. Clin. Microbiol. **30**:1514-1517.

51. Vincent-Lévy-Frébault, V., and F. Portaels. 1992. Proposed minimum standards for the genus *Mycobacterium* and for description of new slowly growing *Mycobacterium* species. Int. J. Syst. Bacteriol. **42**:315-323.

52. Wayne, L. G. 1974. Simple pyrazinamidase and urease tests for routine identification of mycobacteria. Am. Rev. Resp. Dis. **109**:147-151.

53. Wayne, L. G., and G. P. Kubica. 1986. Genus *Mycobacterium* Lehmann and Neumann 1896. p. 1436-1457. *In* P. H. A. Sneath, N. S. Mair, M. E. Sharpe, and J. G. Holt (ed.). Bergey's manual of systematic bacteriology, Vol. 2. Williams & Wilkins, Baltimore.

54. Wayne, L. G., and H. A. Sramek. 1992. Agents of newly recognized or infrequently encountered mycobacterial diseases. Clin. Microbiol. Rev. **5**:1-25.

55. Williams, D. L., T. P. Gillis, R. J. Booth, D. Looker, and J. D. Watson. 1990. The use of a specific DNA probe and polymerase chain reaction for the detection of *Mycobacterium leprae*. J. Infect. Dis. **162**:193-200.

56. Wolinsky, E. 1992. Mycobacterial diseases other than tuberculosis. Clin. Infect. Dis. **15**:1-12.

57. Yagupsky, P., and M. A. Menegus. 1990. Cumulative positivity rates of multiple blood cultures for *Mycobacterium avium-intracellulare and Cryptococcus neoformans* in patients with the acquired immunodeficiency syndrome. Arch. Pathol. Lab. Med. **114**:923-925.

58. Yakrus, M. A., and R. C. Good. 1990. Geographic distribution, frequency, and specimen source of *Mycobacterium avium* complex serotypes isolated from patients with acquired immunodeficiency syndrome. J. Clin. Microbiol. **28**:926-929.

Exercise 21
Data Table 1: *Mycobacterium* Known Culture Results

		M. tuberculosis			M. kansasii			M. avium			M. phlei		
		Age[a]	L-J[b]	7H10	Age	L-J	7H10	Age	L-J	7H10	Age	L-J	7H10
Colony size and Colony Form	mm												
	Punctiform												
	Irregular												
	Circular												
	Rhizoid												
	Filamentous												
	Other												
Colony Surface	Flat												
	Raised												
	Convex												
	Pulvinate												
	Other												
Colony Margin	Entire												
	Undulate												
	Lobate												
	Erose												
	Other												
Colony Consistency	Butyrous			■			■			■			■
	Viscid			■			■			■			■
	Membranous			■			■			■			■
	Brittle			■			■			■			■
	Other			■			■			■			■
Colony Optical Character	Opaque												
	Translucent												
	Dull												
	Glistening												
	Other												
Colony Surface	Smooth												
	Rough												
	Other												
Photo-chromogenic properties	Light-shielded-1[c]	■			■			■			■		
	Light-shielded-2	■			■			■			■		
	Unshielded	■			■			■			■		
	Photochromogenic	■			■			■			■		
	Color	■			■			■			■		
Growth rate													

[a] Culture age at time of observation, in days. [b] L-J = Lowenstein-Jensen slants; 7H10 = Middlebrook 7H10 agar tubes. [c] Tubes shielded from light require two readings, one before light exposure ("Light-shielded-1") a second after light exposure and incubation ("Light shielded-2").

Exercise 21
Data Table 2: *Mycobacterium* Known Culture Results

		M. tuberculosis			M. kansasii			M. avium			M. phlei		
		Age[a]	Medium[b]	Results	Age	Medium	Results	Age	Medium	Results	Age	Medium	Results
Microscopic:													
Auramine O (10X)	Relative No.[c]												
Ziehl-Neelsen	Relative No.												
Stain	Acid fast												
(1000X)	Shape												
	Branching												
	Granules												
	Relative size												
	Other												
Tween 80[d]													
Pyrazinamidase[d]													
Niacin Test[d]													
Nitrate test	(− to +5)												
Catalase test[d]													
Other													

[a] Culture age at time of observation, in days.
[b] Name of medium from which species derived for test.
[c] See *Part 2*A-6.
[d] Record relative intensity of these results as +1 (minimum positive reaction) to +4 (strong reaction), or − (no reaction).

Other Laboratory Notes

Other Descriptions:

Appearance of Auramine O-Rhodamine Fluorochrome Stain:

Exercise 21
Data Table 3: *Mycobacterium* Sputum Isolate Results

A. Microscopic Observations (_____ X magnification):

   1. Acid fast stain of sputum digest   Date: _____

   2. Acid fast stain of Lowenstein-Jensen (L-J) slant culture:
      Date: _____ Culture Age: _____

B. Culture Observations on L-J Medium:

Observation No.	Date	Culture Age (Days)	Results
1			
2			
3			
4			
5			
6			
7			

C. Photochromogenic Property of Isolate:

   Date: _____ Culture Age: _____

   Covered tube: Length of light exposure: _____

   1. Color before light exposure: _____

   2. Color after light exposure: _____

   Uncovered tube: Color _____

D. Catalase Reaction of Isolate:

   Date: _____ Culture Age: _____

   Results:

Exercise 21
Data Table 4: *Mycobacterium* Sputum Culture Description

		Sputum isolate	
		Age[a]	L-J[b]
Colony size and Colony Form	mm		
	Punctiform		
	Irregular		
	Circular		
	Rhizoid		
	Filamentous		
	Other		
Colony Surface	Flat		
	Raised		
	Convex		
	Pulvinate		
	Other		
Colony Margin	Entire		
	Undulate		
	Lobate		
	Erose		
	Other		
Colony Consistency	Butyrous		
	Viscid		
	Membranous		
	Brittle		
	Other		
Colony Optical Character	Opaque		
	Translucent		
	Dull		
	Glistening		
	Other		
Colony Surface	Smooth		
	Rough		
	Other		
Growth rate			

[a] Culture age at time of observation, in days.
[b] L-J = Lowenstein-Jensen slants

Exercise 21
Mycobacterium

Laboratory Notes

EXERCISE 22
Actinomyces, Nocardia, Rhodococcus, and *Streptomyces*

A group of Gram-positive bacteria that form filamentous, branching, somewhat fungal-like growth induce infections that resemble mycotic diseases. Their filaments (or hyphae) easily fragment to form typical bacterial coccoid, bacilli, or diphtheroid forms, these frequently being likened to arthrospores. Sometimes, spores are also formed in separate fruiting structures. These organisms all belong to a group called the actinomycetes, and include, among others, the *Actinomyces, Nocardia, Rhodococcus,* and *Streptomyces.* These will be the subject of this exercise.

An understanding of the present organization of these actinomycetes, and how this relates to their practical clinical study is informative. In the eighth and earlier editions of *Bergey's Manual of Determinative Bacteriology* these bacteria and similar organisms, including the mycobacteria, were phylogenetically grouped in the Order *Actinomycetales.* The families *Actinomycetaceae, Nocardiaceae,* and *Streptomycetaceae* contained the respective genus *Actinomyces, Nocardia,* and *Streptomyces* (11). At that time, the proper taxonomy of *Rhodococcus* was obscure, therefore a genus for it did not exist. With the accumulation of new data, however, phylogeny of families were not as closely related as was once supposed. Thus, in the current Bergey's Manual, *Actinomyces* is one of the "Irregular Nonsporing Gram-positive Rods," *Nocardia* and *Rhodococcus* are "Nocardioform Actinomycetes," and *Streptomyces* are in "Strep-tomycetes and Related Genera." On a practical basis, the *Actinomyces,* having been released from their family ties, are now frequently grouped with their anaerobic counterparts, and have become the responsibility of the Anaerobe Laboratory for study and identification. Historically, also, the study of the actinomycetes, because of their fungal-like characteristics, has been the object of study by the medical mycologists, the reason for the use of mycological terminology as "hyphae" and "arthrospores." (See Section II, page 339 for more mycological vocabulary.) This continues to be true to some extent even today.

Of course, changing taxonomy has no influence on diseases caused by these organisms. In many the infections are slow to develop, and resemble fungal infections. A good example of this is actinomycetoma due to *N. brasiliensis, N. asteroides* (Photo 22-1), *N. otitidiscaviarum,* and *S. somoliensis.* This disease, which occurs in the tropical zone countries as India and Mexico, is manifest early as a papule, usually of the foot, that then develops into a painless, indurated mass. Its characteristics are the same as eumycetoma caused by certain true fungi.

Unlike the tropics, the most common form of nocardia infection in the United States is nocardiosis, a tuberculosis-like pulmonary infection that can disseminate to other organs. Of the 500 to 1000 cases of nocardia cases per year during 1972-1974, *N. asteriodes* was responsible for over 80% of cases, and 53% of the total cases were considered opportunistic (3). In contrast, the incidence of rhodococcal infection, usually due to *R. equi* (formerly called *Corynebacterium equi*) is rare, although it can be expected to increase, especially with the broadening advance of HIV infections. It has been described as a human pathogen only since the late 1960's, occurring as an opportunistic agent in patients with an immune defect, especially now in AIDS. The clinical expression of this organism is usually pneumonia, resembling tuberculosis and nocardiosis (5, 12). *R. equi* also has long been recognized as a common cause of zoonoses, especially bronchopneumonia among foals and lymphadenitis in swine (17).

Among the *Actinomyces* spp., *A. israelii* is the most common cause of an infrequently occurring disease, actinomycosis. In humans this is usually a chronic granulomatous and opportunistic suppurative infection. This species, like the less frequent disease agents *A. naeslundii, A. viscosus, A. odontolyticus,* and *A. meyeri,* is normal flora of mucous membranes, especially of the oral cavity (13). *A. bovis* (Photo 22-2) also causes "lumpy jaw," a common disease of cattle (21). While actinomycetes are uncommon isolates from humans, some are very common in our environment, therefore nocardiae, rhodococci, and streptomycetes contaminants may appear in samples to confuse the issue. Because of this, isolates should be obtained from more than a single specimen to verify laboratory diagnosis implicating one of these as the cause of a clinical condition.

Specimen types from actinomycetous disease can obviously vary depending on the site of infection, which, in part at least, is determined by the species. For pathogenic nocardiae and rhodococci, sputum, spinal fluid, tissue scrapings or biopsy, blood or urine may be obtained. If sputum, it can be handled similar to that described for tuberculosis samples (Exercise 21). Microscopic examination is done following Gram and Kinyoun acid-fast stain, the latter to show their acid-fast character (see Table 22-1). Primary culture can be on media used in previous exercises, as Middlebrook 7H10 and 7H11, brain heart infusion, sheep blood agar, and other types of solid media. (6, 15). Unfortunately, none of these is selective, and growth of contaminating normal flora can obscure the slower growing nocardiae. However, use of modifications of Thayer-Martin medium (1), and buffered charcoal yeast extract medium (8, 14, 22) for these organisms may alleviate this problem. Furthermore, a selective enrichment using "paraffin baiting" can increase the success of isolation (20). Here, a paraffin-coated glass rod is inserted into a carbon-free broth containing the specimen. After incubation, growth on the rod is cultivated as usual. Advantage has also been taken of this nocardial character to metabolize paraffin by development of a selective paraffin agar (19).

Similar procedures of isolation and culture can be employed for *Rhodococcus*. Growth is more rapid, usually appearing within 24 hours, and like nocardiae, these bacteria are partially acid-fast when stained by the Kinyoun method. Microscopically, they form coccoid to bacillary shapes, with branching in filamentous forms especially seen in young broth cultures (15, 17).

In actinomycosis, the most common specimen is purulent discharge from a cervicofacial location. The "sulfur granule," a macroscopically visible aggregate or microcolony of *Actinomyces*, white, yellow, or brown in color, frequently contained in the pus is very useful in diagnosis. Microscopically, these appear as tangled masses of hyphae. After rinsing with sterile water or broth, it

can be used for culture (2, 13) using media and methods previously described for anaerobic bacteria (Section E, page 000).

A battery of identifying assays for several species of actinomycetes is shown in Table 22-1. However, several alternative methods have been used for their identification. For example, the commercially available An-IDENT® and API20A® include *Actinomyces* in their identification databases, as does the Vitek system using the ANI identification card. *Nocardia* spp., both those causing nocardiosis and actinomycetoma, can be identified using the API-ZYM system (4), which readily differentiate these from *S. griseus*, a contaminating non-pathogen that can be confused with other actinomycetes. Finally, detection of siderophore production using an iron-containing medium, β-galactosidase activity, and ethylene glycol degradation, can be used for a rapid presumptive identification of *Nocardia, Streptomyces, Rhodococcus*, and rapidly growing *Mycobacterium* spp. (7).

In the following brief exercise, *A. israelii, N. asteroides, R. equi* and *Streptomyces griseus* will be compared using a limited number of assays.

MATERIALS

Part 1
Per pair of students:
    1 Brain heart infusion agar slant each of *Actinomyces israelii, Nocardia asteroides, Rhodococcus equi*, and *Streptomyces griseus*.
    Catalase reagent
    Kinyoun acid fast stain
Per class:
    Demonstration cultures of *A. israelii, N. asteroides*, and *S. griseus* on or in the following media:
        Gelatin tubes
        Starch agar "Y" plates
        Tyrosine agar plates

LABORATORY PROCEDURES

Part 1
A. Known cultures: Each pair of students is to do the following:
    1. Examine each culture of *A. israelii, N. asteroides, R. equi* and *S. griseus* provided you by doing the following: Describe the colony characteristics, then suspend a small amount of material in a drop of water and

Table 22-1
Characteristics of Some Actinomycetes

	Acid Fast	Catalase	NO$_3$ Reduct.	β-Galactosidase	Lysozyme Resistant	Decomposition of: Cas	Gel	Star[c]	Tyr	Xan	Urease	Acid from: Gal	Inos[c]	Mann	Xyl
Anaerobic Actinomycetes[a]:															
Actinomyces spp. (13, 18)															
A. bovis	—[b]	—	—	—		—	—	+	—	—	—	+	V	—	—
A. israelii	—	—	V	+		—	—	V	—	—	—	+	+	V	+
A. naeslundii	—	—	+	V		—	—	V	—	—	+	+	+	—	V
A. meyeri	—	—	—	—		—	—	—	—	—	V	V	—	—	+
A. odontolyticus	—	—	+	—		—	—	V	—	—	—	V	—	—	V
Aerobic Actinomycetes:															
Nocardia spp. (2, 9)															
N. asteroides	V	+	+	+	+	—	—	V	—	—	+	V	—	—	—
N. brasiliensis	V	+	+	+	+	+	+	V	+	—	+	+	+	+	—
N. otitidiscaviarum (N. caviae)	V	+	+	+	+	—	—	V	V	+	+	—	+	V	—
Rhodococcus spp. (10, 15, 17)															
R. equi	—	+	+	—	—	—	—		—	—	+	—	—	—	—
Streptomyces spp. (15, 16, 23)															
S. griseus[d]	—	+	V		—	+		+	+	+	+		V	+	+
S. somoliensis	—	+	—	+	—	+	+	V	+	—	—	—	—	—	—

[a] All "anaerobic" actinomycetes grow anaerobically in the presence of CO_2; many grow facultatively.

[b] + = usually positive; — = usually negative; V = variable reaction depending on strain.

[c] Abbreviations: Cas = casein; Gel = gelatin; Sta = starch; Tyr = tryosine; and Xan = xanthine; Gal = galactose; Inos = inositol; Mann = mannitol; Xyl = xylose.

[d] In the current Bergey's Manual classification, *S. griseus* is included under the encompassing species *S. anulatus* (23).

prepare two smears. Stain one of these by the Gram and the other by the modified Kinyoun acid-fast method. The procedure for the latter is as follows.

a. Apply Kinyoun's carbol fuchsin to heat-fixed smear for 2 minutes. Do not heat while staining.
b. Decolorize with acid-alcohol for 5-10 seconds.
c. Wash with tap water.
d. Counterstain 30 seconds with methylene blue solution.
e. Wash, blot dry and observe. Acid-fast organisms are stained red; other organisms and background material is blue.

Compare and describe distinguishing characteristics. Following this, test for catalase production.

2. Observe the following demonstration cultures containing *A. israelii, N. asteroides,* and *S. griseus.* These were inoculated seven days before your observation:

a. Three starch agar "Y" plates with each containing the three species. Each plate was incubated under the following conditions:
1 plate under anaerobic conditions at 35-37°C.
1 plate incubated aerobically at 30°C.
1 plate incubated aerobically at room temperature.

It should be noted that while all of the species used in this exercise grow well at 35-37°C, many nocardiae and rhodococci prefer 30°C. (15)

b. One tyrosine agar plate with *N. asteroides* and *S. griseus* incubated at room temperature.

c. Three tubes of gelatin, each stab-inoculated with one of the species. That with *A. israelii* was incubated anaerobically at 35-37°C; the others aerobically at 30°C.

Record your observations from these demonstration cultures. If tyrosine and starch are hydrolyzed, an area of clearing will appear under and perhaps around the colony, this being visible on the latter medium after flooding the plate with Gram iodine. Gelatin liquefaction is observed after cooling the cultures, either in a cold water bath or by placing in a refrigerator for a short period. Compare the amount of growth occurring in the starch agar plates incubated at 30°C and room temperature conditions, and aerobically compared to the anaerobic atmosphere.

If growth is minimal, or expected reactions have not appeared, it will be necessary to re-incubate these cultures for later observations. For clinical isolates, as much as four weeks may be necessary for adequate growth to appear.

Part 2

Demonstration cultures: Reexamine as necessary and record your results.

REFERENCES

1. Ashdown, L. R. 1990. An improved screening technique for isolation of *Nocardia* species from sputum specimens. Pathology **22**:157-161.
2. Baron, E. J., L. R. Peterson, and S. M. Finegold. 1994. Bailey & Scott's diagnostic microbiology, 9th ed. Mosby-Year Book, Inc., St. Louis. p. 467-471.
3. Beaman, B. L., J. Burnside, B. Edwards, and W. Causey. 1976. Nocardial infections in the United States, 1972-1974. J. Infect. Dis. **134**:287-289.
4. Boiron, P., and F. Provost. 1990. Enzymatic characterization of *Nocardia* spp. and related bacteria by API ZYM profile. Mycopathologia **110**:51-56.
5. Brown, A. E.. 1990. Other corynebacteria, p. 1581-1586. *In* G. L. Mandell, R. G. Douglas, Jr., and J. E. Bennett (ed.), Principles and practices of infectious diseases, 3rd ed. Churchill Livingstone, New York.
6. Collins, C. H., M. D. Yates, and A. H. C. Uttley. 1988. Presumptive identification of nocardias in a clinical laboratory. J. Appl. Bacteriol. **65**:55-59.
7. Fiss, E., and G. F. Brooks. 1991. Use of a siderophore detection medium, ethylene glycol degradation, and β-galactosidase activity in the early presumptive differentiation of *Nocardia, Rhodococcus, Streptomyces,* and rapidly growing *Mycobacterium* species. J. Clin. Microbiol. **29**:1533-1535.
8. Garrett, M. A., H. T. Holmes, and F. S. Nolte. 1992. Selective buffered charcoal-yeast extract medium for isolation of nocardiae from mixed culture. J. Clin. Microbiol. **30**:1891-1892.
9. Goodfellow, M., and M. P. Lechevalier. 1989. Genus *Nocardia* Trevisan 1889, p. 2350-2361. *In* S. T. Williams, M. E. Sharpe, and J. G. Holt (ed.), Bergey's manual of systematic bacteriology, Vol. 4, Williams & Wilkins, Baltimore.
10. Goodfellow, M. 1989. Genus *Rhodococcus* Zopf 1891, p. 2362-2371. *In* S. T. Williams, M. E. Sharpe, and J. G. Holt (ed.), Bergey's manual of systematic bacteriology, Vol. 4, Williams & Wilkins, Baltimore.
11. Gottlieb, D. 1974. Order I. *Actinomycetales* Buchanan 1917, p. 657-659. *In* R. E. Buchanan, and N. E. Gibbons (ed.), Bergey's manual of determinative bacteriology, 8th ed. The Williams & Wilkins Co., Baltimore.
12. Harvey, R. L., and J. C. Sunstrum. 1991. *Rhodococcus equi* infection in patients with and without human immunodeficiency virus infection. Rev. Infect. Dis. **13**:139-145.
13. Hillier, S., and B. J. Moncla. 1991. Anaerobic Gram-positive nonsporforming bacilli and cocci, p. 522-537. *In* A. Balows, W. J. Hausler, Jr., K. L. Herrmann, H. D. Isenberg, and H. J. Shadomy (ed.), Manual of clinical microbiology, 5th ed. American Society for Microbiology, Washington, D. C.
14. Kerr, E., H. Snell, B. L. Black, M. Storey, and W. D. Colby. 1992. Isolation of *Nocardia asteroides* from respiratory tract specimens by using selective buffered charcoal-yeast extract agar. J. Clin. Microbiol. **30**:1320-1322.
15. Land, G., M. R. McGinnis, J. Staneck, and A. Gatson. 1991. Aerobic pathogenic *Actinomycetales*, p. 340-359. *In* A. Balows, W. J. Hausler, Jr., K. L. Herrmann, H. D. Isenberg, and H. J. Shadomy (ed.), Manual of clinical microbiology, 5th ed. American Society for Microbiology, Washington, D. C.
16. Mishra, S. K., R. E. Gordon, and D. A. Barnett. 1980. Identification of nocardiae and streptomycetes of medical importance. J. Clin. Microbiol. **11**:728-736.
17. Prescott, J. F. 1991. *Rhodococcus equi*: an animal and human pathogen. Clin. Microbiol. Rev. **4**:20-34.
18. Schaal, K. P. 1986. Genus *Actinomyces* Hartz 1877, p. 1383-1418. *In* P. H. A. Sneath, N. S. Mair, M. E. Sharpe, and J. G. Holt (ed.). Bergey's manual of systematic bacteriology, Vol. 2. Williams & Wilkins, Baltimore.
19. Shawar, R. M., D. G. Moore, and M. T. LaRocco. 1990. Cultivation of *Nocardia* spp. on chemically defined media for selective recovery of isolates from clinical specimens. J. Clin. Microbiol. **28**:508-512.
20. Singh, M., R. S. Sandhu, and H. S. Randhawa. 1987. Comparison of paraffin baiting and conventional culture techniques for isolation of *Nocardia asteroides* from sputum. J. Clin. Microbiol. **25**:176-177.
21. Timoney, J. F., J. H. Gillespie, F. W. Scott, and J. E. Barlough. 1988. Hagan and Bruner's microbiology and infectious diseases of domestic animals, 8th ed. Comstock Publishing Associates, Ithica, NY. p. 259-266.
22. Vickers, R. M., J. D. Rihs, and V. L. Lu. 1992. Clinical demonstration of isolation of *Nocardia asteroides* on buffered charcoal-yeast extract media. J. Clin. Microbiol. **30**:227-228.
23. Williams, S. T., M. Goodfellow, and G. Alderson. 1989. Genus *Streptomyces* Waksman and Henrici 1943, p. 2452-2492. *In* S. T. Williams, M. E. Sharpe, and J. G. Holt (ed.), Bergey's manual of systematic bacteriology, Vol. 4, Williams & Wilkins, Baltimore.

Exercise 22
Data Table 1: *Actinomyces, Nocardia, Rhodococcus* and *Streptomyces* Results

		Culture Age	A. israelii		N. asteroides		R. equi		S. griseus	
			BHI[a]	Other	BHI	Other	BHI	Other	BHI	Other
Colony size and Colony Form	mm									
	Punctiform									
	Irregular									
	Circular									
	Rhizoid									
	Filamentous									
	Other									
Colony Surface	Flat									
	Raised									
	Convex									
	Pulvinate									
	Other									
Colony Margin	Entire									
	Undulate									
	Lobate									
	Erose									
	Other									
Colony Consistency	Butyrous									
	Viscid									
	Membranous									
	Brittle									
	Other									
Colony Optical Character	Opaque									
	Translucent									
	Dull									
	Glistening									
	Other									
Colony Surface	Smooth									
	Rough									
	Other									
Colony odor and color										
Catalase Produced										

[a] Brain heart infusion agar.

Exercise 22
Data Table 2: *Actinomyces, Norcardia,* and *Streptomyces* Demonstration Results

		Culture Age	A. israelii		N. asteroides		S. griseus	
			BHI[a]	Other	BHI	Other	BHI	Other
Kinyoun Acid Fast Stain								
Gram stain	Reaction							
	Morphology							
	Arrangement							
Tyrosine	Decomposition							
Starch	Anaerobic, 35°C							
	Aerobic, 30°C							
Gelatin Liquefaction	Anaerobic, 35°C							
	Aerobic, 30°C							
Other								

Other Laboratory Notes:

NOTES

NOTES

SECTION I - Pathogenic Bacteriology

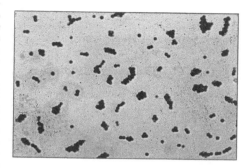

1-1 Gram stain of *Staphylococcus aureus*. Note cells in singles, pairs, short chains, and clusters. Also observe the presence of occasional Gram-negative cells among predominantly Gram-positive cells after overnight incubation. (From: California State University Collection, San Francisco, CA)
←

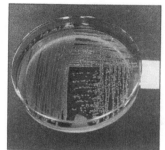

1-2 *Staphylococcus aureus* grown on sheep blood agar (SBA) seen after 18 hours incubation. Red cells have been hemolyzed except for a small area near the last isolation streak. At this age, colonies are only slightly pigmented. (From: California State University Collection, San Francisco, CA)
→

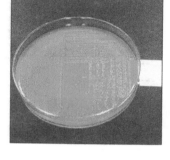

1-3 *Staphylococcus epidermidis* on SBA, 18 hour culture. Note white color and lack of hemolysis. (From: California State University Collection, San Francisco, CA)
←

1-4 *Staphylococcus aureus* on mannitol salt agar, 18 hour culture. Acid production is demonstrated by the yellow color. (From: California State University Collection, San Francisco, CA)
→

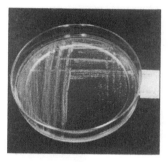

1-5 Staph-Trac™ kit (API Analytab Products, Plainview, NY). Each of 19 cupules contain a different substrate (the twentieth is a negative control). This assay is read after 24 hours incubation. Identification aids consisting of differential charts, profile listings, and identification code book are available.
←

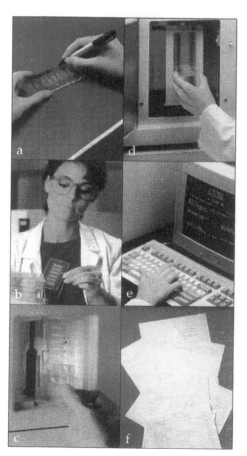

1-6 Vitek systems (Hazelwood, Mo.). This series shows the sequence of testing in this automated system. (a) A test card is filled and sealed (b & c), then inserted into the Reader/Incubator (d). During incubation preliminary results may be obtained from a monitor (e), and final reports printed (f) after the cycle is completed.
→

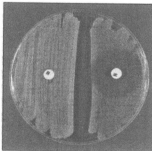

←

1-7 Novobiocin disk inhibition test (Remel, Lenexa, KA). A zone of ≥16 mm is a demonstration of a positive inhibition test.

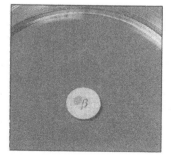

1-8 BBL® Cefinase™ test (Becton Dickinson Microbiology Systems, Cockeysville, MD). This positive test for the presence of β-lactamase is seen by the red color developing on the yellow disk.
←

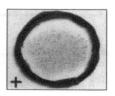 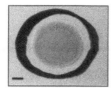

1-9 The BBL® Staphyloslide test (Becton Dickinson Microbiology Systems, Cockeysville, MD). This particular assay uses fibrinogen-coated red cells to detect *S. aureus* producing clumping factor. Its presence causes red cells to aggregate within 15 seconds, a positive test. ←

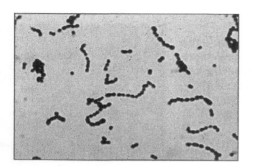

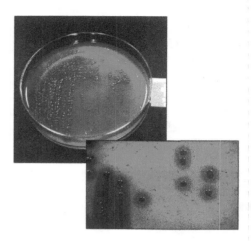

2-1 Gram stain of *Streptococcus pyogenes* showing cells arranged in singles and pairs, but mostly in chains (1000X magnification). This sample was obtained from a BHI agar colony approximately 24 hours of age. (From: California State University Collection, San Francisco, CA) ←

→

2-2 *Streptococcus pneumoniae*, Type 3, grown on sheep blood agar, about 24 hours of age. Alpha hemolysis surrounds each colony. (From: California State University Collection, San Francisco, CA)

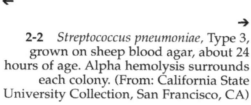

2-3 *Streptococcus pyogenes*, 24-hr. growth on sheep blood agar. These bacteria are beta-hemolytic, forming a zone of complete lysis of red cells. (From: California State University Collection, San Francisco, CA) ←

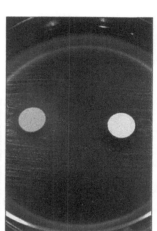

2-4 *S. pyogenes* on SBA showing the inhibitory effects of bacitracin-containing disks (left, brown disk), compared to non-inhibition of optochin (right, white disk). (From: California State University Collection, San Francisco, CA) →

2-5 *S. pneumoniae* on SBA with bacitracin and optochin differentiation disks. Observe the reverse relationship of the effect of these compounds to that of *S. pyogenes* seen in Photo 2-4. Here optochin (white disk) only is inhibitory. (From: California State University Collection, San Francisco, CA.) ←

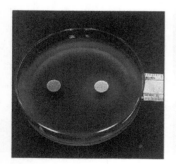

2-6 The bile solubility test with *Streptococcus pneumoniae* and an alpha-hemolytic streptococci. Cell lysis and clearing of the suspension is a property of *S. pneumoniae*. (From collection of R. A. Borichewski, Curtin Matheson Scientific, Inc., Houston, TX.) →

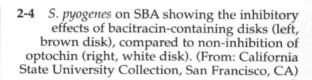

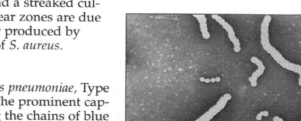

2-7 CAMP test using staphylococcal β-lysin impregnated disks (Remel, Lenexa, KA) and a streaked culture of *Staphylococcus aureus*. The clear zones are due to the interaction of "CAMP" factor produced by *Streptococcus agalactiae* and β-lysin of *S. aureus*. ←

2-8 Negative stain of *Streptococcus pneumoniae*, Type 3, from enriched broth culture. The prominent capsules are clearly seen surrounding the chains of blue bacteria (1000X magnification). (From: California State University Collection, San Francisco, CA.) →

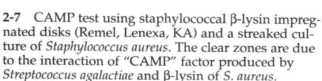

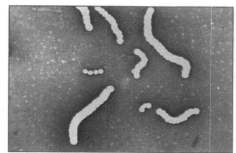

BETA LYSIN DISK

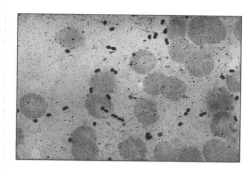

2-9 Gram stain of *Streptococcus pneumoniae* in mouse heart blood. Unlike culture-adapted pneumococci, as seen in Photo 2-8, *in vivo* and freshly-isolated organisms tend to gave a "lancet-shaped" morphology and to be arranged in pairs.
←

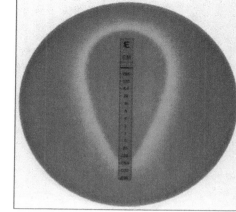

2-10 The AB Biodisk (Solna, Sweden) antimicrobial sensitivity test. This photograph shows the drop-shaped inhibition zone of a β-hemolytic streptococci along the erythromycin concentration gradient.
→

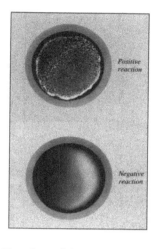

2-11 Example of a slide agglutination reaction using the Wellcogen™ Strep B assay. A positive test is apparent by the aggregation of organisms on the top compared to a smooth suspension of a negative test on the bottom. (Courtesy of Wellcome Diagnostics, Research Triangle Park, NC)
←

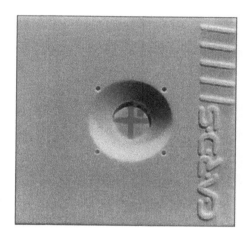

2-12 A positive enzyme-linked test for Group A streptococci as demonstrated using the Cards® Strep A kit (Pacific Biotech, Inc., San Diego, CA). The blue "+" results from Group A antigen reacting with components of the enzyme-linked reagents.
→

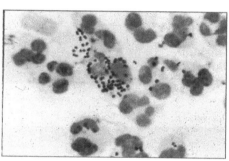

3-1 *Neisseria gonorrhoeae* in leukocytes as viewed in a clinical specimen from a gonorrhea patient. This Gram-stained preparation clearly shows the intracellular location of these cocci, many of which appear kidney-bean shaped and in pairs. (From: Dr. H. Wessenberg collection, San Francisco State University.)
←

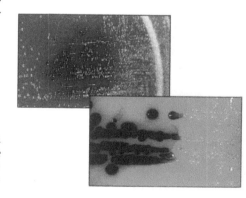

3-2 A positive oxidase test on culture of a *Neisseria* sp. (From: California State University Collection, San Francisco, CA.)
→

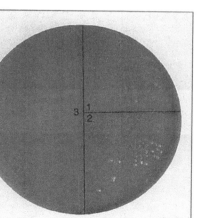

3-3 Approximately twenty-four hour growth of *Neisseria gonorrhoeae* (segment 1) and *N. meningitidis* (segment 2) on Thayer-Martin medium containing lincomycin, colistin, amphotericin B, and trimethoprim (Unipath Co., Oxoid Div., Ogdensburg, NY). This is a selective agar as seen here by the lack of growth of *Proteus vulgaris* in segment 3. (Courtesy Unipath Co., Oxoid Div., Ogdensburg, NY.)
←

3-4 Gonochek™ II (E·Y Laboratories, San Mateo, CA), an example of a rapid culture confirmation test of *Neisseria gonorrhoeae*. This is based upon a chromogenic enzyme substrate released by organisms named in the photograph, each causing a separate color to develop. No color is present in a negative test. This assay can be read following 30 minutes of incubation at 37°C. →

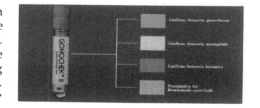

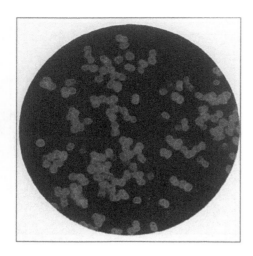

3-5 Microtrack®, an example of a fluorescent antibody test for culture confirmation of *Neisseria gonorrhoeae*. (Courtesy of Syva Co., Palo Alto, CA.)
←

3-6 Directigen® Meningitis Combo kit (Becton Dickinson Microbiology Systems, Cockeysville, Md), an example of a latex bead agglutination rapid identification kit. This can detect *Neisseria meningitidis* Groups A, B, C, W135, and Y, *Streptococcus pneumoniae, S. agalactiae*, and *Haemophilus influenzae* type b, all agents of meningitis. The kit contains positive and negative control reagents (Bottles A, B, P, N), and antigen-containing latex beads for each of the several groups of bacteria (bottles numbered 1-6).
→

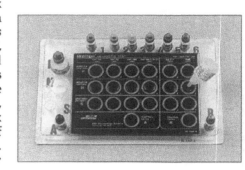

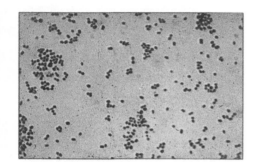

4-1 *Acinetobacter calcoaceticus* Gram stain after 24 hours growth on nutrient agar (1000X magnification). Although considered rods, they may, as here, be coccoid shapes. (From: California State University Collection, San Francisco, CA.)
←

4-2 *Acinetobacter calcoaceticus* growing on nutrient agar after 24 hours incubation at 37°C. This shows the capacity for these bacteria to grow well on an unenriched medium. (From: California State University Collection, San Francisco, CA.)
→

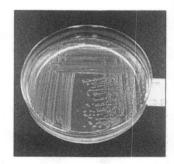

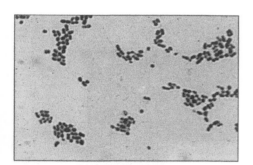

4-3 Gram stain of *Moraxella osloensis* (1000X magnification). Conditions of growth here were similar as described for Photo 4-1. (From: California State University Collection, San Francisco, CA.)
←

5-1 *Haemophilus influenzae* grown on rabbit blood agar and then Gram-stained. (Rabbit blood contains X and V factors.) This shows their typical small, coccoid to rod shapes. (From: California State University Collection, San Francisco, CA.)
→

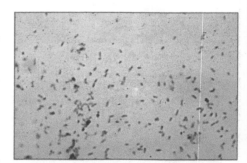

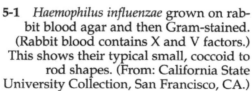

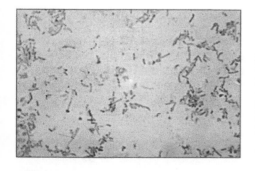

5-2 *Haemophilus parainfluenzae* from rabbit blood agar and Gram-stained (1000X magnification). Note the tendency to form "threads" or chains. These can be very long and may occur in any species of haemophilae. (From: California State University Collection, San Francisco, CA.)
←

5-3 *Bordetella pertussis*, Gram-stained after being grown on B-G agar. While in the same size range as the haemophilae, morphologically these are more rod-like. (From: California State University Collection, San Francisco, CA.)
→

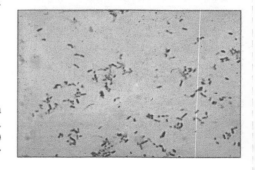

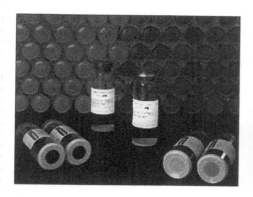

6-1 BacT\Alert blood culture bottles (Organon Teknika, Durham, NC). CO_2 produced by microorganisms growing in the culture bottle is detected by an internal sensor at the bottom of each bottle. This is monitored through a computerized instrument detection system.
←

8-1 Gram stain of *Escherichia coli* (1000X magnification) grown in nutrient broth. This photograph, Photo 8-2, and Photo 8-3 show the typical rod forms of enteric bacteria, arranged singly and in short chains. (From: California State University Collection, San Francisco, CA.)
→

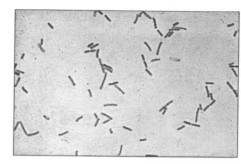

8-2 *Salmonella typhi* from nutrient agar and Gram-stained (1000X magnification). (From: California State University Collection, San Francisco, CA.)
←

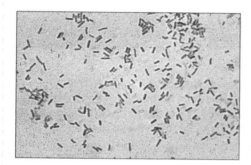

8-3 *Yersinia enterocolitica* grown in BHI broth, then stained with methylene blue. Bipolar staining is apparent in some of the cells. (From: California State University Collection, San Francisco, CA.)
→

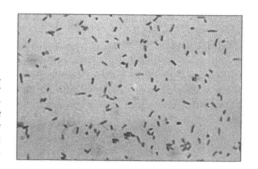

8-4 through 8-7 Appearance of *Escherichia coli* on several selective and differential agars after 24 hours incubation at 37°C. Photo 8-4 presents a full view of the green metallic sheen typical of colonies of this organism on EMB, a result of lactose fermentation. On MacConkey agar (Photo 8-5) pink colonies and precipitated bile in the agar, also pink, develop due to lactose fermentation and consequent acid production. Hektoen Enteric (HE) agar colonies (Photo 8-6) also precipitate bile. In this case, both it and colonies are orange. Photo 8-7, a close-up view of Photo 8-6, show the typical colonies forms of *E. coli* on HE agar. (From: California State University Collection, San Francisco, CA.)

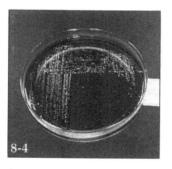
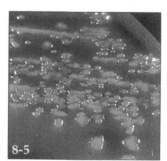
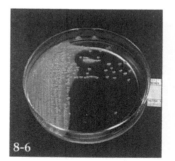
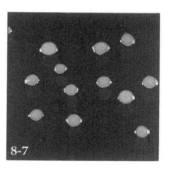

8-8 through 8-10 *Enterobacter cloacae* on EMB, MacConkey, and HE agars after 24 hours at 37°C. In Photo 8-8 the full view of the EMB plate shows this organism's capacity to develop pink colonies due to lactose fermentation without a metallic sheen. On MacConkey agar (Photo 8-9), pink colonies also indicate lactose fermentation, as do orange colonies on HE agar (Photo 8-10). (From: California State University Collection, San Francisco, CA.)

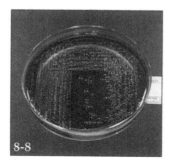
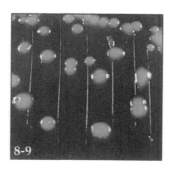
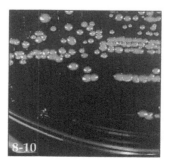

8-11 through 8-14 *Salmonella typhi* grown on four different types of differential and selective agar media 24 hours at 37°C. In Photos 8-11 through 8-13 colonies on EMB, MacConkey, and SS agars appear colorless because of the lack of lactose fermentation. Not seen at this stage of growth, but which usually appears before 48 hours, is the dark center forming in the colony on SS agar due to H_2S production. Dark blue or blue-green colonies are typical of this organism on HE agar (Photo 8-14). Dark centers form in these colonies as well because of H_2S production, but are not visible in this picture. (Photos 8-13 & 8-14 from California State University Collection, San Francisco, CA.; Photos 8-11 & 8-12 from collection of R. A. Borichewski, Curtin Matheson Scientific, Inc., Houston, TX.)

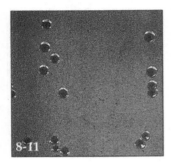 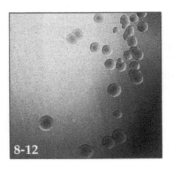 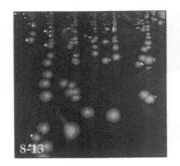 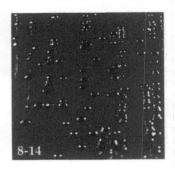

8-15 through 8-17 *Shigella sonnei* grown on EMB, and *S. dysenteriae* on MacConkey, and SS agars (24 hours at 37°C). In this series of photographs, colorless colonies of this non-lactose fermenting species are seen. On SS agar (Photo 8-17), unlike salmonellae, dark colony centers will not form because shigellae do not produce H_2S. (Photo 8-15 from California State University Collection, San Francisco, CA.; Photos 8-16 and 8-17 from collection of R. A. Borichewski, Curtin Matheson Scientific, Inc., Houston, TX.)

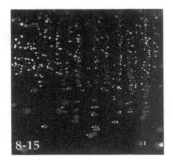 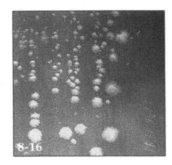 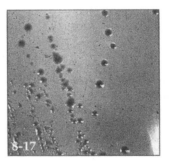

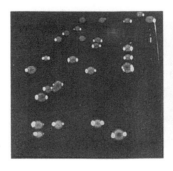

8-18 *Proteus vulgaris* grown on EMB (48 hours at 37°C) form colorless colonies. Because of the spreading nature of the proteae, growth can completely cover the plate surface in a short period. This is frequently inapparent, but can be verified by careful observation or by rubbing the surface with a loop or needle. (From: California State University Collection, San Francisco, CA.)
←

8-19 through 8-21 EMB, MacConkey, and SS agar plates containing a mixture of enteric bacteria (24 hours at 37°C.). The differentiation of lactose-fermenting and lactose non-fermenting bacteria can readily be made. Also, H_2S-producing bacteria (*S. typhi*, in this case) are apparent on SS agar by the black color. (From: California State University Collection, San Francisco, CA.)

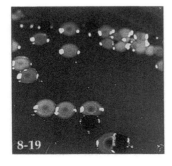 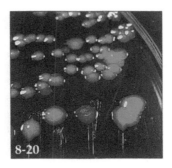 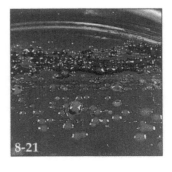

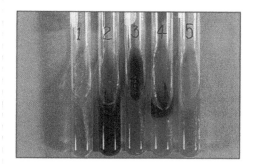

8-22 Triple sugar iron agar reactions with: 1) *Klebsiella pneumoniae*; 2) *Proteus vulgaris*; 3) *Pseudomonas aeruginosa*; 4) *Salmonella typhi*; and 5) *Shigella dysenteriae*. *P. aeruginosa* is a non-fermenting, non-H₂S producing bacteria (see Exercise 12). Interpret the reactions of enteric bacteria seen here with the aid of Table 8-5; for *P. aeruginosa* from Photo 12-2. (From: California State University Collection, San Francisco, CA.)
←

8-23 through 8-28 Examples of alternative methods for identification of enteric bacteria from culture (most can be used to identify other groups as well). Rapid* E (Analytab Products, Plainview, NY) is a 4-hour biochemical assay (Photo 8-23), while Minitek™ (Becton Dickinson Microbiology Systems, Cockeysville, MD) (Photo 8-24) needs 18-24 hours incubation, but offers flexibility in test selection. This is possible because disks containing substrates can be chosen as needed. Photo 8-25 shows a Biolog GN Microplate™ (Biolog, Hayward, CA) that permits testing of 95 carbon substrates in a microplate. The reactions can be directly read on a plate reader and results viewed in a monitor. Spectrum 10 (Austin Biological Laboratories, Austin, TX) for enteric bacteria provides a manual system where from one to three trays (one of which is shown, Photo 8-26) can be used, depending on the need for additional identification assays. Micro-ID® (General Diagnostics, Morris Plains, NJ) (Photo 8-27) utilizes a 15-well panel that can be read in 4 or 24 hours procedures. The Sensititre® Microbiology System (Radiometer America Inc., Westlake, OH) (8-28) is a semi-automated and automated system. Results are available in 5 to 18 hours.

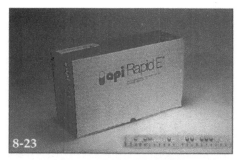

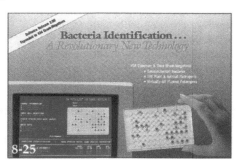

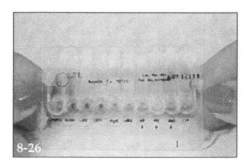

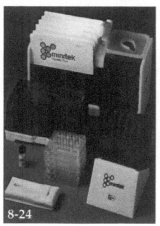

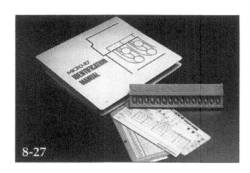

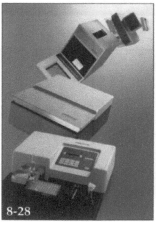

9-1 *Klebsiella pneumoniae* in arginine (Tube 1) and lysine (Tube 2) broths, and *Salmonella typhi* in arginine (Tube 3) and lysine (Tube 4) broths after 48 hours at 37°C. (From: California State University Collection, San Francisco, CA.)
→

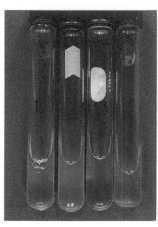

10-1 *Vibrio cholerae* (1) and *Escherichia coli* (2) on TCBS Cholera medium. The differential and selective nature of this medium for the sucrose-fermenting *V. cholerae* is readily seen. (Courtesy of Unipath Co., Oxoid Div., Ogdensburg, NY)
←

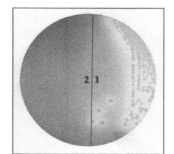

10-2 *Vibrio cholerae.* Note curving cells with monotrichous polar flagella. (Courtesy of Centers for Disease Control, Div. of Medical and Training Services, Atlanta, GA.) →

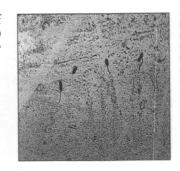

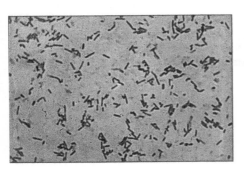

12-1 *Pseudomonas aeruginosa,* Gram stain preparation, observed at 1000X magnification. This organism was cultivated on nutrient agar for 24 hours. (From: California State University Collection, San Francisco, CA.) ←

12-2 *Pseudomonas aeruginosa,* 24-hour culture grown on sheep blood agar. Pigment formation and hemolysis are visible in the heavily streaked areas. (Again observe Photo 8-22. Can you now deduce the source of dark color in the TSI slant of this organism?) (From: California State University Collection, San Francisco, CA.) →

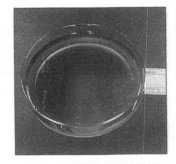

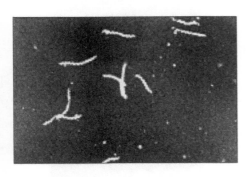

13-1 *Legionella* on unsupplemented buffered charcoal yeast extract agar showing growth only around the *Legionella* differentiation disk. (Courtesy of Remel, Lenexa, KA). ←

LEGIONELLA DIFF. DISK

13-2 *Legionella pneumophilia* in a sputum sample showing specific fluorescence following staining with a labeled monoclonal antibody (Courtesy Sanofi Diagnostics Pasteur, Chaska, MN). →

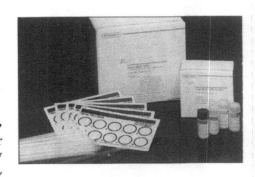

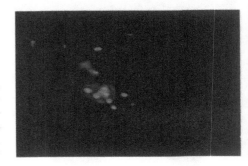

14-1 *Treponema pallidum* subsp. *pallidum* as seen in the darkfield microscope. (Courtesy of Dr. D. Cox, Centers for Disease Control, Atlanta, GA.) ←

→

14-2 Rapid plasma reagin test kit for detection of patient reagin antibody against *Treponema pallidum* (Seradyn, Indianapolis, IN).

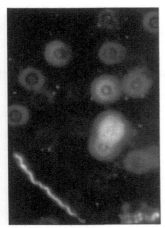

15-1 *Borrelia burgdorferi* seen in a wet mount by dark field microscopy (Courtesy of Dako Corp., Carpinteria, CA). ←

15-2 *Ixodes scapularis,* a Lyme disease tick vector in most of U.S.A. (Courtesy of John Montenieri, Centers For Disease Control, Vector-Borne Infectious Diseases Div., Ft. Collins, CO).

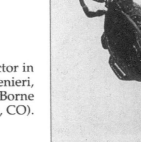

16-1 BBL® GasPak™ system showing both the CampyPak Plus for *Campylobacter* culture and the GasPak Plus for culturing of anaerobic bacteria (Becton Dickinson Microbiology Systems, Cockeysville, MD).
↓

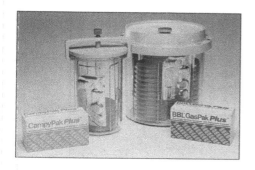

16-2 The BioBag™ Environmental Chamber system (Becton Dickinson Microbiology Systems, Cockeysville, MD), an example of a smaller volume anaerobic container.
→

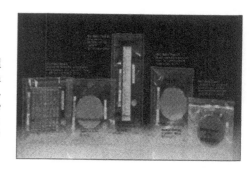

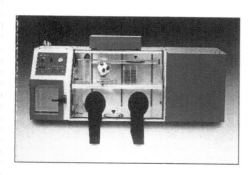

16-3 An anaerobic chamber for large volume anaerobic culture work (Bactron System, Shel-Lab, Cornelius, OR). The chamber is maintained under anaerobic conditions, while a "Pass Through" box, where oxygen removal from in-going materials takes place, permits movement of media and materials in and out of the chamber.
←

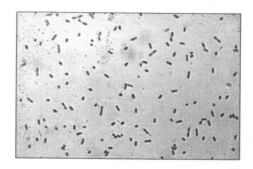

↑
16-4 Gram stain of *Bacteroides fragilis* obtained from a 48-hour culture grown anaerobically on Vitamin K₁-blood agar (K₁BA) (1000X magnification). (From: California State University Collection, San Francisco, CA.)

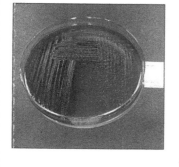

16-5 *Bacteroides fragilis* growing on a K₁BA plate after 48 hours of anaerobic incubation. (From: California State University Collection, San Francisco, CA.)
←

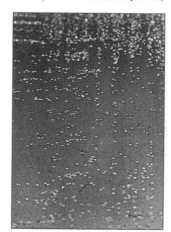

16-6 Close-up photograph of Photo 16-5 showing colony form of *Bacteroides fragilis*. (From: California State University Collection, San Francisco, CA.)
→

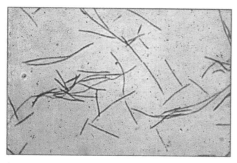

16-7 *Fusobacterium nucleatum,* Gram stain of culture from K₁BA plate incubated anaerobically for 48 hours (1000X magnification). The unique morphology and arrangement of these Gram-negative bacilli are evident. (From: California State University Collection, San Francisco, CA.)
←

16-8 Anaerobically-incubated K₁BA plate (48 hours, 37°C) of *Fusobacterium nucleatum*. (From: California State University Collection, San Francisco, CA.)
→

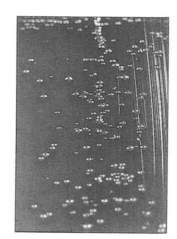

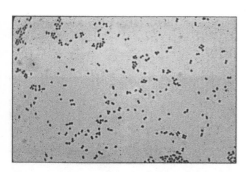

16-9 *Veillonella parvula* seen after Gram-staining growth from an anaerobically-incubated K₁BA plate. (From: California State University Collection, San Francisco, CA.)

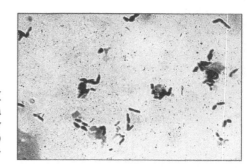

16-10 Gram stain of *Propionibacterium acnes*, 1000X magnification, prepared from a 48 hour culture grown on K₁BA. (From: California State University Collection, San Francisco, CA.) →

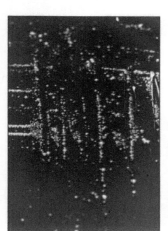

16-11 K₁BA culture growth of *Propionibacterium acnes* after 48 hours of anaerobic incubation. (From: California State University Collection, San Francisco, CA.) ←

17-1 Microscopic observation (1000X magnification) of a Gram-stained preparation of *Clostridium tetani* from cooked meat medium. Note the swollen sporangia at their terminal locations ("drumstick" appearance) due to spore formation. (From: California State University Collection, San Francisco, CA.) →

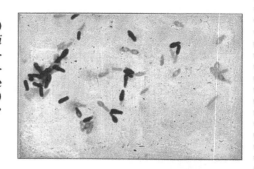

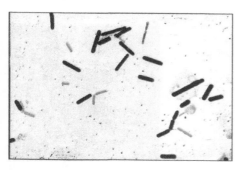

17-2 *Clostridium tetani* prepared similarly to that seen in Photo 17-1, except the Wirtz-Conklin spore stain was used. Spores are stained by the malachite green, and vegetative cells red by the safranin counterstain. (From: California State University Collection, San Francisco, CA.) ←

17-3 *Clostridium botulinum* Gram stain (1000X magnification) prepared from cooked meat medium. Spores are located subterminally. (From: California State University Collection, San Francisco, CA.) →

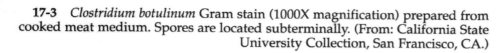

17-4 *Clostridium perfringens* as seen at 1000X magnification. A characteristic of this species, found here after growth in cooked meat medium, is the lack of spores. (From: California State University Collection, San Francisco, CA.) ←

18-1 Gram stain of *Bacillus anthracis* obtained from a 24-hour culture of nutrient broth (1000X magnification). (From: California State University Collection, San Francisco, CA.) →

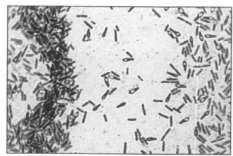

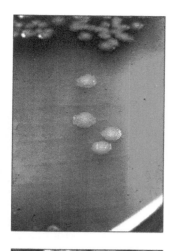

18-2 *Bacillus anthracis* grown on sheep blood agar, seen here after 24 hours at 37°C. (From: California State University Collection, San Francisco, CA.)
←

18-3 *Bacillus cereus*, Gram stain. Conditions of growth were the same as that given for Photo 18-1. (From: California State University Collection, San Francisco, CA.)
→

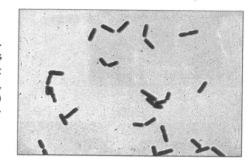

18-4 *Bacillus cereus* on sheep blood agar after 24 hours at 37°C. (From: California State University Collection, San Francisco, CA.)
←

18-5 Spore-stained (Wirtz-Conklin method) *Bacillus subtilus*. This organism was grown on sporulation agar. (From: California State University Collection, San Francisco, CA.)
→

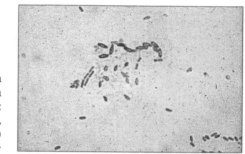

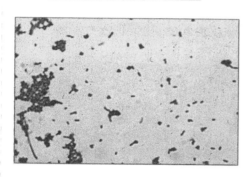

19-1 Microscopic appearance of a methylene blue stained preparation of *Listeria monocytogenes* obtained from 24-hour growth on blood agar (970X magnification). (From: California State University Collection, San Francisco, CA.)
←

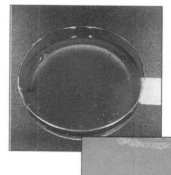

19-2 *Listeria monocytogenes* growth on blood agar after 24 hours. Narrow zones of beta hemolysis around colonies are not visible in this photograph. (From: California State University Collection, San Francisco, CA.)
→

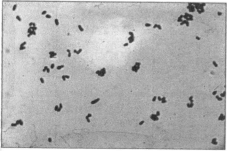

20-1 *Corynebacterium diphtheriae*, biotype *gravis*, grown in thioglycollate broth for 24 hours at 37°C, then Gram stained. Note the presence of "V" arrangements and palisade formation (1000X magnification). (From: California State University Collection, San Francisco, CA.)
←

20-2 *Corynebacterium diphtheriae*, biotype *gravis*, grown under similar conditions as described for Photo 20-1, but stained with methylene blue (1000X magnification). This method enhances the appearance of metachromatic granules. Observe that the uneven staining can give these rods the appearance of cocci. (From: California State University Collection, San Francisco, CA.)
→

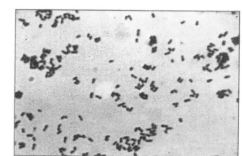

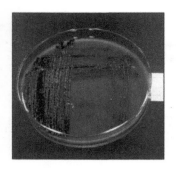

20-3 *Corynebacterium diphtheriae*, biotype *intermedius* on cystine-tellurite agar after incubation at 37°C for 24 hours. (From: California State University Collection, San Francisco, CA.)
←

20-4 *Corynebacterium diphtheriae*, biotype *intermedius* grown on sheep blood agar incubated at 37°C for 24 hours. (From: California State University Collection, San Francisco, CA.)
→

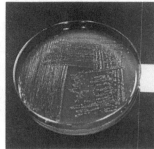

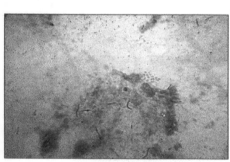

21-1 *Mycobacterium bovis*, acid-fast stained. This culture was derived from Lowenstein-Jensen medium (1000X magnification). (From: California State University Collection, San Francisco, CA.)
←

21-2 *Mycobacterium leprae* in a human skin section stained by the acid-fast method (970X magnification). (From collection of R. A. Borichewski, Curtin Matheson Scientific, Inc., Houston, TX.)
→

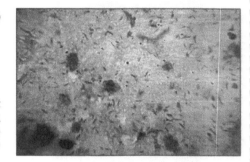

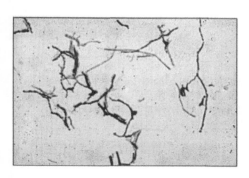

21-3 *Mycobacterium tuberculosis* in a smear prepared from sputum and stained by the acid-fast method (970X magnification). The slender, curving, and thin rods, some with beads, are evident. (From collection of R. A. Borichewski, Curtin Matheson Scientific, Inc., Houston, TX.)
←

21-4 *Mycobacterium tuberculosis* from Lowenstein-Jensen culture and stained by acid-fast stain (1000X magnification). (From: California State University Collection, San Francisco, CA.)
→

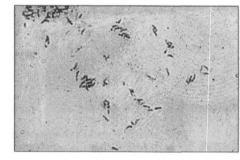

22-1 *Nocardia asteroides* from BHI agar: Gram-stained (1000X magnification). The filamentous and branched structure of these Gram-positive bacteria, along with occasional typical single rod forms are shown. (From: California State University Collection, San Francisco, CA.)
←

22-2 *Actinomyces bovis* seen after anaerobic growth on BHI agar followed by Gram staining. These organisms are filamentous, diphtheroid, Gram-positive rods that can be branched. (From: California State University Collection, San Francisco, CA.)
→

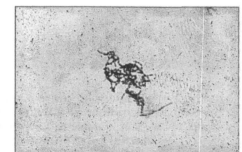

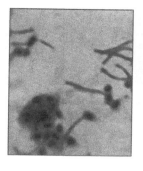
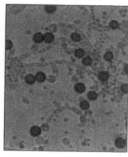

24-1 *Candida albicans* germ tubes (600X magnification) and chlamydoconidia (450X magnification). (Courtesy Upjohn Co., Kalmazoo, MI.) ←

24-2 *Cryptococcus neoformans* colony and yeast cells in an India ink preparation (400X magnification). (Courtesy Upjohn Co., Kalmazoo, MI.) →

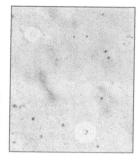

25-1 *Fonsecaea pedrosoi* colony and conidiophores (400X magnification). (Courtesy Upjohn Co., Kalmazoo, MI.)

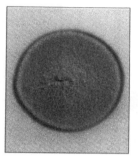
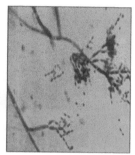

25-2 *Pseudallescheria boydii* colony surface (a) and reverse (b) views, and photograph of conidia (400X magnification). (Courtesy Upjohn Co., Kalmazoo, MI.)

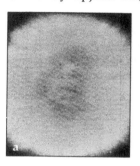
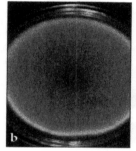
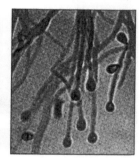

25-3A *Sporothrix schenckii* colony and conidia (400X magnification) when grown at 24°C. (Courtesy Upjohn Co., Kalmazoo, MI.)

25-3B *Sporothrix schenckii* colony and yeast phase cells (1000X magnification) when grown at 37°C. (Courtesy Upjohn Co., Kalmazoo, MI.)

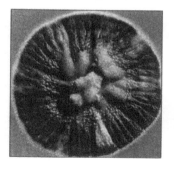
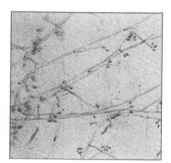
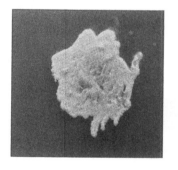
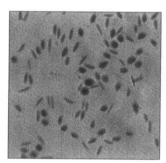

25-4 *Epidermophyton floccosum* macroconidia (800X magnification). (Courtesy Upjohn Co., Kalmazoo, MI.)

25-5 *Microsporum audouinii* macroconidium and chlamydoconidia (400X magnification). (Courtesy Upjohn Co., Kalmazoo, MI.)

25-6 *Trichophyton mentagrophytes* microconidia (400X magnification). (Courtesy Upjohn Co., Kalmazoo, MI.)

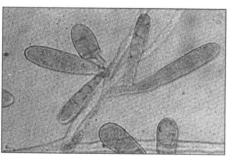
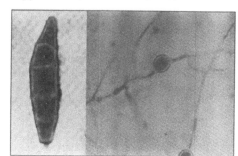
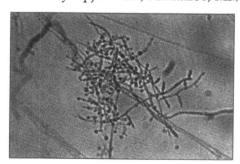

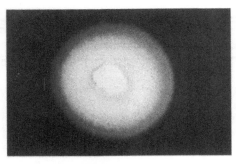
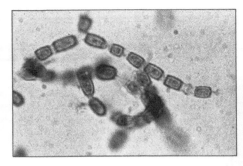

26-1A *Coccidioides immitis* colony and arthroconidia (800X magnification). (Courtesy Upjohn Co., Kalmazoo, MI.)

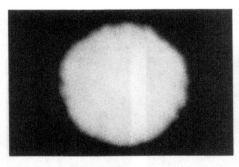

26-1B *Coccidioides immitis* spherules in lymph node preparation (600X magnification). (Courtesy Upjohn Co., Kalmazoo, MI.)

26-2A *Histoplasma capsulatum* colony and macroconidia and microconidia (400X magnification) resulting from growth at 24°C. (Courtesy Upjohn Co., Kalmazoo, MI.)
←

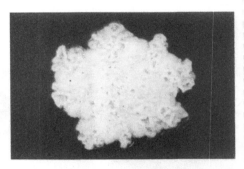

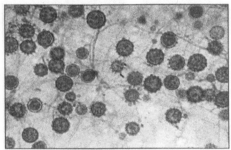

26-2B *Histoplasma capsulatum* colony and yeast phase cells (1200X magnification) when grown at 37°C. (Courtesy Upjohn Co., Kalmazoo, MI.)
→

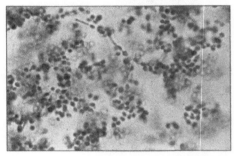

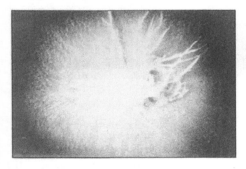

26-3A *Blastomyces dermatitidis* colony and conidia (800X magnification) when grown at 24°C. (Courtesy Upjohn Co., Kalmazoo, MI.)
←

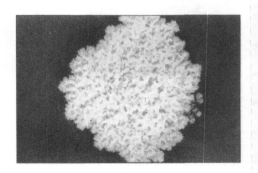

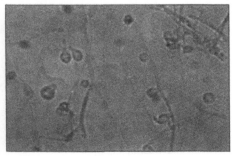

26-3B *Blastomyces dermatitidis* colony and yeast phase cells (1000X magnification) when grown at 37°C. (Courtesy Upjohn Co., Kalmazoo, MI.)
→

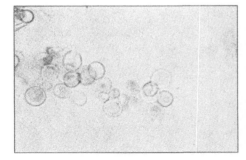

SECTION II
MEDICAL MYCOLOGY

INTRODUCTION

I. Groupings, Taxonomy, and Terminology

The fungi, which comprise a very large taxonomic group of organisms, are frequently placed in the kingdom Fungi (Myceteae) (5, 10). Simply put, they are non-photosynthetic plant-like organisms that are eukaryotic, chemoheterotrophic, obtain their nutrients by absorption, and have chitinous cell walls. Morphologically, those considered of importance in medical mycology fall into two broad informal groups, the yeasts and the filamentous types, or moulds. The former, as used in this manual, are single celled, usually ovoid in shape, that multiply by blastospore (or bud) formation (Figure 23-1), and commonly form butyrous colonies. (Note: This description is not accepted by all mycological taxonomists, who may prefer to restrict "yeasts" to only those that form sexual ascospores, discussed later, but otherwise fit the description used above.) A very common example an organism belonging to this group is *Saccharomyces cerevisiae* used in making bread, wine and other products, and a rare agent of infection. Filamentous types, however, are multicellular, growing by the formation of long filaments, the hypha (see below for definition of mycological terms), which form a colony consisting of a mass of hyphae or mycelium. Mould colonies have various surface textures ranging from floccose (wool-like) to glabrous (smooth), but they form a leathery base that grows into the agar. Both yeasts and moulds may form sexual spores, the characteristics of which weigh heavily in their formal classification, and asexual spores that are important in identification, as we will see below.

The fungi have been grouped in various ways. While a formal classification is used based on botanical conventions, it can be complex and confusing for the non-specialist. Because of this, a clinical grouping is receiving greater emphasis by clinical and medical microbiologists. This includes the superficial (cutaneous or dermatophytic fungi),

subcutaneous, and systemic or deep types (Table 23-1). While organisms within these are not restricted to a particular disease pattern, this grouping does have utilitarian value and is commonly used. The following discussion will provide basic background information on both formal and informal groupings. An expansion of this will follow in Exercises 24 through 26.

A sampling of a few of the less than 100 clinically important species out of an estimated 250,000 total species of fungi (5) is given in Table 23-1. This relates the morphologic type and clinical category of each, and the names of the associated disease. As the name implies, fungi categorized as superficial are restricted to those affecting the cornified area of the body as skin and hair without invasion of tissue. Pityriasis versicolor due to *Malassezia furfur*, for example, can invade the corneum stratum of skin, while *Trichosporon beigelii* infects only the hair shaft. Members of the dermatophytic or cutaneous group infect keratinized tissue as skin, hair and nails. While capable of cutaneous infection, they cannot move into the subcutaneous or systemic locations because of host defenses and their own nutritional deficiencies (21).

Subcutaneous fungi induce a variety of conditions as eumycotic mycetoma (see Exercise 22, page 327 for a discussion on the clinically similar disease actinomycetoma), sporotrichosis, and other slow-developing conditions. These infections arise due to tissue trauma, but do not disseminate to deeper locations. This is contrasted to the systemic (or deep) types, whether due to true pathogenic species that infect immunocompetent individuals, as *Histoplasma capsulatum* (teleomorph name: *Ajellomyces capsulatus*), or opportunistic species as *Aspergillus fumigatus* (teleomorph name: *Sortorya fumigata*). These organisms can infect at a primary site, as the lung, establish infection, then disseminate to other organs producing potentially life-threatening infections.

Table 23-1
Clinical Grouping of Some Medically Important Fungal Species (2, 4, 16)

Group	Selected Genera	Morphology Group	Disease
Superficial	*Malassezia furfur*	Yeast	Pityriasis versicolor
	Phaeoannellomyces werneckii	Yeast	Superficial phaeohyphomycosis
	Pedraia hortae	Filamentous	Black piedra
	Trichosporon beigelii	Yeast	White piedra
Cutaneous	*Epidermophyton floccosum*	Filamentous	Dermatophytosis
	Microsporum spp. (Anam)[a]		
	(*Arthroderma* spp. (Teleo)[a]	Filamentous	Dermatophytosis
	Trichophyton spp. (Anam.)		
	(*Arthroderma* spp.) (Teleo)	Filamentous	Dermatophytosis
Subcutaneous	*Candida albicans*	Yeast	Candidiasis
	Exophiala jeanselmei	Filamentous	Mycotic mycetoma and phaeohyphomycosis
	Fonsecaea verrucosa	Filamentous	Chromoblastomycosis
	Pseudallescheria boydii (Teleo)		
	(*Scedosporium apiospermum*) (Anam)	Filamentous	Mycotic mycetoma
	Sporothrix schenckii	Dimorphic	Sporotrichosis
Systemic: Pathogenic	*Coccidioides immitis*	Dimorphic	Coccidioidomycosis
	Histoplasma capsulatum (Anam)		
	(*Ajellomyces capsulatus*) (Teleo)	Dimorphic	Histoplasmosis
	Blastomyces dermatitidis (Anam)		
	(*Ajellomyces dermatitidis*) (Teleo)	Dimorphic	Blastomycosis
Opportunist	*Aspergillus* spp.	Filamentous	Aspergillosis
	Candida albicans	Yeast	Candidiasis
	Cryptococcus neoformans (Anam)		
	(*Filobasidiella neoformans*) (Teleo)	Yeast	Cryptococcosis
	Geotrichum candidum (Anam.)		
	(*Endomyces candidum*) (Teleo.)	Yeastlike	Geotrichosis

[a] Anam = name of anamorph, the asexual form; Teleo = name of teleomorph, the perfect or sexual form. See text for further details.

It also should be pointed out that there is a group of fungi that form black or brown colonies that are sometimes referred to as the dematiaceous fungi. These can be responsible for "phaeohyphomycoses," and may occur in any of the site-related categories (11). These will be discussed further in Exercise 24.

An abbreviated formal classification of fungi emphasizing the medically-important species is shown below. It is apparent from this abbreviated scheme that many fungi have more than one formal name. This arose in part because they were originally described as not having a sexual stage (i.e. an anamorph) and therefore placed in the Subdivision Deuteromycotina (the "imperfect fungi"). When a sexual stage (teleomorph form) was identified, these were then reclassified into a group based upon the type of sexual spore formed and other characteristics (i.e. Ascomycotina if ascospores produced; Basidiomycotina if basidiospores produced, etc.) and given an appropriate name. Nomenclaturally the teleomorph name is applied when sexual spores are identified, an uncommon occurrence in most clinical laboratory situations. From a practical standpoint, though both are acceptable, the anamorph names are most commonly used by the clinical mycologist. However, in this manual, to acquaint students with both, the most commonly used name will be given followed by the teleomorph or anamorph name, if any.

KINGDOM MYCETEAE
DIVISION: *AMASTIGOMYCOTINA* (1, 5)

SUBDIVISION: Zygomycotina. Have coenocytic, hyphae with few septa.

CLASS: Zygomycetes. Form asexual sporangiospores and sexual zygospores.

FAMILY: Mucoraceae

GENUS: *Mucor, Rhizopus, Absidia,* and others.

SUBDIVISION: Ascomycotina. When hypha are present, they are coenocytic with perforated septa. Form asexual ascospores within ascus.

CLASS: Ascomycetes. Sexually reproduce by various methods; asexual reproduction usually by conidia.

SUBCLASS: Hemiascomycetidae. Yeast or yeast-like without ascocarp (i.e. lack structure supporting or housing asci).

FAMILY: Endomycetaceae. Asexual reproduction by blastospores or arthrospores; forms typical hyphae.

GENUS: *Endomyces geotrichum* (anamorph: *Geotrichum candidum*).

FAMILY: Saccharomycetaceae. The unicellular yeasts that asexually reproduce by fission or budding.

GENUS: *Saccharomyces, Pichia guilliermondii* (anamorph name: *Candida guilliermondii*).

SUBCLASS: Plectomycetidae. Usually form unicellular ascospores in a true ascoma or ascocarp.

FAMILY: Gymnoascaceae

GENUS: *Ajellomyces dermatitidis* (anamorph: *Blastomyces dermatitidis*), *Arthroderma benhamiae* (anamorph: *Trichophyton mentagrophytes*), *Ajellomyces capsulatus* (anamorph: *Histoplasma capsulatum*), *Nannizzia gypsea* and *N. incurvata* (anamorph of both: *Microsporum gypseum*), and others.

FAMILY: Eurotiaceae

GENUS: *Sartorya fumigata* (anamorph: *Aspergillus fumigatus*); *Talaromyces* and *Eupenicillium* (anamorph: *Penicillium*)

SUBDIVISION: Basidiomycotina. Form sexual spores (basidiospores) on a basidium. Includes smuts, rusts, and mushrooms.

CLASS: Basidiomycetes

SUBCLASS: Teliomycetidae (basidiomycetous yeasts, rusts, smuts)

FAMILY: Ustilaginaceae

GENUS: *Filobasidiella neoformans* (anamorph: *Cryptococcus neoformans*)

SUBDIVISION: Deuteromycotina. No sexual phase. Reproduce by asexual conidia, coenocytic hyphae with perforated septa. The imperfect fungi.

CLASS: Deuteromycetes

SUBCLASS: Blastomycetidae. Asexual yeastlike organisms.

FAMILY: Cryptococcaceae (20)

GENUS: *Cryptococcus neoformans* (teleomorph name: *Filobasidiella neoformans*), *Candida* spp., *Rhodotorula* spp., *Trichosporon* spp., and others.

SUBCLASS: Hyphomycetidae. Conidia borne on hyphae in open.

FAMILY: Moniliaceae (Conidia formed directly on hyphum or on conidiophores that are poorly organized).

GENUS: *Trichophyton* spp., *Microsporum* spp. (but see family *Gymnoascaceae* above), *Epidermophyton floccosum, Geotrichum candidum* (teleomorph: *Endomyces geotrichum*), *Sporothrix schenckii, Coccidioides immitis, Aspergillus fumigatus* (teleomorph: *Sartorya fumigata*), *Penicillium* spp. (teleomorph: *Talaromyces* and *Eupenicillium* spp.) and many others.

FAMILY: Dematiaceae (usually dark hyphae and conidia; no organized fruiting body produced).

GENUS: *Phialophora* spp., *Cladosporium* spp., *Fonsecaea, Alternaria, Exophiala* spp., and others.

Identification of the genus and species of the pathogenic fungi and distinguishing these from saprophytic (saprobic) contaminants is generally accomplished based on morphological and cultural characteristics. Unlike most pathogenic bacteria, these organisms may differentiate, forming identifying morphologic structures. For the beginning student, one difficulty with studying the fungi is using the proper descriptive term. Many are defined at the end of this introductory section. Since these are important in communicating your findings to others (and vise versa), you should become acquainted with them. To relate some of the terms to structures, refer to Figure 23-1.

II. General Approaches to Fungal Identification.

Laboratory identification of the fungi will begin with the specimen, which, like that of other microorganisms, may be sputum, tissue biopsy, cerebrospinal fluid, stools, urine, blood, etc. However, unlike other microorganisms, specimens may include hair, skin scraping, and nail samples. No special care is required to collect or maintain samples aside from good techniques and common sense. Collection methods to avoid contamination are important because fungi, especially moulds, are slow-growing. Transport from patient to laboratory should be done as quickly as possible; if a delay is encountered, refrigeration is necessary. As should be expected, the sample type and organism contained in it influences its recovery with passage of time. Generally, yeasts or yeastlike dimorphic fungi are more sensitive to environmental conditions than moulds, and organisms in urine and blood specimens are less stable to holding than other types (2, 12). Once isolated, however, most can be stored for extended periods at -70°C if needed (5).

Subsequent steps generally follow those used in bacteriology and include microscopic examination, culture, and serology. Microscopic observation of the sample can provide data of great importance in diagnosis. Observation of yeasts, conidial or hyphal elements can be critical as a early indicator of whether a mycotic infection is present, and, if so, what type.

Microscopic examination using appropriate stains is presently the most-used type of direct sample examination. Stains as Calcofluor white, Giemsa, Gram, acid fast, negative stains, or one of many other possibilities can be used, depending on the type of sample and expected organism. The application of clearing agents as 10 to 20% KOH mixed with methylene blue will aid in distinguishing hyphal elements in strands of hair and in nail scrapings (8, 12).

Most fungi can be cultured on simple media. However, advantage has been taken of their characteristics in attempts to provide isolation media to obtain pure cultures and/or differentiation from other organisms. Moulds especially are unaffected by many antibacterial compounds, therefore one or more can be added to agar to inhibit bacterial contaminants if these are believed to be present. Sabouraud dextrose-brain heart infusion (SABHI) agar can be supplemented with chloramphenicol, gentamicin, penicillin, streptomycin, and other compounds. Similarly, BHI and inhibitory mold agar may be made more selective by similar or other additions. Cycloheximide has been frequently used to inhibit the growth of many saprobic fungal strains, however, care is advised since this compound also inhibits many yeasts. Sabouraud's dextrose agar containing chloramphenicol and cycloheximide is recommended for isolation of dermatophytic fungi. Blood enhances the growth of some fungi, particularly the dimorphic forms, therefore, for these it may be added in a 5-10% concentration (2, 12).

Some types of media directed toward differentiation are also available. Birdseed and caffeic acid agar for pigment production of *Cryptococcus neoformans* (teleomorph: *Filobasidiella neoformans*), and cornmeal agar for *Candida albicans* chlamydoconidia formation are examples. Some of these will be used in Exercise 24.

At this point the identification procedure for yeast forms and moulds may diverge. The former lends themself to physiological testing, much like the bacteria. Therefore, as we will see in Exercise 24 concerning the yeasts, assimilation and fermentation testing can be done as an aid in identification. Also, commercially-available rapid tests based on assaying these characteristics are usable among these organisms, and will be addressed in that exercise.

For the moulds, slide cultures may be required to accomplish a full morphological description (procedure described later in this exercise). This, then, along with information obtained from agar culture should provide all the descriptive information required for identification.

Antibody responses are weak in mycotic infections, therefore serological assay of patient antibodies do not have an important role in diagnosis of most fungal infections It is used for some, however. An example is the use of the complement fixation test to detect patient antibodies in histoplasmosis and coccidioidomycosis where the presence of titers of 1:8-1:16 and higher are suggestive of active infection (2, 9).

Detection of fungal antigens by serological methods is much more widely used. A latex agglutination test for detection of cryptococcal polysaccharide directly in spinal fluid is one such test. Also, other methods as CIE for detection of *Aspergillus*, *Candida*, and *Sporotrichum* antigens, agglutination for *C. albicans* and *Cryptococcus neoformans* (*F. neoformans*), immunofluorescence for *Candida*, and double diffusion for the fungi are among those used (9). Exoantigen detection using the latter methods has proven valuable for identification of dimorphic fungi and aspergilli (7). This method involves extraction of slant or broth culture filtrates to obtain exoantigen. Antiserum against the suspect antigen is then used for the assay in a double diffusion test, along with proper controls.

Commercially-available DNA probe tests are available from Gen-Probe for some fungi. These Accuprobe™ System assays are available for three systemic group fungi *H. capsulatum* (*A. capsulatus*), *B.* (*A.) dermatitidis*, and *C. immitis*, and for the yeast *C.* (*F.) neoformans*. These will be discussed further later.

Exercises 23-26 are designed to introduce you to some of the medically important fungi, and methods used in their identification. Becoming acquainted with these, along with proper applied terminology will be necessary for the continued study of these important organisms.

III. Laboratory Safety.

Relatively few fungi are life-threatening in the non-immunocompromised individual. Of the true pathogenic fungi, the dimorphic group of systemic fungi has been the major offenders. This picture is changing, however, with the increasing number of opportunistic type of mycotic infections, many by organisms that were once considered saprobic (e.g. 15, 16). Furthermore, the moulds form conidia of various types that may readily detach from their parent structures. Therefore, without a containment device, the chance of increasing spore contamination in the immediate environment is very high. This can lead to an increase in culture contamination throughout the laboratory. Of course, if the organism is pathogenic, the hazard to health should be apparent.

It is for these reasons that clinical specimens examined for fungi, and especially mould cultures, are handled in a containment device as a laminar flow biohazard hood (2, 12). Of all fungi, *Coccidioides immitis* is most notorious for its capacity to "escape" and cause infection, therefore, it should only be handled not only under containment, but also only after being formalinized (16). All fungal stages of the dimorphic fungi or materials suspected of containing the conidial form of these should follow Biosafety Level 3 practices (19). Yeast phase growth of these, though, and of other yeasts do not present the same problems. Therefore, these can be worked with on the open bench following good microbiological practices.

IMPORTANT MYCOLOGICAL TERMS (6, 8, 16)

Aleurioconidium (pl. aleurioconidia): Conidium attached laterally or terminally to hyphae or conidiophore formed by expansion of hyphal branch or conidiogenous cell. It separates from the hyphae by breaking of the wall of the hyphae below the conidium. (Syn. Aleuriospore.)

Anamorph: The asexual reproductive or imperfect form of a fungus.

Anthropophilic: Preference for humans as a host.

Arthroconidium (pl. arthroconidia): Conidium formation by hyphal segmentation of the septa. Release occurs by separation at the septum. (Syn: Arthrospore.)

Ascospore: A sexual spore formed within an ascus.

Ascus: A sac-like structure containing ascospores characteristic of Ascomycotina.

Basidiospore: A sexual spore formed on a basidium of the Subdivision Basidiomycotina.

Basidium (pl. basidia): A specialized structure producing basidiospores.

Blastoconidium (pl. blastoconidia): An asexual conidium produced through budding from a parent cell. It is a characteristic method of yeast reproduction. (Syn. Blastospore.)

Chlamydoconidium (pl. chlamydoconidia): A large, round, thick-walled resting cell produced by differentiation of the hyphae, and containing nutrient material. It may be intercalary (between cells of the hypha) or terminal. (Syn. Chlamydospore.)

Clavate: Shape in the form of a club.

Coenocytic: Hyphae having few septa and many nuclei, as in Zygomycotina hyphae.

Columella: The sterile part of a sporangiophore within the sporangium, as exemplified in the Zygomycotina.

Conidiogenous cell: Conidium-producing cell.

Conidiophore: A specialized hyphal branch, usually erect and aerial, containing cells (i.e. conidiogenous cell) upon which conidia develop.

Conidium (pl. conidia): An external asexual reproductive unit or propagule.

Dematiaceous: Having hypha and/or conidia that are pigmented black to brown (Also see Phaeo-).

Denticle: Small projection upon which a conidium arises.

Dimorphic: Having two forms (e. g. yeast form and hyphal form).

Echinulate: Presence of surface spines.

Ectothrix: Fungal invasion of the hair shaft with arthroconidia forming a sheath on the outside surface of the shaft.

Endospore: Spores formed within a structure (e. g. spores within a spherule or sporaniospores within a sporangium).

Endothrix: Fungal invasion and formation of arthroconidia within the hair shaft.

Floccose: Wool- or cotton-like.

Fusiform: Having a spindle shape.

Geophilic: Soil-associated as a habitat.

Germ-tube: Initial tube-like structure from yeast cell conidium or spore that develop into hypha.

Glabrous: Smooth.

Hypha (pl. hyphae): A single mycelial filament.

Intercalary: Formed between cells along the hypha (as chlamydoconidia).

Macroconidium (pl. macroconidia): A large, usually multiseptate conidium.

Metula (pl. metulae): Conidiophore branches that are sterile upon which conidia-bearing phialides are borne, as exemplified by *Aspergillus* and *Penicillium.*

Microconidium (pl. microconidia): A small, single celled conidium.

Mycelium (pl. mycelia): A mass of growth formed by the elongation, branching, and intertwining of the hyphae.

Nodular bodies: An intertwining mass of hyphae forming a ball-like structure.

Pectinate bodies: Narrow projections along one side of a hyphae giving the hyphal element an appearance of a comb.

Phaeo-: Prefix meaning dark pigmentation.

Phialide: A conidiogenous cell, typically bottle-shaped, producing conidium (specifically referred to as phialoconidium) in sequence without change in its own length or apical diameter.

Phialoconidium (pl. phialoconidia): Conidium formed from a phialide.

Pleomorphism: The occurrence of more than one form by an organism. In the fungi this frequently is used to describe the loss of spore-forming capacity and formation of sterile aerial mycelium.

Propagule: A cellular unit that can grow into another individual.

Pseudohyphae: Hyphal-like, elongated, filamentous blastoconidia formed from yeast-like parent cells. (Syn. pseudomycelium.)

Racquet (or racket) hyphae: Hypha consisting of a series of club-shaped cells in which the smaller end is attached to the larger end of a adjacent cell.

Rhizoid: Hypha that has the appearance of a root and grows into the medium, as seen in *Rhizopus.*

Saprobe: Saprophyte.

Septum: (pl. septa): Cross walls that divide the hypha into a multicellular structure.

Spiral hyphae: Mycelium showing cork-screw or coiled convolutions.

Sporangiospore: An asexual propagule produced within a sporangium.

Sporangium (pl. sporangia): A terminal sac-like structure within which sporangiospores are produced, and that is usually borne on a hyphal structure, the sporangiophore.

Sterigma (pl. Sterigmata): A structure from which basidiospores develop on the basidium.

Stolen: Hyphae that form root-like rhizoids; runners.

Sympodial: Condiogenesis at apices along a cell, alternately forming on side of the cell then the other.

Teleomorph: The sexual or perfect form of a fungus.

Thallus: The vegetative portion of a fungus; the mycelium.

Truncate: Abrupt or sharply ended, as if cut off.

Tuberculate: Having surface nodular projections.

Vesicle: An expanded or swollen tip of the conidiophore bearing phialides.

Zoophilic: Preference for animal hosts other than humans.

Zygospore: Thick-walled, large, multinucleate sexual propagules formed through the fusion of nuclei of specialized hyphae (gametangia). These are the characteristic sexual spores of the Zygomycotina.

EXERCISE 23
The Ubiquitous Filamentous Fungi

The fungi, like bacteria, are found as normal inhabitants of our environment. It is from this source, especially soil, that conidia cause infection in plants and animals. Among the filamentous fungi, only the anthropophilic dermatophytes, which are very common disease agents, spread from person to person (16).

The purpose of this exercise is to acquaint you with some of the procedures associated with isolation and identification of all filamentous fungi. Also, it will suggest to you some of the fungi that occur as airborne contaminants. Keeping in mind that disease-causing fungi come from soil, it is possible you may isolate one of these, especially those that cause opportunistic infections. *Aspergillus, Mucor, Rhizopus, Phialophora,* and others are frequently encountered from this source (2, 3). While non-infectious for the majority, use appropriate precautions outlined in "Laboratory Safety" in the introduction to this section.

The ubiquitous fungi such as those you isolate here are probably most important, from the standpoint of medical microbiology, by the confusion that they may cause in determination of the agent of disease. This is especially true in mycotic infections where the actual disease-causing agent may have been isolated, yet it is classified as a fungal contaminant. Therefore, it is always important to consider this possibility when fungi appear on cultures from clinical material.

MATERIALS

Part 1
Per student:
    1 plate Inhibitory Mold agar (deep poured)
    1 Parafilm strip

Part 2
Per student:
    2 culture dishes, each with sterile slide and cover slip
    1 Scalpel with No. 11 Baird-Parker blade
    5 ml sterile water
    1 5 ml pipette, sterile
    2 Parafilm strips
    2 dissecting needles

Per group of three students:
    1 Inhibitory Mold agar plate (standard depth)
    1 beaker 95% ethanol
Per Bench:
    1 bottle Lactophenol cotton blue (LCB)
    1 bottle clear fingernail polish
        95% ethanol
Optional, Per Bench:
    1 bottle Calcofluor White stain
    1 bottle 15% KOH solution

LABORATORY PROCEDURE

Part 1
A. Each student do the following for the isolation of filamentous fungi:
    1. Expose one Inhibitory Mold agar plate to the open air for 30-45 minutes. (This may be done anywhere you choose, but reduce the time if done in a dusty location, as on the floor where there is heavy foot traffic.) Note that this plate is "deep poured" and therefore contains extra agar to compensate for drying that may occur over the lengthy incubation period.
    2. Seal the plate with a Parafilm strip to reduce drying of the medium.
    3. Incubate plate in an inverted position at room temperature until medium sized mature colonies of fungi appear. At this time place the cultures in the refrigerator. Do not allow the colonies to overgrow each other, but do allow them to form reproductive structures, generally seen by a change from white to another color.
    4. Turn in 2 slides and 2 coverslips for sterilization.

Part 2
Note: To avoid excessive spore contamination in the laboratory, do all live and open culture work in a biohazard hood.
A. Airborne isolates: Each student is to carry out the following, using at least two isolated colonies from your Inhibitory Mold agar plate that appear to differ in color and/or morphology:

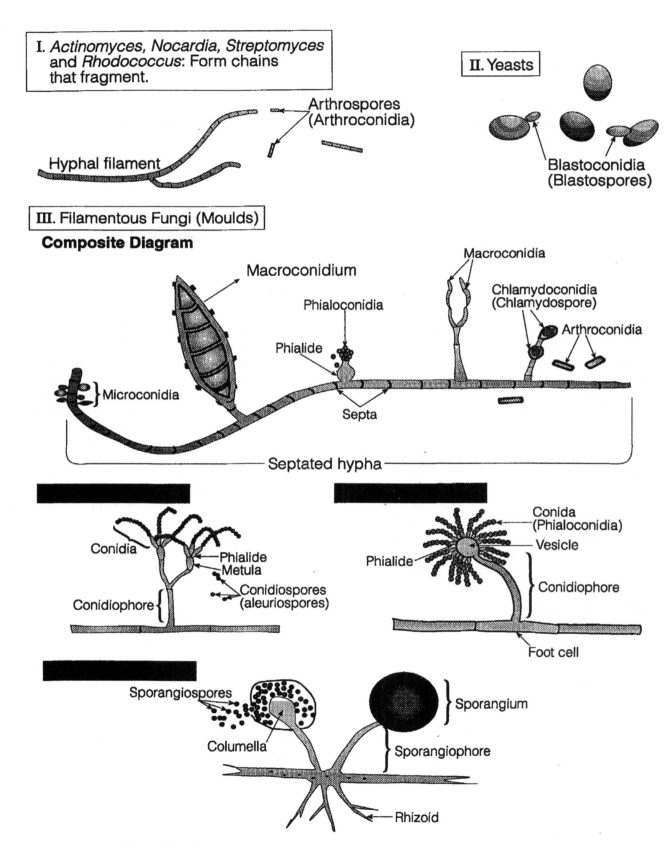

Figure 23-1: Diagram of fungal-like bacteria and true fungi showing their parts.

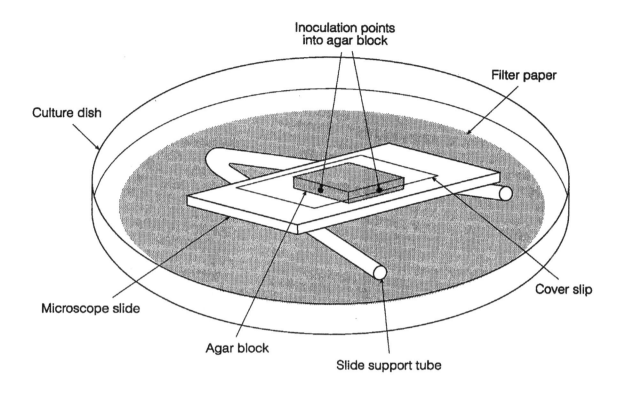

Figure 23-2: Slide culture for microscopic study of filamentous fungi.

1. Using the dissecting microscope, examine the fringes and upper surfaces of each colony. Especially observe isolated conidia or sporangia. Note the arrangement of the various mold parts. Also observe the general colony characteristics. Describe its texture (powdery, cottony. glabrous, yeast-like, velvety), surface and underside color, diffusible pigment and color, if any. Also, note the nature of surface topography (as folded, flat, heaped, or concentric rings), and any other characterstics that may be useful in identification.

2. Prepare a tease mount of your two isolates by the following method:

   a. Sterilize a scalpel blade by flaming off twice using 95% ethanol. Allow the blade to cool, then cut out a small, *thin* amount of agar with a portion of a colony containing mycelium with conidia or sporangium. Use care not to brush over the hyphae with the blade as this will break off and disorganize the fruiting structures.

   b. Transfer to a slide containing lactophenol cotton blue (LCB) and carefully tease the mycelium apart with 2 sterile dissecting needles, then place a cover slip on top and gently press into place. Resterilize needles and scalpel by flaming off twice with 95% ethanol.

   c. Examine with low and high-dry objectives of the microscope. LCB causes wall material containing chitin to stain light blue. This medium also aids in clearing hyphal material, as well as acting as a preservative.

3. Alternately, the transparent adhesive tape method can be used. This is done by touching the top of each of the two colony surfaces with the adhesive side of short lengths of tape. It is then flattened against a clean slide containing a small drop of LCB with adhesive side toward the glass and microscopically examined.

An improved variation of this (17) is to place an adhesive on one side of glass cover slips using the Pelikan Roll-Fix device (The Gillette Co., Boston, MA). Holding the cover slips with sterile forceps, the adhesive surface of each cover slip is now gently touched to the surface of separate colonies and each mounted over a small drop of LCB. Unlike the adhesive tape method, these can be sealed with fingernail polish to give a semi-permanent preparation.

4. When making your microscopic examination, note and record the following:
   a. Mycelium: Septate or non-septate; hyaline or dark; fine or course; pseudo-hyphae or true mycelium, and other notable properties.
   b. Fruiting structure: Type, as chlamydoconidia, arthroconidia, microconidia, macroconidia, sporangiospores, or other forms, and descriptions of each (color, shape, size, arrangement of its parts, and other features).
   c. Conidium or sporangiospores: Shape, relative size, color, thin or thick walls, and smooth or rough.

5. Sketch a diagram that realistically represents the fungus you see, and label each part. Can you make a tentative identification of your two isolates at the genus level?

B. Microslide cultures (5, 8): Commonly, material examined by tease or adhesive tape mounts as in *Part 2* A, fail to provide sufficient information to identify the isolate because of disorientation of the fungal parts. If this occurs it is necessary to grow the organism such that its structural features are intact yet microscopically observable. This can best be done by microslide cultures. One such procedure is given below. (Also see Figure 23-2).

1. Obtain a petri dish containing a sterile slide resting on a bent glass tubing, both situated on a piece of filter paper.

2. Using a scalpel flamed in 95% ethanol, slice Inhibitory Mold agar of standard depth so as to obtain pieces with surface dimensions of approximately 0.5-1.0 cm square.

3. Place the agar square on top of the slide contained within the petri dish (Figure 23-2).

4. Working within a containment hood, obtain an inoculum (a small piece of the colony is preferable) with a sterile loop or needle using one of the colonies studied above. With this, inoculate the agar square near the center of each of the four exposed sides, but not on top.

5. Cover the agar square with a sterile cover slip. Add 1-1.5 ml sterile distilled water to the bottom of the dish. The filter paper will absorb the moisture and provide a humid atmosphere within the culture dish. Seal the plate with Parafilm and incubate at room temperature. If necessary, add more water during the incubation period to prevent becoming dry.

6. Repeat steps 1-5 using the second isolate you previously described in *Part 2* A.

7. Examine the slide cultures at 2-3 day intervals (if necessary, scan with the dissecting microscope) until conidia or sporangia appear. These must be present before moving on to Step 8.

8. After the appearance of fruiting structures, the organisms can be prepared for examination. Since these were isolated from the air, it is most probable that they are saprobes. However, if a pathogenic filamentous fungous is suspected to be present, it must be killed. Do so by exposing the microculture, still contained within the Petri dish, to formaldehyde. This is done by placing 5 ml formaldehyde in a small beaker into an air-tight jar, then inserting the microculture dish, and sealing the container. This is allowed to stand at room temperature for three days (18). Following this, proceed with Step 9.

9. Again working within the confines of a biohazard hood, carefully remove the cover slip of one culture and set aside with fungal growth facing upward. Remove the agar square from the slide and discard in an appropriate container with disinfectant.

10. With cover slip: Place a small drop of lactophenol cotton blue in the center of a clean slide. Invert the cover slip so fungal growth faces downward and lower it on to the mounting medium.

11. With slide: Place a small drop of lactophenol cotton blue on slide over the area of growth. Cover with clean cover slip.

12. Seal both preparations with clear fingernail polish and examine.

   Alternately, if a fluorescent microscope equipped with a mercury vapor lamp and 250-400 nM-transmitting filter is available for your use, carry out the calcofluor white staining procedure as follows (13, 14):

   a. Place one drop of Fungi-Fluor™ or fluorescent brightener (calcofluor white; see Appendix 2 for formulation) to the slide over the area of growth.

   b. Add a drop of 15% KOH, which serves as a clearing agent.

   c. Cover with a glass cover slip, and seal with clear fingernail polish.

   d. Observe your preparation by bright field or phase contrast optics, then by fluorescent microscopy. In the latter fungi will fluoresce apple green or blue white. The major advantage of calcofluor white fluorescence is that it allows rapid scanning of a preparation under low power of the microscope.

13. Repeat Steps 9-12 with the second slide culture.

14. Describe your findings. Draw an accurate illustration of your organism. Compare observations using LCB and calcofluor white, if the latter was done. Attempt to identify your isolates using one of the references available for your use.

REFERENCES

1. Alexopoulos, C. J., and C. W. Mims. 1979. Introductory mycology, 3rd ed. John Wiley & Sons, New York. 632 p.

2. Baron, E. J., L. R. Peterson, and S. M. Finegold. 1994. Bailey & Scott's diagnostic microbiology, 9th ed. Mosby-Year Book, Inc., St. Louis. p. 689-710.

3. Campbell. C. K. 1989. Identification of common culture contaminants, p. 171-185. In E. G. V. Evans, and M. D. Richardson (ed.), Medical mycology: a practical approach. IRL Press, Oxford.

4. Davis, B. D., R. Dulbecco, H. N. Eisen, and H. S. Ginsberg. 1990. Microbiology, 4th ed. J. B. Lippincott Co., Philadelphia. p. 737-765.

5. Dixon, D. M., and R. A. Fromtling. 1991. Morphology, taxonomy and classification of the fungi, p. 579-587. In A. Balows, W. J. Hausler, Jr., K. L. Herrmann, H. D. Isenberg, and H. J. Shadomy (ed.), Manual of clinical microbiology, 5th ed. American Society for Microbiology, Washington, D. C.

6. Evans, E. G. V., and M. D. Richardson (ed.). 1989. Medical mycology: a practical approach. IRL Press, Oxford. p. 285-287.

7. Kaufman, L., and P. G. Standard. 1987. Specific and rapid identification of medically important fungi by exoantigen detection. Ann. Rev. Microbiol. **41**:209-225.

8. Larone, D. H. 1987. Medically important fungi: a guide to identification. Elsevier Science Publishing Co., Inc., New York. p. 173-220.

9. Mackenzie, D. W. R. 1989. Serological tests, p. 201-233. In E. G. V. Evans, and M. D. Richardson (ed.). Medical mycology: a practical approach. IRL Press, Oxford.

10. McGinnis, M. R. 1980. Recent taxonomic developments and changes in medical mycology. Ann. Rev. Microbiol. **34**:109-135.

11. McGinnis, M. R. 1983. Chromoblastomycosis and phaeohyphomycosis: new concepts, diagnosis, and mycology. J. Am. Acad. Dermatol. **8**:1-16.

12. Merz, W. G., and G. D. Roberts. 1991. Detection and recovery of fungi from clinical specimens, p. 588-600. In A. Balows, W. J. Hausler, Jr., K. L. Herrmann, H. D. Isenberg, and H. J. Shadomy (ed.), Manual of clinical microbiology, 5th ed. American Society for Microbiology, Washington, D. C.

13. Milne, L. J. R. 1989. Direct microscopy, p. 17-45. In E. G. V. Evans, and M. D. Richardson (ed.), Medical mycology: a practical approach. IRL Press, Oxford.

14. Pasarell, L., and W. A. Schell. 1992. Potassium hydroxide-calcofluor white procedure, p. 6.4.1-6.4.2. In H. D. Isenberg (ed.), Clinical microbiology procedures handbook, Vol. 1: M. R. McGinnis (sect. ed.), Mycology. American Society for Microbiology, Washington, DC.

15. Rinaldi, M. G. 1991. Problems in the diagnosis of invasive fungal diseases. Rev. Infect. Dis. **13**:493-495.

16. Rippon, J. W. 1988. Medical mycology, 3rd ed. W. B. Saunders Co., Philadelphia, p. 1-11; 779-784.

17. Rodriguez-Tuela, J. L., and P. Aviles. 1991. Improved adhesive method for microscopic examination of fungi in culture. J. Clin. Microbiol. **29**:2604-2605.

18. Sigler, L. 1992. Preparing and mounting slide cultures, p. 6.12.1-6.12.4. In H. D. Isenberg (ed.), Clinical microbiology procedures handbook, Vol. 1: M. R. McGinnis (sect. ed.), Mycology. American Society for Microbiology, Washington, DC.

19. U. S. Public Health Service, Centers for Disease Control and National Institutes of Health. 1988. Biosafety in microbiological and biomedical laboratories, 2nd ed. Publication No. (NIH) 88-8395. Dept. of Health and Human Services, Washington, DC. p. 45-55.

20. Warren, N. G., and H. J. Shadomy. 1991. Yeasts of medical importance, p. 617-629. In A. Balows, W. J. Hausler, Jr., K. L. Herrmann, H. D. Isenberg, and H. J. Shadomy (ed.), Manual of clinical microbiology, 5th ed. American Society for Microbiology, Washington, D. C.

21. Weitzman, I., and J. Kane. 1991. Dermatophytes and agents of superficial mycoses, p. 601-616. In A. Balows, W. J. Hausler, Jr., K. L. Herrmann, H. D. Isenberg, and H. J. Shadomy (ed.), Manual of clinical microbiology, 5th ed. American Society for Microbiology, Washington, D. C.

Exercise 23: Ubiquitous Fungi Results
Data Table 1: Isolate No. 1

Isolation Data:

Date of Exposure: _____ Location of Exposure _____

Time of Exposure: _____

Date of First Reading: _____ Culture Age _____

Date of Second Reading: _____ Culture Age _____

Colony Characteristics		First Reading	Second Reading
Size, mm			
Surface Texture	Velvet-like		
	Granular		
	Floccose		
	Glabrous		
Topography	Flat		
	Folded		
	Radial furrows		
	Heaped		
	Other		
Color (describe)	Surface		
	Underside		
	Soluble pigment		
	Other		
Other	(Describe)		
Properties			

Exercise 23: Ubiquitous Fungi Results
Data Table 1: Isolate No. 1 (Cont'd)

Microscopic Observations:

Culture Age of Tease Preparation: _____ Of Slide Culture: _____

Character		Tease Preparation	Slide Culture	
			CW[b]	LCB[b]
Hyphae	Septate or nonseptate			
	Hyaline or dark			
	Course or fine			
	Other (describe)			
Spores	Type(s)[a]			
	Size			
	Shape			
	Color			
	Surface appearance			
	Wall thickness			
	Other (describe)			

[a] Types = chlamydoconidia, arthroconidia, etc.
[b] CW = calcofluor white; LCB = lactophenol cotton blue

Drawing with Labeled Parts:

Tease Preparation

Magnification: _____

Culture Age: _____

Slide Culture Preparation

Magnification: _____

Stain: _____

Culture Age: _____

Probable Name of Isolate No. 1: _____

Exercise 23: Ubiquitous Fungi Results
Data Table 2: Isolate No. 2

Isolation Data:

Date of Exposure: _____ Location of Exposure _____

Time of Exposure: _____

Date of First Reading: _____ Culture Age _____

Date of Second Reading: _____ Culture Age _____

Colony Characteristics		First Reading	Second Reading
Size, mm			
Surface Texture	Velvet-like		
	Granular		
	Floccose		
	Glabrous		
Topography	Flat		
	Folded		
	Radial furrows		
	Heaped		
	Other		
Color (describe)	Surface		
	Underside		
	Soluble pigment		
	Other		
Other	(Describe)		
Properties			

Exercise 23: Ubiquitous Fungi Results
Data Table 2: Isolate No. 2 (Cont'd)

Microscopic Observations:
Culture Age of Tease Preparation: _____ Of Slide Culture: _____

	Character	Tease Preparation	Slide Culture	
			CW[b]	LCB[b]
Hyphae	Septate or nonseptate			
	Hyaline or dark			
	Course or fine			
	Other (describe)			
Spores	Type(s)[a]			
	Size			
	Shape			
	Color			
	Surface appearance			
	Wall thickness			
	Other (describe)			

[a] Types = chlamydoconidia, arthroconidia, etc.
[b] CW = calcofluor white; LCB = lactophenol cotton blue

Drawing with Labeled Parts:

Tease Preparation

Magnification: _____

Culture Age: _____

Slide Culture Preparation

Magnification: _____

Stain: _____

Culture Age: _____

Probable Name of Isolate No. 2: _____

Other Laboratory Notes

EXERCISE 24
Pathogenic Yeasts

I. Disease Associations.

Yeasts are usually considered to be fungi that are single cells during at least a part of their vegetative cycle and that reproduce by budding, although there are exceptions. Most of those that have life cycles including a sexual stage are found in the Ascomycotina, but some are also classified in the Basidiomycotina.

The yeasts that cause infection are found in many genera. One of the most common in humans are species of *Candida,* and among these, the predominant species, both as an infectious agent and as normal flora, is *C. albicans*. These organisms can be found in the gastrointestinal tract and mucocutaneous membranes. It is also widely distributed in our environment, as soil, food, and fomites. In disease, it is an opportunist capable of causing a host of systemic disease, as endocarditis, pneumonia, arthritis, and meningitis. It also causes subcutaneous disease, especially of the mucocutaneous types, including vaginitis, thrush (oral infection), gastrointestinal candidiasis, and others. It is evident that this organism has a versatility to attack various host tissue beyond most other organisms we have studied up to this time. Yet, interestingly, most cases of disease are derived from the endogenous flora of the patient, usually due to a decrease in normal host defenses (8, 27). In the oral cavity, for example, 60-70% of the normal yeast flora in healthy individuals consists of *C. albicans,* followed by lesser concentrations of *C. glabrata* and *C. tropicalis* (22). In laboratory diagnosis of a yeast infection, this can have an obvious impact since now a separation of normal flora *C. albicans* must be made from one that is the agent of disease.

Approximately twelve species of *Candida* of the more than 150 total are thought capable of causing opportunistic disease, several of which are shown in Table 24-1, along with *C. albicans*. There is general agreement that the incidence of infection due to all opportunistic *Candida* is increasing. In fact, this is generally true of all fungal infections (2), and especially in nosocomial environments. This can be expected to continue with the increased sizes of high risk populations and expanded use of medical interventions (26).

Another important yeast is *Cryptococcus (Filobasidiella) neoformans,* the primary agent of cryptococcosis (older names include European blastomycosis and torulosis). This agent is categorized as an opportunist capable of causing systemic infections (Table 23-1). It is saprobic, especially in soil enriched with bird droppings, and found on plants and animals. While the disease occurs in a variety of conditions as corticosteroid therapy, diabetes mellitus, and cancer, it has been particularly troublesome in AIDS patients. It is the most frequent fungal infection here, leading to life threatening circumstances. In the U. S., 5-10% of HIV-infected patients develop meningitis due to *C. (F.) neoformans* (24), and is one of the key disease indicators of AIDS (5). While this species is, for practical purposes, the only infectious agent among the many species of *Cryptococcus, C. albidus* and some others have also been rarely implicated as disease agents (27).

Many other species of yeast have been obtained from clinical specimens, but of less frequency than *Candida* and *Cryptococcus,* are also given in Table 23-1 and in Table 24-1. They are all opportunistic and systemic types. (As an aside, it should be noted that *Geotrichum candidum* is not actually a yeast, but generally included as such because its colony characteristics are yeast-like, and its method of study is similar to that applied to yeasts.) *S. cerevisiae,* as an example, while commonly found in the human respiratory, urinary, and gastrointestinal tracts as a commensal, also has been implicated as a systemic agent. However, it is rare with only 17 cases of infection reported in the English literature through mid-1990 (1).

Other pathogenic fungi have yeast-like phases. These are typified by *Histoplasma capsulatum (Ajellomyces capsulatus)* and *Blastomyces (Ajellomyces) dermatitidis*. Despite having, at least in part, a form that is yeastlike, they are generally not compatible with the study of yeasts. These will therefore be covered separately in Exercise 26.

II. Clinical Specimens.

Based upon the preceding discussion, clinical samples for isolation of yeasts can come from a variety of sources. Cerebrospinal fluid, especially containing *C. (F.) neoformans*, pus, blood, oropharyngeal, urine, stools, and others are potential types. Because of the normal flora aspect for many of these, caution is required concerning which samples actually to process for yeast isolation. Sandven (20) recommends that minimally all samples from serious mycotic infection (e.g. systemic and CNS), pus, and those that are normally sterile should be analyzed. Aside from these, each facility must make a judgment based on their own situation.

Primary isolation, as discussed in the Introduction to Medical Mycology, can be done on several types of media. Cycloheximide inhibits many yeasts, including *C. (F.) neoformans*, but not *C. albicans* (27). Candida Bromcresol Green (BCG) agar, a differential medium, is used by some for primary isolation or for secondary culture (12, 20). Birdseed agar, a differential medium for *C. (F.) neoformans*, is also useful when processing sputum from AIDS patients (6). This species alone in its genus forms brown colonies on this agar containing an extract of a common component of birdseed, *Guizotia abyssinia* (Indian thistle plant) seeds.

On most agars, yeasts will typically have a butyrous consistency, with a smooth to rough surface, dull appearance, with pigmentation. If a capsule is present, as with cryptococci, a mucoid appearance will be seen. The optimal growth temperature for saprobic types is less than 37°C, while infectious strains grow well at this temperature and this can therefore be useful in differentiation of some species (27).

III. Identification.

Identification of yeasts is based upon several tests including cultural assays such as induction of sexual spores; biochemical tests encompassing fermentation, assimilation, and urease tests; animal inoculation tests; and serological techniques. Table 24-1 provides some selective differential data concerning those discussed here. Some additional comments will be helpful, however.

Microscopic examination of clinical or other material will show that yeasts are generally larger in size than bacteria. *S. cerevisiae* approximates 3-9 X 5-20 μm, *C. albicans* are 3-7 X 3-14 μm, and *C. (F.) neoformans* 4-8 μm in diameter (16). Because of their size, as with many fungi, they frequently can be examined at less than 1000X magnifi-

cation. When making such examinations, in addition to the general size and shape of the parent cell, the appearance of blastospore attachment should be noted, as well as the number of blastospores per parent cell. The presence of capsules (Photo 24-2) also can be significant, as can the presence of chlamydospores, germ tubes, and pseudohyphae, all structures that will be seen in this exercise. Examples of the importance of these is seen with *C. albicans* and *C. (F.) neoformans* where identification to the genus level can be made based on microscopic examination alone. *C. albicans*, as seen in Table 24-1 and Photo 24-1, forms pseudohyphae, chlamydoconidia, and especially germ tubes. *C. (F.) neoformans*, on the other hand, produces none of these structures, but commonly forms a capsule, and, not shown in Table 24-1, produces buds that are narrow at the point of attachment to its parent cell.

Metabolic tests are very important in speciation of the yeasts. Fermentation tests are commonly a part of the identification scheme, where gas (CO_2) production is the indicator, not a change in the color indicator as commonly observed with the bacteria. Substrate assimilation is, however, more significant in measuring the capacity of a yeast to use a compound as its sole carbon source. In the standard tube test, the presence of growth tells whether an organism's enzyme system is capable of using a particular compound (20, 27). Assimilation assays also can be accomplished by using filter paper disks containing single substrates placed on (or in) substrate-free medium containing the isolate. Growth around any disk is indicative of substrate being used. The BBL® Minitek™ Yeast Identification System is based upon this type of arrangement.

Several commercially available rapid tests are made for yeast identification. The API 20C is one of the most widely used, and yields results comparable to the standard tube system. It consists of a tray with 20 cupules, 19 of which contain various substrates, the last serving as a substrate-free growth control. The presence or absence of growth is, as in the standard tube test, the indicator of substrate utilization. Results, which in most cases are available in 48 hours, are compared to a reference data base provided by the manufacturer to reach an identification of the isolate (2, 27). Other examples of miniaturized

**Table 24-1
Identifying characteristics of Selected Yeast Species (4, 20, 27)**

Genus-species[a]	Growth at 37°C	Capsule	Chlamydoconidia	Pseudohypha	Germ tubes	Fermentation Glu[c]	Lac	Malt	Raf	Suc	Treh	Assimilation Glu	Lac	Malt	Mel	Raf	Suc	Treh	Urease	Nitrate Utilizat.
Candida albicans	+[b]	−	+	+	+	+	−	+	−	−	+	+	−	+	−	−	+	+	−	−
C. (Pichia) guilliermondii	+	−	−	+	−	+	−	−	+	+	+	+	−	+	+	+	+	+	−	−
C. (Clavispora) lusitaniae	+	−	−	+	−	+	−	−	−	+	+	+	−	+	−	−	+	+	−	−
C. parapsilosis (Lodderomyces elongisporus)	+	−	−	+	−	+	−	−	−	−	−	+	−	+	−	−	+	+	−	−
C. tropicalis	+	−	−	+[d]	−	+	−	+	−	+	+	+	−	+	−	−	+	+	−	−
Torulopsis glabrata	+	−	−	−	−	+	−	−	ND	−	+	+	−	−	−	−	−	+	−	−
Cryptococcus (Filobasidiella) neoformans	+[e]	+	−	−	−	−	−	−	−	−	−	+	−	+	−	V	+	+	+	−
C. albidus (F. fluoriforme)	V	+	−	−	−	−	−	−	−	−	−	+	V	+	+	+	+	+	+	+
C. laurentii	+	+	−	−	−	−	−	−	−	−	−	+	+	+	+	+	+	+	+	−
Geotrichum (Endomyces) candidum	V	−	−	+[d]	−	−	−	−	−	−	−	+	−	−	−	−	−	−	−	−
Rhodotorula rubra	+	−	−	−	V	−	−	−	−	−	−	+	−	+	−	+	+	+	+	−
Saccharomyces cerevisiae	+	−	−	V	−	+	−	+	+	+	V	+	−	+	−	+	+	V	−	−

[a] Six of 12 *Candida* spp., one of three *Torulopsis*, two of six *Cryptococcus* spp., and one of two *Rhodotorula* spp. frequently isolated from clinical specimens shown. Teleomorph names of anamorphs, if any, given in parenthesis.

[b] Designations: + = usually positive; − = usually negative; V = variable; ND = No data.

[c] Abbreviations for carbohydrates: Glu = glucose; Lac = Lactose; Malt = maltose; mel = melibiose; Raf = raffinose; Suc = sucrose; Treh = trehalose.

[d] Also forms true hyphae.

[e] Forms brown colonies on Birdseed agar.

manufactured systems include the API Yeast Ident™, which can be read in 4 hours, and the Uni-Yeast Tek™ plate and tube system. The automated Vitek system also includes a yeast data base, and has been evaluated for this purpose (e.g. 2, 9), as has the Microscan System (15, 23). Finally, the SOC™ Yeast Identification System takes another approach. Here identification is based on incubation of slide plates at 38-39°C for 3 hours with the test yeast. These are examined microscopically for germ tubes, pseudomycelium, and arthroconidia. After an added 24 hours at room temperature the development of a dark brown color also shows the presence of *C. (F.) neoformans*, or chlamydoconidia formation will verify the presence of *C. albicans*.

Antigen detection methods using commercially available kits can be used, especially for the detection of *C. (F.) neoformans* capsular antigen in CSF and blood. Latex agglutination (LA) tests are found from several sources. Such tests for detection of *C. (F.) neoformans* antigen have proven to be very effective, although cross reactions with rheumatoid factor occur and therefore must be carefully controlled for this (7). *C. albicans* LA tests have suffered from varying specificity and sensitivities (reviewed by reference 14). Therefore, these have not achieved the diagnostic usefulness seen with the cryptococcal LA tests. Agglutination, double diffusion, and ELISA tests also can be used for these organisms. In the latter case, Meridian Diagnostics Premier™ EIA kit has been shown to be more sensitive and equal in specificity for detection of cryptococcal antigen as the Meridian LA test (11). Immuno-Mycologics, Inc. also markets an EIA kit for the detection of *Candida*.

In molecular methods, Gen-Probe Accuprobe™ system has become commercially available for culture confirmation of *C. (F.) neoformans*. Others are also actively being investigated for application toward yeast identification. For *Candida albicans*, DNA probes (e.g. 10), PCR (e. g. 3, 18), and restriction fragment analysis (17) have been applied, as have DNA probes for *C. (F.) neoformans* (19, 21, 25).

For epidemiological purposes, the typing scheme of *C. (F.) neoformans* is straight-forward. These organisms fall into one of four serotypes, A, B, C, or D. Types A and D correspond to *F. neoformans* var. *neoformans*; types B and C to *F. neoformans* var. *gatti*. Type A is most common worldwide, B has been isolated from the far Western U. S., and from AIDS patients throughout the U. S. (27). A typing system for *C. albicans* remains to be perfected, despite a large number of attempts by many approaches (review by reference 13).

MATERIALS

Part 1

A. Per pair of students:
  - 1 each 2-3 day old brain heart infusion (BHI) agar slant cultures of *C. albicans*, *C. (P.) guilliermondii*, and *S. cerevisiae*
  - 1 plate corn meal Tween 80 agar
  - 2 tubes fetal bovine serum or bovine serum, 0.5 ml/tube
  - 3 tubes with 5 ml sterile distilled water
  - 3 tubes each of the following fermentation media with Durham tubes:
    Glucose
    Maltose
    Raffinose
  - 3 tubes each modified Wickerham medium containing:
    Glucose
    Maltose
    Raffinose
    No carbohydrate
  - 1 sterile 10 ml pipette
    20 ml sterile mineral oil
    95% ethanol in 125 ml beaker
B. Per bench:
  Cryptococcus (Filobasidiella) neoformans stock culture
  - 1 bottle India ink
  - 1 tube Vaspar
    Applicator stick

LABORATORY PROCEDURES

Part 1

A. Known cultures: Each pair of students will be provided with 2-3 day old BHI plate cultures of *Candida albicans*, *C. (P.) guilliermondii*, and *Saccharomyces cerevisiae*. Carry out the following steps with these:
  1. Prepare smears of *C albicans* and *S. cerevisiae*. Gram stain and observe microscopically. Sketch and describe. Note the relative sizes of these organisms. Are there blastoconidia? If present, are there more than one per cell? Are the blastoconidia broad or narrow at the apex? Dark or hyaline? What is their shape?
  2. Carry out the germ tube test as follows using *C. albicans* and *C. (P.) guilliermondii*.
    a. Prepare a light suspension of organisms in separate tubes of bovine serum containing 0.5 ml per tube.
    b. Incubate tubes at 37°C water bath for two hours.
    c. Prepare a wet mount of each organism and microscopically observe. This is done by scanning each area under the cover slips with the low power objective of the microscope. The high power (400X) objective can be used to confirm their presence, but use of the oil immersion objective should be unnecessary. Germ tubes will be noted as a thin, hyphal-like projection from the yeast cell, *unconstricted* at its base. Draw a diagram of a germ-tube producing organism that you observe. If none are seen at this time, repeat the observation with a new wet mount preparation after 1 or 2 hours of additional incubation. If still none is seen, the test is negative (27).
    d. Record the results of this assay.
  3. Carry out a colony examination for each organism on the stock culture plate. Use the same descriptive procedures as that used for bacteria.
  4. For the production of chlamydoconidia, do the following:
    Inoculate each organism onto ⅓ plate of corn meal Tween 80 agar. Do so by

streaking each in three or four short parallel lines with a needle, then cut across these with a sterile loop (27). Slice the agar to the depth of the medium and about 1.5 to 2 cm long. Prepare the cut at a 45° angle relative to the agar surface. Also, while the loop is inserted into the agar, lift the agar slightly so as to separate a small area of it from the bottom of the dish allowing some of the inoculum to move between that surface and the agar. Place a sterile cover slip over the streaked and cut agar (cover slip may be sterilized by flaming off with 95% ethanol). Incubate at room temperature for 24-72 hours.

5. Prepare a very dilute suspension of each organism in separate tubes containing 5 ml sterile distilled water. Do so by placing a small amount of inoculum from a loop or needle into the water. Now, working in a biohazard hood, gently aspirate the tube contents several times with a sterile Pasteur pipette and bulb. After the inoculum is thoroughly suspended, transfer *one* drop to each:

   a. Glucose, maltose and raffinose fermentation broths. Overlay each tube with 2 ml mineral oil and incubate at room temperature. Positive cultures may be discarded, but negative cultures should be incubated up to 10 days.

   b. Glucose, maltose, and trehalose Wickerham medium slants to determine assimilation patterns. If necessary, use a loop to spread the inoculum over the slant surface. Also, inoculate a control slant of medium containing no sugar. Incubate at room temperature for up to 2 weeks. Positive cultures may be discarded as incubation progresses.

B. *Cryptococcus (Filobasidiella) neoformans*

1. Each pair of student prepare an India ink wet mount for capsule observation from a stock culture of C. (F.) neoformans made available for this purpose. This can be done by placing a small drop of water on a clean slide, then transferring and emulsifying a minute amount of organisms into this. After placing a cover slip over the preparation, allow a drop of India ink to diffuse under it from the outer edge. Excess liquid may be blotted with absorbent material (and then

discarded in disinfectant). Seal the preparation with vaspar.

Repeat this procedure using your stock culture of *S. cerevisiae*. Microscopically observe for the presence of capsules around both of the organisms (also see Photo 24-2). While observing the cryptococci, also find whether it has blastoconidia, and if so, the number per cell, and its appearance at the attachment site. Are pseudohyphae and chlamydoconidia present? Record your findings (Data Table 3) and diagram your observations.

2. Observe the demonstration of C. (F.) neoformans inoculated into the same fermentation and assimilation media used above. Also, it has been placed on Caffeic acid agar or on Birdseed agar and onto a Christensen urea agar slant. Note the incubation time and temperature. Record your observations.

Part 2

A. *Candida* spp. and *Saccharomyces*:

1. Observe corn meal Tween 80 agar plate for presence of chlamydoconidia. These should appear (on species that are capable of producing them) within 24 hours, but some may be delayed. Start by examining growth under the cover slip on top of the agar or under the surface of the inverted plate. Use the low power objective of your microscope, being careful not to break the cover slip or to touch the agar. Chlamydospores are morphologically circular, thick walled, and larger in diameter than blastoconidia (Photo 24-1). In most instances, these will be readily found, along with blastoconidia, and, for many, pseudohyphae. Occasionally, however, both top and bottom of plates will need to be examined to locate an "environmental nitch" that permits chlamydoconidia formation.

   Diagram the typical morphology of structures observed for each species. Label the parts of your drawing.

2. Observe fermentation and assimilation tests. Remember that the former is positive only if gas is present in ample amounts. Do the two types of assays give similar results? Should they?

3. Record and discuss your results (Data Tables 1-3).

B. Observe prepared slides of *Saccharomyces cerevisiae* ascospores grown on Ascospore medium (Remel) (16). Note the relative size of asci and the number and arrangement of ascospores. Record your observations.

QUESTIONS

1. In the assimilation test (*Part 1* A-5b), what is the purpose of diluting the yeasts before inoculation of Wickerham medium? Is this step also important for fermentation tests (*Part 1* A-5a)? Why?

2. Speculate about the purpose of inoculating *C. albicans* and other yeasts to induce chlamydoconidia formation by slicing the agar and either allowing the inoculum to flow beneath it, or covering the organisms with a cover slip (*Part 1* A-4)? (Note: To facilitate microscopic examination is only part of the answer.)

REFERENCES

1. Aucott, J. N., J. Fayen, H. Grossnicklas, A. Morrissey, M. J. Lederman, and R. A. Salata. 1990. Invasive infection with *Saccharomyces cerevisiae*: report of three cases and review. Rev. Infect. Dis. 12:406-411.

2. Baron, E. J., L. R. Peterson, and S. M. Finegold. 1994. Bailey & Scott's diagnostic microbiology, 9th ed. Mosby-Year Book, Inc., St. Louis. p. 689-775.

3. Buchman, T. G., M. Rossier, W. G. Merz, and P. Charache. 1990. Detection of surgical pathogens by in vitro DNA amplification. Part I. Rapid identification of *Candida albicans* by in vitro amplification of a fungus-specific gene. Surgery 108:338-347.

4. Campbell, M. C., and J. C. Stewart. 1980. The medical mycology handbook. John Wiley & Sons, New York. p. 3-10, 85-209, 244-252.

5. Centers for Disease Control. 1987. Revision of the CDC Surveillance case definition for acquired immunodeficiency syndrome. MMWR 36 (Suppl.):1S-15S.

6. Denning, D. W., D. A. Stevens, and J. R. Hamilton. 1990. Comparison of *Guizotia abyssinica* seed extract (birdseed) agar with conventional media for selective identification of *Cryptococcus neoformans* in patients with acquired immunodeficiency syndrome. J. Clin. Microbiol. 28:2565-2567.

7. Diamond, R. D. 1990. Crytpococcus neoformans, p. 1980-1989. *In* G. L. Mandell, R. G. Douglas, Jr., and J. E. Bennett (ed.), Principles and practices of infectious diseases, 3rd ed. Churchill Livingstone, New York.

8. Edwards, J. E., Jr. 1990. Candida species, p. 1943-1958. *In* G. L. Mandell, R. G. Douglas, Jr., and J. E. Bennett (ed.), Principles and practices of infectious diseases, 3rd ed. Churchill Livingstone, New York.

9. El-Zaatari, M., L. Pasarell, M. R. McGinnis, J. Buckner, G. A. Land, and I. F. Salkin. 1990. Evaluation of the updated Vitek yeast identification data base. J. Clin. Microbiol. 28: 1938-1941.

10. Fox, B. C., H. L. T. Mobley, and J. C. Wade. 1989. The use of a DNA probe for epidemiological studies of candidiasis in immunocompromised hosts. J. Infect. Dis. 159:488-494.

11. Gade, W., S. W. Hinnefeld, L. S. Babcock, P. Gilligan, W. Kelly, K. Wait, D. Greer, M. Pinilla, and R. L. Kaplan. 1991. Comparion of the PREMIER cryptococcal antigen enzyme immunoassay and the latex agglutination assay for detection of cryptococcal antigens. J. Clin. Microbiol. 29:1616-1619.

12. Haley, L. D., J. Trandel, and M. B. Coyle. 1980. Cumitech 11. Practical methods for culture and identification of fungi in the clinical microbiology laboratory. Coord. ed., J. C. Sherris. American Society for Microbiology, Washington, DC. 17 p.

13. Hunter, P. R. 1991. A critical review of typing methods for *Candida albicans* and their applications. Crit. Rev. Microbiol. 17:417-434.

14. Jones, J. M. 1990. Laboratory diagnosis of invasive candidiasis. Clin. Microbiol Rev. 3:32-45.

15. Land, G. A., I. F. Salkin, M. El-Zaatari, M. R. McGinnis, and G. Hashem. 1991. Evaluation of the Baxter-MicroScan 4-hour enzyme-based yeast identification system. J. Clin. Microbiol. 29:718-722.

16. Larone, D. H. 1987. Medically important fungi: a guide to identification. Elsevier Science Publishing Co., Inc., New York. p. 53-75, 193-211.

17. Magee, P. T., L. Bowdin, and J. Staudinger. 1992. Comparison of molecular typing methods for *Candida albicans*. J. Clin. Microbiol. 30:2674-2679.

18. Miyakawa. Y., T. Mabuchi, K. Kagaya, and Y. Fukazawa. 1992. Isolation and characterization of a species-specific DNA fragment for detection of *Candida albicans* by polymerase chain reaction. J. Clin. Microbiol. 30:894-900.

19. Polacheck, I., G. Lebans, and J. B. Hicks. 1992. Development of DNA probes for early diagnosis and epidemiological study of cryptococcosis in AIDS patients. J. Clin. Microbiol. 30:925-930.

20. Sendven, P. 1990. Laboratory identification and sensitivity testing of yeast isolates. Acta Odontol. Scand. 48:27-36.

21. Spitzer, E. D., and S. G. Spitzer. 1992. Use of dispersed repetitive DNA element to distinguish clinical isolates of *Cryptococcus neoformans*. J. Clin. Microbiol. 30:1094-1097.

22. Stenderup, A. 1990. Oral mycology. Acta Odonol. Scand. 48:3-10.

23. St.-Germain, G., and D. Beauchesne. 1991. Evaluation of the MicroScan rapid yeast identification panel. J. Clin. Microbiol. 29: 2296-2299.

24. Sugar, A. M. 1991. Overview: cryptococcosis in the patient with AIDS. Mycopathologia 114:153-157.

25. Varma, A., and K. J. Kwon-Chung. 1992. DNA probe for strain typing of *Cryptococcus neoformans*. J. Clin. Microbiol. 30:2960-2967.

26. Walsh, T. J., and P. A. Pizzo. 1988. Nosocomial fungal infections: a classification for hospital-acquired fungal infections and mycoses arising from endogenous flora or reactivation. Ann. Rev. Microbiol. 42:517-545.

27. Warren, N. G., and H. J. Shadomy. 1991. Yeasts of medical importance, p. 617-629. *In* A. Balows, W. J. Hausler, Jr., K. L. Herrmann, H. D. Isenberg, and H. J. Shadomy (ed.), Manual of clinical microbiology, 5th ed. American Society for Microbiology, Washington, D. C.

Exercise 24
Data Table 1: Yeast Results

		Culture Age (Days)	Candida albicans		C. (P.) guilliermondii		Saccharomyces cerevisiae		Cryptococcus (Filobasidiella) neoformans	
			BHI[a]	Other	BHI	Other	BHI	Other	Caffeic agar	Other
Colony size and Colony Form	mm									
	Punctiform								■	■
	Irregular								■	■
	Circular								■	■
	Rhizoid								■	■
	Filamentous								■	■
	Other									
Colony Surface	Flat									
	Raised									
	Convex									
	Pulvinate									
	Smooth									
	Rough									
	Color (Describe)									
	Other									
Colony Margin	Entire								■	■
	Undulate								■	■
	Lobate								■	■
	Erose								■	■
	Other								■	■
Colony Consistency	Butyrous								■	■
	Viscid								■	■
	Membranous								■	■
	Brittle								■	■
	Other								■	■
Colony Optical Character	Opaque									
	Translucent									
	Dull									
	Glistening									
	Other									
Other										

[a] Brain heart infusion agar.

Exercise 24
Data Table 2: Yeast Results

		Culture Age (Days)	Candida albicans	C. (P.) guilliermondii	Saccharomyces cerevisiae	Cryptococcus (Filobasidiella) neoformans
Gram stain	Reaction					████
	Morphology					████
	Arrangement					████
Fermentation	Glucose					
	Maltose					
	Trehalose					
Assimilation	Glucose					
	Maltose					
	Trehalose					
Urease			████	████	████	
Other						

Exercise 24
Data Table 3: Summary of Microscopic Observations

	Culture Age (Days)	Candida albicans	C. (P.) guilliermondii	Saccharomyces cerevisiae	Cryptococcus (Filobasidiella) neoformans
Blastocondia present					
No./cell					
Type of base[a]					
Chlamydoconidia present					████
Pseudohyphae seen					
Germ tubes seen					████
Capsule present		████	████		

[a] Describe attachment site as broad or narrow.

Exercise 24
Diagrams and Other Laboratory Data

Labeled Diagrams of Yeast on Corn Meal Tween 80 Agar:

Culture Age: _____ Observation Date: _____

Candida albicans	Candida (Pichia) guilliermondii	Saccharomyces cerevisiae

Diagrams of Germ Tube Test: Magnification _____ Culture Age (hrs.) _____

Candida albicans	Candida (Pichia) guilliermondii

Diagrams of India Ink Wet Mount Observations:

Magnification _____ Culture Age (hrs.) _____ Culture medium: _____

Cryptococcus (Filobasidiella) neoformans	Saccharomyces cerevisiae

***Saccharomyces cerevisiae* Ascospores:** Culture age: _____ Magnification: _____ Stain: _____

Other Laboratory Notes

EXERCISE 25
Fungi Associated With Superficial, Subcutaneous, and Cutaneous Mycoses

I. Introduction.

The clinical categories of superficial, cutaneous, and subcutaneous fungi were introduced to you earlier (Introduction, Medical Mycology). The three categories differ because of the tissue sites these organisms choose to infect and grow. In the aggregate there are many species involved, however, only a few will be studied in this exercise to provide introductory information for them.

Before proceeding, additional background on the clinical organization of these fungi would be profitable (also see Table 23-1). Within the three clinical categories given above, reference is frequently made to the groups of diseases mycetoma, chromoblastomycosis, dermatophytosis, and phaeohyphomycosis. These are also groups of diseases caused by more than one species. Table 25-1 shows the relationship of selected species in the various categories.

A. Subcutaneous Fungi and Their Infections.

Phaeohyphomycosis is a relatively recently coined term designating a broad spectrum of disease in the superficial, cutaneous, subcutaneous, and systemic categories (2). It arose out of a need to distinguish those opportunistic infections caused by any dematiaceous fungi from the clinically distinct mycetoma and chromoblastomycosis. However, as seen in Table 25-1, non-phaeohyphomycotic infection can be produced by dematiaceous fungi (e. g. *Sporothrix schenckii*). Distinguishing characteristics of phaeohyphomycosis are the observation of fragments of hyphae, pseudohyphal-like, and/or yeast-like cells that are typically dematiaceous in tissue (13). Infections by *Piedraia hortae* and *Phaeoannellomyces werneckii*, which are superficial fungi (and, in the latter case, a yeast), are phaeohyphomycotic agents, while *Exophiala jeanselmei* and *Phialophora verrucosa* can cause subcutaneous phaeohyphomycosis, as well as eumycetoma and chromoblastomycosis, respectively. The latter diseases do not fit the criteria for phaeohyphomycosis, hence are separate clinical entities.

It also should be noted that, while not shown on Table 25-1 nor discussed further as a group, "halohyphomycosis" agents represent non-dematiaceous fungi whose tissue form is hyaline mycelial fragments (15). These therefore represent the complementary opposite group to the phaeohyphomycotic agents and include species of *Aspergillus, Penicillium, Fusarium, Paecilomyces,* and many others.

Clinically, each of the organisms given in Table 25-1 (and others), while being categorized as superficial, cutaneous, or subcutaneous fungi, may have a separate disease name. *P. hortae*, for example, causes black piedra, while *T. beigelii* is the agent of white piedra. Both cause nodular growth along the hair shaft. *P. werneckii*, the agent of tinea nigra, is characteristically a superficial infection of the palmar surfaces leading to a dark coloration (11).

In subcutaneous infections *E. jeanselmei* probably is the most common agent of the phaeohyphomycoses, usually causing subcutaneous nodules that eventually become an encapsulated abscess (13). Other organisms that cause this clinical entity usually appear as subcutaneous granulomas or cystic abscesses (7).

Chromoblastomycosis, caused most frequently by *Fonsecaea pedrosoi*, but also can be due to *P. verrucosa* and other species, slowly develops from a traumatic wound of the foot or leg. Papular development is eventually followed by formation of wart-like lesions. Eumycetoma is similar in its clinical characteristics to actinomycetoma described in Exercise 22 (p. 327), with about 50% of cases falling into each type. In the U. S. *Pseudallescheria boydii* (anamorph: *Scedosporium apiospermum*) is the usual cause of the mycotic form (11).

Finally, among the subcutaneous fungi, *Sporothrix schenckii* is the agent of sporotrichosis, the most common clinical form being a lymphatic involvement following an initial infection of the skin, usually of the hand. Without treatment, chronic infection can develop to produce nodular and ulcerating lesions along the affected lymphatic channel (7, 11). Like other organisms discussed above, *S. schenckii* is found in our environment. As an example, an outbreak of

Table 25-1
Clinical Groupings of Selected Superficial, Cutaneous, and Subcutaneous Fungi (11, 13, 14)

Name of Fungus	Clinical Group	Phaeohyphomycosis	Chromoblastomycosis	Eumycetoma	Dermatophytosis or Ringworm Group
Malassezia furfur	Superficial				
Phaeoannellomyces werneckii	"	+			
Piedraia hortae	"	+			
Trichosporon beigelii	"				
Epidermophyton floccosum	Cutaneous				+
Microsporum (Arthroderma)	"				+
Trichophyton (Arthroderma)	"				+
Exophilia jeanselmei	Subcutaneous[a]	+		+	
Fonsecaea pedrosoi	"		+		
Phialophora verrucosa	"	+	+		
Pseudallescheria boydii	"			+	
Scedosporium apiospermum	"				
Sporothrix schenckii	"				

[a] E. jeanselmei also causes systemic phaeohyphomycosis.

sporotrichosis occurred in 1988 in the U. S. involving 84 cases that had handled tree seedlings wrapped in sphagnum moss (6). The latter had previously been implicated as a source of the organism causing this disease (5).

B. Cutaneous Fungi and Their Infections.

While the cutaneous fungi can include *Candida albicans* infecting skin and nails (onychomycosis), *Aspergillus fumigatus,* also an agent of onychomycosis, and several other species, the emphasis of this exercise will be on the dermatophytes. These organisms, also referred to as the ringworm or tinea (meaning worm or moth (4)) group encompass three genera, *Trichophyton* (teleomorph: *Arthroderma*), *Microsporum* (*Arthroderma*), and *Epidermophyton*. Their normal habitat varies from that of humans (i.e. anthropophilic) and lower animals (zoophilic) to soil (geophilic). In infection, one or more members of *Trichophyton* (*Arthroderma*) can invade nails, skin, and hair; those of the *Microsporum* (*Arthroderma*) attack skin and hair, but not nails; while *Epidermophyton* infect skin and, less frequently, nails, but not hair. The clinical designation for the affected body area is made by using the term "tinea" as a synonym for

dermatophytosis. Thus, tinea corporis indicates dermatophytosis of the body skin; tinea capitis, infection of the scalp; tinea manum, of the hands, and so on (4).

II. Laboratory Study.

As for the ubiquitous fungi studied in Exercise 23, morphological characteristics have a major role in the identification of superficial, cutaneous, and subcutaneous moulds. Therefore, as discussed earlier, microscopic examination of the clinical specimen will be an important starting point, followed by culture on, in this case, Sabouraud dextrose agar (SDA). While Inhibitory mold agar also can be used for the subcutaneous fungi, the typical colony characteristics are best seen on SDA (9). Following growth and maturation of the colony, microscopic morphology is established using methods outlined in Exercise 23.

The conidia of the moulds is distinctive for the various species, as shown by diagram and colony descriptions in Tables 25-2 and 25-3 and Photos 25-1 through 25-6 of fungi used in this exercise. Other *in vitro* tests are also available for identifying dermatophytes. These include the hair

Table 25-2
Characteristics of Some Fungi Associated with
Subcutaneous Infections (11, 12, 14)

Organism	Characteristics
Fonsecaea pedrosoi	**Colony:** Dark olive-gray to black (dematiaceous), flat colony which may show zones of color. Black underside. Wide variation in characteristics between strains. Mature growth in two weeks. **Microscopic:** Septate, branching hyphae. Three conidial arrangements: (i) *Cladisporium* type: blastoconidia in chains; (ii) *Phialophora* type: vase-like phialides with conidia that collect at the flared collarette; and (iii) *Rhinocladiella* type: single-celled, fusiform conidia that form sympodial along an erect conidiophore.

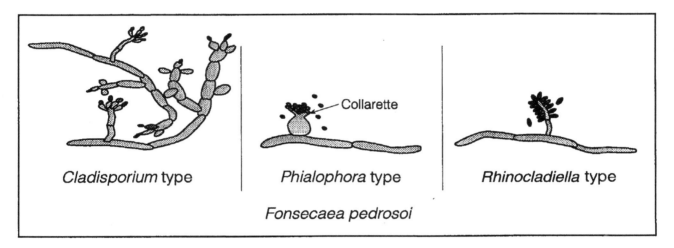

Cladisporium type   *Phialophora* type   *Rhinocladiella* type

Collarette

Fonsecaea pedrosoi

Pseudallescheria boydii	**Colony:** Dark, smoky-gray. Rapid growing. Floccose hyphae. White underside turning gray to black. Mature growth in about one week. **Microscopic:** Clavate and truncated conidia borne singly along hyphae. Forms eight ascospores per cleistothecium.

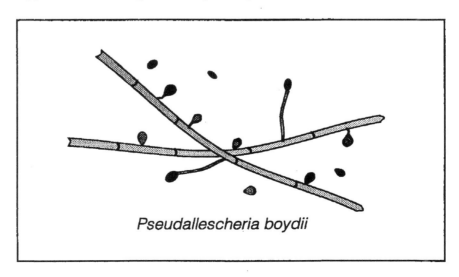

Pseudallescheria boydii

Sporothrix schenckii

Colony: Dimorphic; yeast phase in tissue and at 35-37°C on a high glucose containing medium. Colonies pasty, tan, and glabrous in yeast phase. At room temperature, a rapid growing, moist, leathery, folded colony occurs. Early growth is white, turning brown to black in old cultures.

Microscopic: Yeast phase: Fusiform to spherical cells that reproduce by blastoconidia formation. Filamentous phase: Septate, thin hyphae. Elliptical conidium borne along side and at tip of the conidiophore. Conidia may be borne along hyphae as thick-walled, dark, single cells, or hyaline, clavate to oval cells arising from a denticle (short, thin stalk bearing a conidium) borne singly along the hyphae.

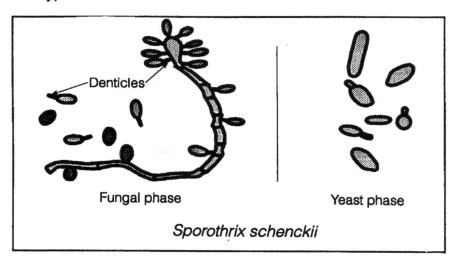

Fungal phase

Yeast phase

Sporothrix schenckii

---

perforation test (microscopic wedge-shaped perforation of the hair shaft when incubated with the proper organism) that differentiate certain species of *Trichophyton* and *Microsporum,* the urease test to differentiate *Trichophyton* spp., and growth on rice grain medium to distinguish *M. audouinii* from others of *Microsporum.* Also, temperature tolerance and nutritional assays are available (17).

There are a lack of miniaturized and rapid assay methods for the fungi being studied in this exercise. The API 20C Yeast Identification System has been applied to the dematiaceous fungi and shows potential usefulness in identifying most *Cladosporium* and *Phialophora* species and distinguishing some paired species that are difficult to separate by traditional assays (10). DNA typing by electrophoresis of restriction fragments from *S. schenckii* (6), and immunoblot of antibody responses to this species (16) have been done on an experimental basis, however, there does not

appear to be a concerted effort to apply these to diagnostic procedures.

MATERIALS

Per Bench:

Selection of cultures from the following on Sabouraud dextrose agar incubated as given below will be available for your observation:

Incubated for 10 days at room temperature:
Sporothrix schenckii
Microsporum audouinii
Fonsecaea pedrosoi
Trichophyton mentagrophytes
    (*Arthroderma benhamiae*)
Pseudallescheria boydii
Epidermophyton floccosum

Incubated at 37°C for 5 days:
Sporothrix schenckii

One microslide culture preparation of each of the above per bench

Table 25-3
Characteristics of Some Dermatophytes (9, 11, 17)

Organism	Characteristics
idermophyton floccosum	**Colony:** Shades of yellow to tan with radial furrows and folds. Powdery in texture. Floccose tufts of sterile mycelium may appear on the colony surface in older cultures. Yellow to light brown reverse. Growth takes 1.5-2 weeks. **Microscopic:** Macroconidia: clavate, septate with rounded distal tips, in singles or in clusters. Also glabrous and thick-walled. These usually attached directly to hyphae. Microconidia: None. Racket and spiral hyphae, and nodular bodies may be found.

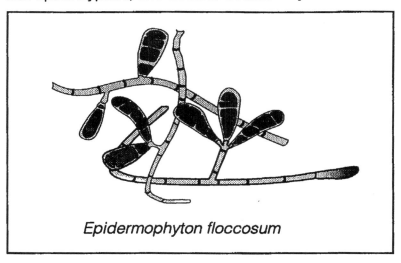

Epidermophyton floccosum

icrosporum audouinii	**Colony:** Gray to tan with radially folded velvety surface. Underside usually red-brown. Grows in 1 to 1.5 weeks. **Microscopic:** Macroconidia: rare; narrow, echinulate or smooth, with or without septa. Microconidia: occasional, usually clavate borne terminally or laterally on short conidiophores. Hyphae septate and may have abnormal shapes such as racket shapes or pectinate and nodular bodies. Terminal chlamydoconidia are frequently noted.

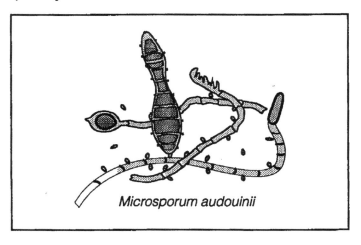

Microsporum audouinii

Trichophyton
mentagrophytes

Colony: Variable features. Grows in 1-1.5 weeks. Flat, powdery to dense growth. Dull yellow to tan colored surface and off white to deep red reverse color. May have a diffusible pigment.
Microscopic: Macroconidia: Clavate to cigar-like, thin-walled, with up to seven septa. Microconidia: Small, pyriform to clavate, and hyaline.

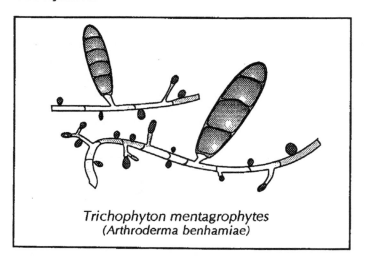

Trichophyton mentagrophytes
(Arthroderma benhamiae)

LABORATORY PROCEDURE

Part 1

A selection of cultures shown in the "Materials" section will be made available for observation, along with a microslide culture of each. With these, each pair of students carry out the following:
A. First Observation Period.
  1. Plate Cultures: Describe colony form, texture, surface morphology, and surface and underside color. Is a soluble pigment produced? (Note: Do not open plates.)
  2. Slide cultures: Describe microscopic morphology for each of the available species. Especially note the presence of conidia. Describe their size, morphology, and arrangement. Also, note whether hyphae are septate or non-septate. Are racket hyphae, pectinate bodies, or other structures helpful in identification present?
B. Second Observation Period.
Reexamine plate cultures of filamentous forms following an additional 5-7 days of incubation at room temperature. (It is unnecessary to reobserve

the *S. schenckii* that had been incubated at 37°C.) Record changes in any of the morphological characteristics previously examined in *Part 1*A.

Discuss your results. Do microscopic and colony characteristics confirm the species identification for these cultures? What are outstanding features that you observed that allow you to make such a confirmation and separate the six species observed here?

Part 2

Demonstration: The Hair Perforation Test (1).

Microscopically observe the two slides with strands of hair mounted in lactophenol cotton blue. These were prepared by using either the method of Ajello and Georg (1) or that described by Baron, Peterson, and Finegold (3). In the former, strands of sterilized hair (autoclaved at 121°C for 10 minutes) are incubated in 25 ml distilled water with 0.1 ml filter-sterilized 10% yeast extract solution. In the latter method, these are placed on top of sterile wetted filter paper circle in a petri dish. In both procedures, *T. mentagrophytes* (*A. benhamiae*) culture fragments are then added to one dish, *T. rubrum* to the other. Your observations are being made after incubation at room temperature for the period specified by your instructor.

From your observations, is either *T. mentagrophytes* (*A. benhamiae*) or *T. rubrum* capable of penetrating the shafts of hair. A positive test is seen by the presence of wedge-shaped perforations due to hyphal invasion into the hair (1, 11).

REFERENCES

1. Ajello, L., and L. K. Georg. 1957. In vitro cultures for differentiating between atypical isolates of *Trichophyton mentagrophytes* and *Trichophyton rubrum*. Mycopathol. Mycol. Appl. **8**:3-17.

2. Ajello, L., L. K. Georg, R. T. Steigbigel, and C. J. K. Wang. 1974. A case of phaeohyphomycosis caused by a new species of *Phialophora*. Mycologia **66**:490-498.

3. Baron, E. J., L. R. Peterson, and S. M. Finegold. 1994. Bailey & Scott's diagnostic microbiology, 9th ed. Mosby-Year Book, Inc., St. Louis. pp. 710-775.

4. Campbell, M. C., and J. L. Stewart. 1980. The medical mycology handbook. John Wiley & Sons, New York. p. 31-81.

5. Centers for Disease Control. 1982. Sporotrichosis associated with Wisconsin sphagnum moss. MMWR **31**:542-544.

6. Cooper, C. R., Jr., B. J. Breslin, D. M. Dixon, and I. F. Salkin. 1992. DNA typing of isolates associated wth the 1988 sporotrichosis epidemic. J. Clin. Microbiol. **30**:1631-1635.

7. De Vroey, C. 1989. Identification of agents of subcutaneous mycoses, p. 111-139. *In* E. G. V. Evans, and M. D. Richardson (ed.), Medical mycology: a practical approach. IRL Press, Oxford.

8. Dixon, D. M., and R. A. Fromtling. 1991. Morphology, taxonomy and classification of the fungi, p. 579-587. *In* A. Balows, W. J. Hausler, Jr., K. L. Herrmann, H. D. Isenberg, and H. J. Shadomy (ed.), Manual of clinical microbiology, 5th ed. American Society for Microbiology, Washington, D. C.

9. Elewski, B. E., and P. G. Hazen. 1989. The superficial mycoses and the dermatophytes. J. Am. Acad. Dermatol. **21**:655-673.

10. Espinel-Ingroff, A., M. R. McGinnis, D. H. Pincus, P. R. Goldson, and T. M. Kerkering. 1989. Evaluation of the API 20C yeast identification system for the differentiation of some dematiaceous fungi. J. Clin. Microbiol. **27**:2565-2569.

11. Howard, B. J., J. Klass II, S. J. Rubin, A. S. Weissfeld, and R. C. Tilton. 1987. Clinical and pathogenic microbiology. The C. V. Mosby Co., St. Louis. p. 559-584.

12. Larone, D. H. 1987. Medically important fungi: a guide to identification. Elsevier Science Publishing Co., Inc., New York. p. 173-220.

13. McGinnis, M. R. 1983. Chromoblastomycosis and phaeohyphomycosis: new concepts, diagnosis, and mycology. J. Am. Acad. Dermatol. **8**:1-16.

14. McGinnis, M. R., I. F. Salkin, W. A. Schell, and L. Pasarell. 1991. Dematiaceous fungi, p. 644-658. *In* A. Balows, W. J. Hausler, Jr., K. L. Herrmann, H. D. Isenberg, and H. J. Shadomy (ed.), Manual of clinical microbiology, 5th ed. American Society for Microbiology. Washington, D. C.

15. Rogers, A. L., and M. J. Kennedy. 1991. Opportunistic hyaline hyphomycetes, p. 659-673. *In* A. Balows, W. J. Hausler, Jr., K. L. Herrmann, H. D. Isenberg, and H. J. Shadomy (ed.), Manual of clinical microbiology, 5th ed. American Society for Microbiology, Washington, D. C.

16. Scott, E. N., and H. G. Muchmore. 1989. Immunoblot analysis of antibody responses to *Sporothrix schenckii*. J. Clin. Microbiol. **27**:300-304.

17. Weitzman, I., and J. Kane. 1991. Dermatophytes and agents of superficial mycoses, p. 601-616. *In* A. Balows, W. J. Hausler, Jr., K. L. Herrmann, H. D. Isenberg, and H. J. Shadomy (ed.), Manual of clinical microbiology, 5th ed. American Society for Microbiology, Washington, D. C.

Exercise 25: Results
Data Table 1: *Fonsecaea pedrosoi*

Date of First Reading: _____ Culture Age _____

Date of Second Reading: _____ Culture Age _____

Colony Characteristics		First Reading	Second Reading
Size, mm			
Surface Texture	Velvet-like		
	Granular		
	Floccose		
	Glabrous		
Topography	Flat		
	Folded		
	Radial furrows		
	Heaped		
	Other		
Color (describe)	Surface		
	Underside		
	Soluble pigment		
	Other		
Other	(Describe)		
Properties			

Exercise 25: Results
Data Table 2: *Pseudallescheria boydii*

Date of First Reading: _____ Culture Age _____

Date of Second Reading: _____ Culture Age _____

Colony Characteristics		First Reading	Second Reading
Size, mm			
Surface Texture	Velvet-like		
	Granular		
	Floccose		
	Glabrous		
Topography	Flat		
	Folded		
	Radial furrows		
	Heaped		
	Other		
Color (describe)	Surface		
	Underside		
	Soluble pigment		
	Other		
Other(Describe)			
Properties			

Exercise 25: Results
Data Table 3: *Sporothrix schenckii* Grown at Room Temperature

Date of First Reading: _____ Culture Age _____

Date of Second Reading: _____ Culture Age _____

Colony Characteristics		First Reading	Second Reading
Size, mm			
Surface Texture	Velvet-like		
	Granular		
	Floccose		
	Glabrous		
Topography	Flat		
	Folded		
	Radial furrows		
	Heaped		
	Other		
Color (describe)	Surface		
	Underside		
	Soluble pigment		
	Other		
Other(Describe)			
Properties			

Exercise 25: Results
Data Table 4: *Sporothrix schenckii* Grown at 37°C

		Culture Age (Days)			
Colony size and Colony Form	mm				
	Punctiform				
	Irregular				
	Circular				
	Rhizoid				
	Filamentous				
	Other				
Colony Surface	Flat				
	Raised				
	Convex				
	Pulvinate				
	Smooth				
	Rough				
	Color (Describe)				
	Other				
Colony Margin	Entire				
	Undulate				
	Lobate				
	Erose				
	Other				
Colony Consistency	Butyrous				
	Viscid				
	Membranous				
	Brittle				
	Other				
Colony Optical Character	Opaque				
	Translucent				
	Dull				
	Glistening				
	Other				
Other					

Exercise 25: Results
Data Table 5: *Epidermophyton floccosum*

Date of First Reading: _____ Culture Age _____

Date of Second Reading: _____ Culture Age _____

Colony Characteristics		First Reading	Second Reading
Size, mm			
Surface Texture	Velvet-like		
	Granular		
	Floccose		
	Glabrous		
Topography	Flat		
	Folded		
	Radial furrows		
	Heaped		
	Other		
Color (describe)	Surface		
	Underside		
	Soluble pigment		
	Other		
Other(Describe)			
Properties			

Exercise 25: Results
Data Table 6: *Microsporum audouinii*

Date of First Reading: _____ Culture Age _____

Date of Second Reading: _____ Culture Age _____

Colony Characteristics		First Reading	Second Reading
Size, mm			
Surface Texture	Velvet-like		
	Granular		
	Floccose		
	Glabrous		
Topography	Flat		
	Folded		
	Radial furrows		
	Heaped		
	Other		
Color (describe)	Surface		
	Underside		
	Soluble pigment		
	Other		
Other (Describe)			
Properties			

Exercise 25: Results
Data Table 7: *Trichophyton mentagrophytes*

Date of First Reading: _____ Culture Age _____

Date of Second Reading: _____ Culture Age _____

Colony Characteristics		First Reading	Second Reading
Size, mm			
Surface Texture	Velvet-like		
	Granular		
	Floccose		
	Glabrous		
Topography	Flat		
	Folded		
	Radial furrows		
	Heaped		
	Other		
Color (describe)	Surface		
	Underside		
	Soluble pigment		
	Other		
Other (Describe)			
Properties			

Exercise 25: Results
Data Table 8: Microscopic Observations on Microslide Culture

	Character	*Fonsecaea pedrosoi*	*Pseudallescheria boydii*
Hyphae	Septate or nonseptate		
	Hyaline or dark		
	Course or fine		
	Other (describe)		
Spores	Type(s)[a]		
	Size		
	Shape		
	Color		
	Surface appearance		
	Wall thickness		
	Other (describe)		

[a] Types = chlamydoconidia, arthroconidia, etc.

Drawing with Labeled Parts:

Fonsecaea pedrosoi

Magnification: _____

Culture Age: _____

Pseudallescheria boydii

Magnification: _____

Culture Age: _____

Exercise 25: Results
Data Table 9: Microscopic Observations on Microslide Culture

	Character	*Sporothrix schenckii* Room Temperature	37°C
Hyphae	Septate or nonseptate		
	Hyaline or dark		
	Course or fine		
	Other (describe)		
Spores	Type(s)[a]		
	Size		
	Shape		
	Color		
	Surface appearance		
	Wall thickness		
	Other (describe)		

[a] Types = chlamydoconidia, arthroconidia, etc.

Drawing with Labeled Parts:

Sporothrix schenckii

Room Temperature

Magnification: _____

Culture Age: _____

37°C

Magnification: _____

Culture Age: _____

Exercise 25: Results
Data Table 10: Microscopic Observations on Microslide Culture

	Character	Epidermophyton floccosum	Microsporum audouinii
Hyphae	Septate or nonseptate		
	Hyaline or dark		
	Course or fine		
	Other (describe)		
Spores	Type(s)[a]		
	Size		
	Shape		
	Color		
	Surface appearance		
	Wall thickness		
	Other (describe)		

[a] Types = chlamydoconidia, arthroconidia, etc.

Drawing with Labeled Parts:

Epidermophyton floccosum

Magnification: _____

Culture Age: _____

Microsporum audouinii

Magnification: _____

Culture Age: _____

Exercise 25: Results
Data Table 11: Microscopic Observations on Microslide Culture

	Character	Trichophyton mentagrophytes	
Hyphae	Septate or nonseptate		
	Hyaline or dark		
	Course or fine		
	Other (describe)		
Spores	Type(s)[a]		
	Size		
	Shape		
	Color		
	Surface appearance		
	Wall thickness		
	Other (describe)		

[a] Types = chlamydoconidia, arthroconidia, etc.

Drawing with Labeled Parts:

Trichophyton mentagrophytes

Magnification: _____

Culture Age: _____

Exercise 25
Other Laboratory Notes

EXERCISE 26
The Dimorphic Fungi of Systemic Infections

As introduced earlier, several species of fungi can be categorized as systemic, especially those that are opportunistic (Table 23-1). However, our focus in the exercise will be on the true pathogens, namely *Histoplasma capsulatum* (Teleomorph: *Ajellomyces capsulatus*), *Blastomyces dermatitidis* (teleomorph: *Ajellomyces dermatitidis*), and *Coccidioides immitis*. These, along with *Paracoccidioides brasiliensis*, a species only found in South America, share certain properties including that they are all dimorphic, residing in soil in their filamentous stage, but not while *in vivo*; they are not contagious, with practically all infections arising from soil-borne organisms; they most frequently infect by the pulmonary route; and their endemic areas are somewhat circumscribed. The latter is important since the incidence of disease due to resident species is much higher within those areas, therefore laboratory diagnosis of these organisms is logically more frequent there. However, it must be remembered that in an age of high mobility, these infections can be seen in individuals that have only visited, sometimes only briefly, an endemic area (12, 19, 24). Epidemiologically, histoplasmosis (and therefore *H. capsulatum* (*A. capsulatus*) var. *capsulatum*) occurs mostly in the Central U.S., particularly in the Mississippi River valley. Cases have also been reported, for example, in Asia and Russia. *H. capsulatum* var. *duboisii* occurs only in central Africa (13, 25). In the U.S., blastomycosis overlaps with the region endemic for histoplasmosis, but extends further north and east to include the Ohio River and St. Lawrence River valleys, the Great Lakes region, and South Central States. It also occurs in Central and South America and in Africa (4). In contrast to these, coccidioidomycosis occurs in the Lower Sonoran Life Zone, the semi-arid region located in the Southwestern States of the U.S., and in areas of Central and South America (20).

The incidence of infection of each of these within their endemic regions can be high. Using coccidioidomycosis as an example, between 50,000 and 100,000 new cases per year occur in the U.S. endemic areas (5, 20). Most of these, as is true for histoplasmosis and blastomycosis, are self-limiting pulmonary infections. However, they all have the potential to produce symptomatic pulmonary infection, and to disseminate to infect other organs, as skin, reticuloendothelial system (especially histoplasmosis), meninges, and to many other locations (1, 2, 3). Fortunately, the incidence of dissemination is low, being less than 1% for coccidioidomycisos (1), and only 0.05% for histoplasmosis in Indianapolis where several outbreaks have occurred since 1978 (26). Conversely, there is ample evidence that a deficiency of the immune system, as caused by an HIV infection, can markedly increase the likelihood of severe clinical consequences, especially in progressive disseminated histoplasmosis (18).

Dimorphism of the pathogenic agents of systemic fungal infection is one of the important clues showing their presence. *H. capsulatum* (*A. capsulatus*) and *B.* (*A.*) *dermatitidis* are found as yeasts *in vivo* and can be grown in their yeast phase at 37°C (Photo 26-2A, 26-3A). *Coccidioides immitis* does not have a yeast form, but it is still diphasic. Its tissue phase consists of spherules (sporangia filled with endospores, Photo 26-1B). In its common *in vitro* culture form it is filamentous in character and forms highly infectious arthroconidia that readily detach from their parent hyphae (Photo 26-1A). Because of this, it is extremely hazardous to work with in its mycelial phase and, as cautioned earlier, it should only be done after killing with formaldehyde (see Introduction to Medical Mycology, Section III, p. 339). In identification it is therefore important that spherule formation is shown by careful observation of clinical material or by inoculation of animals with such specimens, thus avoiding the use of *in vitro* culture beyond growth of the initial mycelial colony in a bottle slant (24). Also, while not routinely done, an *in vitro* culture medium is available for the rapid conversion of the mycelial phase to the spherule phase to allow demonstration of this organism's diphasic nature (21).

The types of specimens expected for analysis of the three dimorphic pathogenic fungi are usually of pulmonary origin, as sputum, transtracheal aspirates, and lung biopsy. Blood, urine, spinal fluid, and extrapulmonary tissue biopsy also may be received for analysis. Microscopic examination is done following an appropriate chemical staining procedure, fluorescent antibody staining, or wet mount to discern the presence of yeast phase *H. capsulatum* (*A. capsulatus*) and *B. (A.) dermatitidis*, or spherules of *C. immitis* (see Table 26-1 for a more detailed description of these) (2, 24).

In their filamentous phase, the dimorphic fungi will grow on many types of media. Normally sterile specimens can be placed on BHI, Inhibitory Mold agar, Sabouraud dextrose agar, or other types. If bacterial contamination is suspected, then antimicrobial compounds should be incorporated into the medium of one culture, recalling that moulds are at a competitive disadvantage because of their relatively slow growth. A second culture should not include inhibitory antimicrobials as a precaution to allow growth of sensitive forms. Both are incubated at 25°-30°C. If a dimorphic yeast phase organism is suspected, the organism also should be inoculated on an enriched blood medium and incubated at 37°C (17), a temperature preferable to 35°C because conversion is temperature dependent (24). If conversion is to be done after filamentous growth, cottonseed agar also can be used as a conversion medium for *B. (A.) dermatitidis* (6), as can Kelley's medium (14, 17).

Following growth, colony examinations are done in the usual manner. Descriptions are given in Table 26-1, however, it must be cautioned that characteristics can be highly variable. Note that any open culture work with filamentous form must be handled under Biosafety Level 3 standards, while yeast phase can be worked with under Biosafety Level 2 conditions (23). Therefore, while yeasts can be prepared and examined for microscopic examination, microslide culture preparation for closer examination of filamentous forms is not recommended.

Fungal growth and demonstration of the diphasic nature of these organisms may take several weeks. It is therefore both faster and less hazardous to identify them using other methods. Exoantigen detection has been particularly useful, and has a high level of accuracy. Extracted antigens from cultures, when assayed by the agar double diffusion method using specific antiserum, yields identifying precipitin bands. For example, *C. immitis* contains TP (heat stable Tube Precipitin), HS (Heat Stable at 100°C for 10 minutes), and HL or F (Heat Labile at 60°C) antigens that are extractable and concentrated from merthiolate-treated filamentous cultures. Formation of precipitin bands using antiserum specific for any of these identifies the organism, assuming proper controls are included (8, 9). Obviously, time is still required to grow the culture (7-10 days), but the exoantigen test only requires an additional 2-3 days. Similar procedures can be used to identify *H. capsulatum* (*A. capsulatus*), which contains distinct H and M antigens, while *B. (A.) dermatitidis* contains A and K (Type 1 organism) or only K (Type 2 organism) antigens. Type 2 is prevalent in Africa and not found in North America (10).

Gen-Probe Accu-Probe™ tests have been developed for culture identification of *H. capsulatum* (*A. capsulatus*), *C. immitis,* and *B. (A.) dermatitidis*. In the former, a high level of accuracy is obtained with no cross-reaction with *B. (A.) dermatitidis*. Also, it can be used with either yeast or filamentous organisms, and it can be accomplished within 2 hours with less growth than needed for the exoantigen assay (15). However, it is more expensive to do than the exoantigen test (7) and bacterial contamination may interfere with the probe test causing equivocal results (15). The probe test sensitivity for *C. immitis* and *B. (A.) dermatitidis* also equals that of the exoantigen test (10).

Several serological assays can be used to assess the serum antibody response of patients with systemic mycotic infection. These include the complement fixation test, immunodiffusion, enzyme-linked immunoassay, and others. These are discussed in depth in several references as Kaufman (10), and Pappagianis (16) and therefore will not be taken up further here.

MATERIALS

Demonstration cultures of *Histoplasma capsulatum* (*Ajellomyces capsulatus*) and *Blastomyces (Ajellomyces) dermatitidis* grown as follows:

a. Each species grown on thick-poured Sabouraud dextrose agar and incubated at room temperature for 7 days before observation.

Table 26-1
Characteristics of Asexual Forms of Dimorphic Fungi of Systemic Infections (2, 11, 24)

Organism	Characteristics
Coccidioides immitis	**Room Temperature Growth** Colony: Floccose, white mycelium turning yellow to tan, or even darker. White reverse. Usually grows to maturity within 7 days. Microscopic: Abundant thick-walled, barrel-shaped arthroconidia joined to empty cells (disjunctors).

***In vivo* or at 37-40°C on special medium**

Microscopic: Spherules, 20-200μm in diameter, containing endospores and granular material. Spherules do not have, nor are they joined to hypae.

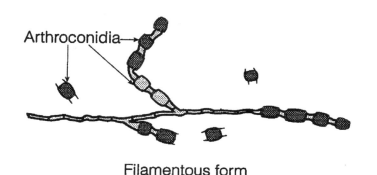 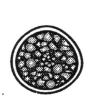

Arthroconidia→

Filamentous form   Spherules formed *in vivo*

Organism	Characteristics
Histoplasma capsulatum (*Ajellomyces capsulatus*)	**Room Temperature Growth** Colony: White surface, turning tan to brown with age. Usually white reverse, but may be yellow to tan. Slow growing, requiring 2 to 8 weeks for maturity. Microscopic: Identifying non-septate, tuberculate ("watch gear-like") or smooth macroconidia, 7-15 μm in diameter. Microconidia are spherical to pyriform, borne sessile to hyphae or on short condiophores. **37°C Growth *In vitro*** Yeast-like. Smooth, butyrous, dull and moist. Surface varies from glabrous to rough and heaped. Color usually cream to light tan, but may be pink. May have a prickly appearance due to short hyphal projections. Microscopic: Small, oval to spherical yeast cells, 2-5μm in diameter, with blastoconidia that have a narrow base.

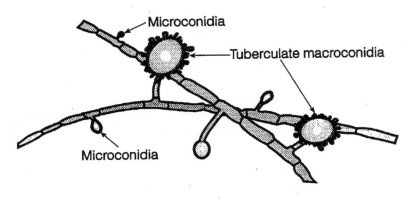

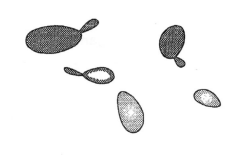

Mycelial phase at room temperature

Yeast phase at 37°C

Blastomyces dermatitidis
(*A. dermatitidis*)

Room Temperature Growth

Colony: Variable characteristics. Fluffy white to glabrous, tan or brown with concentric rings. Growth may take up to 4 weeks.

Microscopic: Delicate, septate hyphae, bearing pyriform to globose (round) conidia 2-10 μm in diameter on conidiophores.

37°C *In vitro* Growth

Colony: Glabrous, folded, heaped, and butyrous, white to brown in color yeast-like colonies. May have prickly appearance due to short hyphal projections.

Microscopic: Thick-walled, spherical yeast cells, 8-15μm in diameter, with broad-based buds. Maximum of one blastoconidia/cell (differential character from *Paracoccidioides brasiliensis* that can have multiple buds/cell).

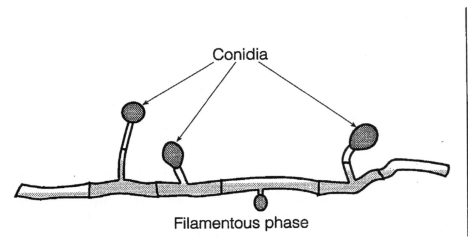

Filamentous phase

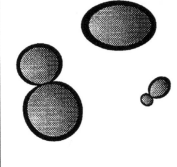

Yeast phase

Well No.	Contents	Band Designation and location
1 2	Anti-*Histoplasma* *Histoplasma* antigen	H, M, with H located nearest antibody well
3 4	Anti-*Blastomyces* *Blastomyces* antigen	A
5 6	Anti-*Coccidioides* *Coccidioides* antigen	F, TP, with TP nearest antibody well
7 8	Antigen for unknown preparation Physiological saline solution	

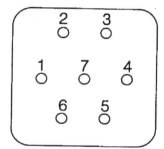 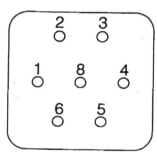

Figure 26-1: Arrangement of additions to double diffusion plates for the exoantigen test.

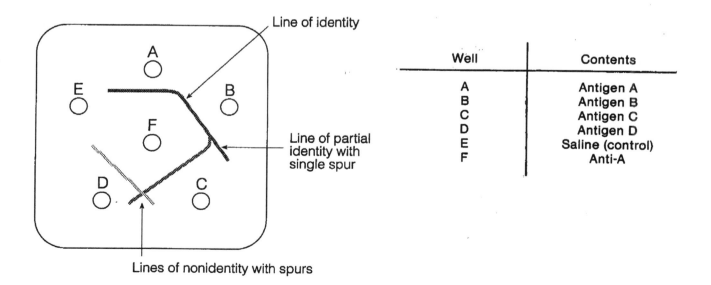

Well	Contents
A	Antigen A
B	Antigen B
C	Antigen C
D	Antigen D
E	Saline (control)
F	Anti-A

Line of identity

Line of partial identity with single spur

Lines of nonidentity with spurs

Figure 26-2: Double diffusion plate with well contents as shown. In this example, Antigens A and B are identical; Antigens B and C are partially identical; and Antigens C and D are different. Well E contains physiological saline and, as expected, shows no reaction with anti-A in the center well, Well F.

b. Each culture grown on thick-poured 10% blood agar supplemented with 1% glucose and 0.1% cysteine and incubated at 37°C for 7 days before observation.

LABORATORY PROCEDURE

Part 1: Culture Observations.

Demonstration cultures of the fungal cultures given under the "Materials" will be placed on display following one week of incubation. Observe colony characteristics of these organisms, Compare growth characteristics of those cultures at 37°C with those grown at room temperature. (Note: Plates are sealed. *Do not open.*)

After these observations, if mature colonies have not yet formed, the cultures will be returned to their respective incubation conditions. Continue to follow their growth on a weekly basis until they have matured. Especially note the relative growth rate of the yeast phase of *H. capsulatum* (*A. capsulatus*) with its own mycelial phase, and with the yeast phase of *B. (A.) dermatitidis.* Make similar comparisons of the latter with its filamentous phase. Record and discuss your findings.

Part 2: Exoantigen Test.

An exoantigen assay using commercially-available reagents, has been set up for your observation and analysis. This double diffusion test includes antigens extracted from *H. capsulatum* (*A. capsulatus*), *B. (A.) dermatitidis,* and *C. immitis* with their respective known antisera. These have been placed into appropriate wells in plates in an arrangement similar to that shown in Figure 26-1. Also given are the possible bands and their location relative to their antibody wells if there is a possibility of more than a single band.

In interpreting band relationships, if an unknown antigen (with known antiserum) produces a "line of identity" connecting a band formed with known antigen-antibody, then the unknown antigen is the same as the known antigen. If, however, a band is formed by the unknown antigen that crosses (i.e. forms "spurs") the band formed by the known antigen-antibody, the former is a different antigen from the known. One other possibility exists, that of partial identity. Here, a partial melding of the bands is seen along with a spur (22). These general relationships are shown in Figure 26-2.

In this test, for example, the unknown antigen, assuming it is an extract of one of the three fungal species, is identifiable by the line of identity it forms with one of the known antigen-antibody bands. If it melds with the A band of *B. (A.) dermatitidis,* it is also antigen A of this organism; if with H and M, then it is *H. capsulatum* (*A. capsulatus*), and so on.

Observe the demonstration plate(s) using strong transmitted light. Locate the precipitin bands and diagram their locations, labeling according to their proper designations (for example, F and/or TP of *C. immitis,* or A of *Blastomyces*). Also, identify the unknown antigen and show the name of the fungal organism from which it was derived. Discuss.

QUESTIONS

1. Skin test antigens are available for systemic fungi. How are these prepared, and what is their usefulness?

REFERENCES

1. Ampel, N. M., M. A. Wieden, and J. N. Galgiani. 1989. Coccidioidomycosis: clinical update. Rev. Infect. Dis. **11**:897-911.
2. Baron, E. J., L. R. Peterson, and S. M. Finegold. 1994. Bailey & Scott's diagnostic microbiology, 9th ed. Mosby-Year Book, Inc., St. Louis. p. 689-775.
3. Bradsher, R. W. 1991. Blastomycosis Clin. Infect. Dis. **14** (Suppl. 1):S82-S90.
4. Chapman, S. W. 1990. Blastomyces dermatitidis, p. 1999-2008. *In* G. L. Mandell, R. G. Douglas, Jr., and J. E. Bennett (ed.), Principles and practices of infectious diseases, 3rd ed. Churchill Livingstone, New York.
5. Galgiani, J. N., and N. M. Ampel. 1990. Coccidioidomycosis in human immunodeficiency virus-infected patients. J. Infect. Dis. **162**:1165-1169.
6. Haley, L. D., and C. S. Callaway. 1978. Laboratory methods in medical mycology, 4th ed. U. S. Dept. of Health, Education, and Welfare, Public Health Service, Center for Disease Control (HEW Pub. No. (CDC) 78-8361), Atlanta, GA, p. 187-198.
7. Hall, G. S., K. Pratt-Rippin, and J. A. Washington. 1992. Evaluation of a chemiluminescent probe assay for identification of *Histoplasma capsulatum* isolates. J. Clin. Microbiol. **30**:3003-3004.
8. Kaufman, L., and P. Standard. 1978. Improved version of the exoantigen test for identification of *Coccidioides immitis* and *Histoplasma capsulatum* cultures. J. Clin. Microbiol. **8**:42-45.
9. Kaufman, L., and P. G. Standard. 1987. Specific and rapid identification of medically important fungi by exoantigen detection. Ann. Rev. Microbiol. **41**:209-225.
10. Kaufman, L. 1992. Laboratory methods for the diagnosis and confirmation of systemic mycoses. Clin. Infect. Dis. **14** (Suppl. 1):S23-S29.
11. Larone, D. H. 1987. Medically important fungi: a guide to identification. Elsevier Science Publishing Co., Inc., New York. p. 173-220.

12. Lefler, E., D. Weiler-Ravell, D. Merzbach, O. Ben-Izhak, and L. A. Best. 1992. Traveler's coccidioidomycosis: case report of pulmonary infection diagnosed in Israel. J. Clin. Microbiol. **30**:1304-1306.

13. Loyd, J. E., R. M. Des Prez, and R. A. Goodwin, Jr. 1990. Histoplasma capsulatum. p. 1989-1999. *In* G. L. Mandell, R. G. Douglas, Jr., and J. E. Bennett (ed.), Principles and practices of infectious diseases, 3rd ed. Churchill Livingstone, New York.

14. McGinnis, M. R., and L. Pasarell. 1992. Mould identification. p. 6.11.1-6.11.17. *In* H. D. Isenberg (ed.), Clinical microbiology procedures handbook. Vol. 1: M. R. McGinnis (Sect. ed.), Mycology. American Society for Microbiology, Washington, D. C.

15. Padhye, A. A., G. Smith, D. McLaughlin, P. G. Standard, and L. Kaufman. 1992. Comparative evaluation of a chemiluminescent DNA probe and an exoantigen test for rapid identification of *Histoplasma capsulatum*. J. Clin. Microbiol. **30**:3108-3111.

16. Pappagianis, D., and B. L. Zimmer. 1990. Serology of coccidioidomycosis. Clin. Microbiol. Rev. **3**:247-268.

17. Rhodes, J. C., and K. J. Kwon-Chung. 1989. Identification of agents of systemic mycoses, p. 141-170. *In* E. G. V. Evans, and M. D. Richardson (ed.), Medical mycology: a practical approach. IRL Press, Oxford.

18. Sarosi, G. A., and P. C. Johnson. 1992. Disseminated histoplasmosis in patients infected with human immunodeficiency virus. Clin. Infect. Dis. **14** (Suppl. 1):S60-S67.

19. Sekhon, A. S., J. Isaac-Renton, J. M. S. Dixon, L. Stein, and H. V. Sims. 1991. Review of human and animal cases of coccidioidomycosis diagnosed in Canada. Mycopathologia **113**:1-10.

20. Stevens, D. A. 1990. Coccidioides immitis, p. 2008-2017. *In* G. L. Mandell, R. G. Douglas, Jr., and J. E. Bennett (ed.), Principles and practices of infectious diseases, 3rd ed. Churchill Livingstone, New York.

21. Sun, S. H., M. Huppert, and K. R. Vukovich. 1976. Rapid *in vitro* conversion and identification of *Coccidioides immitis*. J. Clin. Microbiol. **3**:186-190.

22. Turgeon, M. L. 1990. Immunology and serology in laboratory medicine. The C. V. Mosby Co., St. Louis, p. 114-122.

23. U. S. Public Health Service, Centers for Disease Control and National Institutes of Health. 1988. Biosafety in microbiological and biomedical laboratories, 2nd ed. Publication No. (NIH) 88-8395. Dept. of Health and Human Services, Washington, DC. p. 52-55.

24. Walsh, T. J., and T. G. Mitchell. 1991. Dimorphic fungi causing systemic mycoses, p. 630-643. *In* A. Balows, W. J. Hausler, Jr., K. L. Herrmann, H. D. Isenberg, and H. J. Shadomy (ed.), Manual of clinical microbiology, 5th ed. American Society for Microbiology, Washington, D. C.

25. Wheat, L. J. 1989. Diagnosis and management of histoplasmosis. Eur. J. Clin. Microbiol. Infect. Dis. **8**:480-490.

26. Wheat, L. J. 1992. Histoplasmosis in Indianapolis. Clin. Infect. Dis. **14** (Suppl. 1):S91-S99.

Exercise 26: Dimorphic Fungi Results

Part 1: Culture Observations

Histoplasma capsulatum (Ajellomyces capsulatus):

Date	Culture Age, Days	Incubation Temperature	Description of Growth

Blastomyces (Ajellomyces) dermatitidis

Exercise 26: Dimorphic Fungi Results (Cont'd)

Part 2: Exoantigen Test Results

Well No.	Contents
1	
2	
3	
4	
5	
6	
7	

Date: _____ Incubation Time: _____

Labelled diagram showing precipitin bands and their positions:

Exercise 26: Dimorphic Fungi Results
Other Laboratory Notes

SECTION III
VIROLOGY

INTRODUCTION

The field of virology encompasses a study of infectious agents which range in size from about 250 nm down to 20 nm. The viruses require living cells for their proliferation. They may generally be divided into broad groups by the hosts that naturally support their replication. These include the bacterial viruses (bacteriophage), animal viruses, and plant viruses. Our major concern here, of course, is the animal viruses.

A virus, as described by Lwoff (12) is a strictly intracellular entity with an organized infectious phase, containing protein, possessing one type of nucleic acid, either RNA or DNA, which is unable to undergo binary fission. Furthermore, they lack metabolic activity, being entirely dependent on host cell machinery for synthesis of new virus materials and for energy. The animal viruses may contain either RNA or DNA depending on the virus. Organisms with both types of nucleic acids such as rickettsiae and chamydiae (psittacosis, lymphogranuloma venereum, trachoma group) are not viruses according to Lwoff's description, a fact that is now well accepted. Those groups also have other properties not common to viruses, including multiplication by binary fission.

Viruses always contain nucleic acid and protein, the latter forming a coat around the RNA or DNA. The protein shell is made up of subunits called capsomeres; the entire coat is called the capsid; and the nucleic acid-protein complex is the nucleocapsid. The nucleocapsid may be surrounded by another structure, the envelope, which consists of proteins and lipid. Both the envelope and capsid serve to protect the nucleic acid and contain attachment receptors for the host cell. In overall symmetry, the particle (the virion) may be helical, icosohedral, or complex.

Great strides have been made in the formal classification of the viruses. The initial division for animal viruses is based upon whether the virion contains RNA or DNA. Further features include capsid symmetry, whether an envelope is present, the number of capsomeres in the capsid, molecular weight of the nucleic acid, and other parameters. Even from this brief set of characteristics, it is apparent that unlike other organisms, viral classification is based upon the molecular makeup of these organisms. The basic outcome is that member viruses are placed into a genus of a family and perhaps a formal species, though informal common names are frequently used. An example is influenza virus, which will be studied in Exercise 27. It is an RNA enveloped virus 80-120 nm in diameter belonging to the family *Orthomyxoviridae* ("true myxovirus"; myxo=Gr. mucous, slime: pertaining to mucous of the respiratory tract where the virus infects), genus *Influenzavirus*. There are three species: influenza virus Type A, Type B, and Type C. These and other relationships are presented for this virus and a selection of others in Table 27-1. For those given, herpes simplex virus is generally the most commonly isolated by the diagnostic virus laboratory. Conversely, smallpox virus is now only of historical interest since the disease caused by it was eradicated in the late 1970s.

Specimens used for the identification of viruses do not markedly differ from those used in bacteriology. Blood, spinal fluid, urine, stools, swabs taken from various locations, and others are used, depending on the type of infection. However, some types of samples also may be used that are uncommon for bacterial isolation. These include washes from various locations of the upper respiratory tract (e. g. nasal, nasopharyngeal, bronchial, etc.), saliva, and semen. Specimen storage and transport usually requires nothing beyond their being kept at refrigeration temperature if culture is to be done within 3 days, or at -70°C if for longer periods. Freezing and storing in a frost-free freezer or one at the usual home freezer temperature (about -15 to -20°C) is unsatisfactory (10, 11). If swabs are used, it is important that they are not stored or transported dry, but placed into broth or transport medium (10).

Table 27-1
Some Characteristics of Selected Animal Viruses Causing Human Infection (5, 13)

Family	Physical Characteristics of Family				Genus	Example Species or Common Name	Disease Name and [Target Tissue]
	Size, nm diameter	Shape[a]	N.A.[b] mol. wt × 10^6	Enveloped			
RNA Viruses							
Picornaviridae	24-30	Icosoh.	2.3-2.8	No	Enterovirus	Poliovirus	Poliomyelitis [Oropharyngeal & intestinal mucosa, then central nervous system]
					Heparnavirus	Hepatitis A virus	Hepatitis [GI tract, then liver, spleen, kidney]
					Rhinovirus	Rhinovirus	Common cold [Upper respiratory tract]
Reoviridae	50-60	Icosoh.	12-15	No	Rotavirus	Rotavirus	Gastroenteritis, especially in young children [Duodenal mucosa]
Togaviridae	70	Icosoh.	3-4	Yes	Rubivirus	Rubella virus	Rubella [Skin and many other organs]
Orthomyxoviridae	80-120	Helical	4-5	Yes	Influenzavirus	Influenza Types A, B, and C	Influenza [Respiratory tract]
Paramyxoviridae	50-300	Helical	5-8	Yes	Paramyxovirus	Mumps virus	Mumps [Respiratory tract, lymph nodes, then salivary glands]
					Morbillivirus	Measles virus	Measles (or morbilli) [Upper respiratory tract, then others]
Retroviridae	About 100	Icosoh.	6-7	Yes	Lentivirus	Human immunodeficiency virus	HIV infection, AIDS [T-cells, especially T4]
DNA Viruses							
Papovaviridae	45-55	Icosoh.	3-5	No	Papillomavirus	Papilloma virus	Warts [Skin]
Hepadnaviridae	40-50	Icosoh.	2.1	Yes	Hepadnavirus	Hepatitis B virus	Hepatitis B [Liver]
Herpesviridae	100	Icosoh.	80-150	Yes	Simplexvirus	Herpes simplex virus Types 1, 2	Herpes simplex [Mucous membranes, lymph nodes]
					Varicellavirus	Varicella-Zoster virus	Chicken pox (Varicella) [Respiratory tract, then ectodermal tissue] Shingles (Herpes zoster) [Nerve tissue]
Poxviridae	230 x 300	Complex	160	Complex	Orthopoxvirus	Smallpox virus	Smallpox [Upper respiratory tract & lymph nodes, then liver, spleen, lungs]

[a] Icosoh. = icosohedron, with capsomers assembled to form 5:3:2-fold rotational symmetry appearing as a multifaceted sphere; helical appear as rod-like structures; and complex are brick-like in shape.
[b] N.A. mol. wt = nucleic acid molecular weight.

Virus culture had its beginning in inoculation of animals, including embryonated eggs. A major advance was made in 1949 when it was reported by Enders, Weller, and Robbins (6) that poliomyelitis virus could be cultivated *in vitro* in non-neural human tissue, showing that tissue host range of viruses was broader than previously believed. This type of methodology has now developed into the standard method for practically all animal viruses.

Procedurally, whether susceptible animals or cell cultures are used, clinical specimens that contain non-viral contaminants must be treated to kill or remove these. A common treatment is to add an antimicrobial solution to the sample, as penicillin, streptomycin, gentamicin, and amphotericin B, all contained in Hank's balanced salt solution (HBSS)*. Some specimen types may require centrifugation to clarify them (e. g. stool samples, ground tissue specimens, etc.), or filtration to remove debris, bacteria, or other types of cells (e. g. a clarified stool specimen).

The appropriate animals or cell lines must be selected for virus growth since they are usually selective as to hosts in which they will multiply. Embryonated eggs and sucking mice are among the most common animals that have been used, although animals are now rarely used in diagnostic virology. These have been replaced with cell cultures (also referred to as tissue cultures or monolayer cultures; see Exercise 28 for further information), as primary monkey kidney and human diploid fibroblasts. Use of these two particular cell lines allow the replication of a broad range of viruses (3, 9). Since herpes simplex virus is one of the most common isolates, and may not do well on these, primary kidney or mink lung cells, which are particularly susceptible for this virus, can be included (1). If, however, influenza virus is suspected, then Madin-Darby canine kidney (MDCK) cells has been widely used (7). Centrifugation of a specimen onto a cell monolayer in a shell vial can reduce the time required to observe viral infection for several viruses, as HSV, influenza virus, measles virus, and others (16, 19).

Detection of virus in cell cultures is made primarily through their cytopathic effect (CPE), which is visible by use of light microscopy or seen macroscopically. This alteration in cell mor-

phology, and frequently cell death, may be evident within one or two days to a week or more. In fact, the rate of CPE, as well as the range of cell culture types can be important in giving an early indication of what the virus might be. However, other effects on cell cultures also can be produced by viruses, as hemadsorption of guinea pig red cells onto infected monolayers due to virus-directed attachment glycoproteins on the surface of cultured cells (18).

Definitive virus identification usually requires the use of known antibody. Here, several methods may be used. Fluorescent antibody can, for instance, detect cells infected by many types of viruses (e.g. HIV, rabies, rotavirus, etc.), whether directly from an infected human or animal, as from tissue scraping, biopsy, or other sources; or from a cell monolayer. Virus neutralizing antibody is also commonly used to detect isolated viruses by acting specifically to prevent virus infection of susceptible cells or from exhibiting other activity. Exercise 27 will involve such a test where influenza virus is neutralized by antibody preventing it from causing hemagglutination. Enzyme-linked immunoassays, radioimmunoassays, latex agglutination, and to a lesser extent, immunoelectron microscopy are also used. These are particularly important for viruses that are difficult to culture, as human rotaviruses and varicella-zoster virus (4, 5). The EIA especially has been adapted to rapid tests, many of which can be used to identify viruses directly from a clinical specimen. Kits based on this technology, fluorescent antibody, and latex agglutination for the detection of influenza virus, rotaviruses, herpes simplex virus, and hepatitis B antigen are a few of those that are commercially available.

While many reports of application of genetic probes (e.g. 8, 15) and polymerase chain reaction (e.g. 2, 14, 20) to viral identification appear in the literature, no commercial rapid assay is yet available. It is not difficult to predict, however, that these will become available for the more commonly encountered viruses in the future.

Serological detection of antibodies from patients exposed to viral infection is also widely used in clinical diagnosis. Types of protocols to accomplish this include latex agglutination (for example, anti-varicella-zoster virus, rubella, and others), EIA (Anti-HIV, rubella, hepatitis A and B, etc.), Western blot (for anti-HIV), and complement fixation. The latter has been a standard

---

* Other combinations can be used. Here, as in other situations in this general review, only common examples will be used, rather than a comprehensive coverage of methods.

serological assay for detection of anti-viral antibodies for many years, and reagents are available for many genera.

Similar principles of laboratory safety apply to study and handling of viruses as previously outlined for other microorganisms. Proper containment hoods, as a Class II laminar flow hood, good laboratory techniques, and protective clothing are needed for the general virology laboratory. Also, immunizations against measles, rubella, polio, mumps, influenza, and hepatitis B viruses may be required depending on the nature of specimens being handled (18). Biosafety 2 or 3 levels of containment are recommended for most viruses that have the potential to infect humans (17).

In the following exercise, virus culture will be done using the embryonated chicken (Exercise 27) and in cell culture (Exercise 28). In the former, standard methods for the hemagglutination test to detect virus, and the hemagglutination inhibition test to identify virus are included. These will provide added general insight into culture and identification of viruses. However, circumstances do not permit more than an introduction here into virological studies. It is therefore suggested that you extend that learned here by outside study in this important discipline.

REFERENCES

1. Arvin, A. M., and C. G. Prober. 1991. Herpes simplex viruses, p. 822-828. *In* A. Balows, W. J. Hausler, Jr., K. L. Herrmann, H. D. Isenberg, and H. J. Shadomy (ed.), Manual of clinical microbiology, 5th ed. American Society for Microbiology, Washington, D. C.
2. Bressoud, A., J. Whitcomb, C. Pourzand, O. Haller, and P. Cerutti. 1990. Rapid detection of influenza virus H1 by the polymerase chain reaction. Biochem. Biophys. Res. Comm. **167**:425-430.
3. Clarke, L. M., J. M. McPhee, and R. V. Cummings. 1992. Isolation of viruses in conventional tube culture: selection and inoculation of cell cultures, p. 8.5.1-8.5.13. *In* H. D. Isenberg (ed.), Clinical microbiology procedures handbook, Vol. 2: L. M. Clarke (Sect. ed.), Viruses, rickettsiae, chlamydiae, and mycoplasmas. American Society for Microbiology, Washington, DC.
4. Colmer, J. 1989. Rapid viral testing methods: an overview. Clin. Lab. Sci. **2**:95-98.
5. Davis, B. D., R. Dulbecco, H. N. Eisen, and H. S. Ginsberg. 1990. Microbiology, 4th ed. J. B. Lippincott Co., Philadelphia. p. 769-1151.
6. Enders, J. F., T. H. Weller, and F. C. Robbins. 1949. Cultivation of the Lansing strain of poliomyelitis virus in cultures of various human embryonic tissues. Science **109**:85-87.
7. Harmon, M. W., and A. P. Kendal. 1991. Influenza viruses, p. 868-877. *In* A. Balows, W. J. Hausler, Jr., K. L. Herrmann, H. D. Isenberg, and H. J. Shadomy (ed.), Manual of clinical microbiology, 5th ed. American Society for Microbiology, Washington, D. C.

8. Kallajoki, M., H. Kalimo, L. Wesslén, P. Auvinen, and T. Hyypiä. 1990. *In situ* detection of enterovirus genmones in mouse myocardial tissue by ribonucleic acid probes. Lab. Invest. **63**:669-675.
9. Landry, M. L., and G. D. Hsiung. 1986. Primary isolation of viruses, p. 31-51. *In* S. Specter, and G. J. Lancz, Clinical virology manual. Elsevier Science Publishing Co., Inc., New York.
10. Lennette, D. A. 1991. Preparation of specimens for virological examination, p. 818-821. *In* A. Balows, W. J. Hausler, Jr., K. L. Herrmann, H. D. Isenberg, and H. J. Shadomy (ed.), Manual of clinical microbiology, 5th ed. American Society for Microbiology, Washington, D. C.
11. Leonardi, G. P., and C. A. Gleaves. 1992. Selection, collection and transport of specimens for viral and rickettsial cultures, p. 8.2.1-8.2.10. *In* H. D. Isenberg (ed.), Clinical microbiology procedures handbook, Vol. 2: L. M. Clarke (Sect. ed.), Viruses, rickettsiae, chlamydiae, and mycoplasmas. American Society for Microbiology, Washington, DC.
12. Lwoff, A. 1957. The concept of virus. J. Gen. Microbiol. **17**:239-253.
13. Melnick, J. L. 1991. Taxonomy of viruses, p. 811-817. *In* A. Balows, W. J. Hausler, Jr., K. L. Herrmann, H. D. Isenberg, and H. J. Shadomy (ed.), Manual of clinical microbiology, 5th ed. American Society for Microbiology, Washington, D. C.
14. Olive, D. M., S. Al-Mufti, W. Al-Mulla, M. A. Khan, A. Pasca, G. Stanway, and W. Al-Nakib. 1990. Detection and differentiation of picornaviruses in clinical samples following genomic amplification. J. Gen. Virol. **71**:2141-2147.
15. Petitjean, J., M. Quibriac, F. Freymuth, F. Fuchs, N. Laconche, M. Aymard, and H. Kopecka. 1990. Specific detection of enteroviruses in clinical samples by molecular hybridization using poliovirus subgenomic riboprobes. J. Clin. Microbiol. **28**:307-311.
16. Salmon. V. C., R. B. Turner, M. J. Speranza, and J. C. Overall, Jr. 1986. Rapid detection of herpes simplex virus in clinical specimens by centrifugation and immunoperoxidase staining. J. Clin. Microbiol. **23**:683-686.
17. U. S. Public Health Service, Centers for Disease Control and National Institutes of Health. 1988. Biosafety in microbiological and biomedical laboratories, 2nd ed. Publication No. (NIH) 88-8395. Dept. of Health and Human Services, Washington, DC. p. 72-87.
18. Wiedbrauk, D. L., and S. L. G. Johnston. 1993. Manual of clinical virology. Raven Press, Ltd., New York, p. 11-17.
19. Wold, A. D. 1992. Shell vial assay for rapid detection of viral infections, p. 8.6.1-8.6.10. *In* H. D. Isenberg (ed.), Clinical microbiology procedures handbook, Vol. 2: L. M. Clarke (Sect. ed.), Viruses, rickettsiae, chlamydiae, and mycoplasmas. American Society for Microbiology, Washington, DC.
20. Zhang, W., and D. H. Evans. 1991. Detection and identification of human influenza viruses by the polymerase chain reaction. J. Virolog. Methods **33**:165-189.

EXERCISE 27
Influenzavirus Culture and Assay

Influenzavirus, the only member of the *Ortho-myxoviridae,* is found as three types, A, B, and C (Table 27-1). Its genomic RNA codes for 10 proteins required for its replication and structure. Proteins (actually, glycoproteins) that are particularly pertinent to our discussion here are those called "H," or hemagglutination, that bind to cell receptors containing sialic (or neuramic) acid, and "N," for neuraminidase. Both of these are antigens, and therefore referred to as HA and NA, respectively. These are located in the surface envelope of the virion, and have key roles in virus attachment to host tissue in infection and to red cells in the commonly used assays used to detect the virus, and in designation of viral subtypes (2).

While influenza virus exists in three types, in terms of the disease influenza, Type A is most significant causing morbidity and mortality in both epidemics and in pandemics. Type B also causes epidemics, but less frequently, and usually are less widespread and less severe than those caused by Type A (occasional exceptions occur, as in the 1990-91 influenza season, disease due to Type B exceeded Type A in the U. S.). Type C is not known to cause human disease. For Type A, especially, it is well-known that HA and NA routinely undergo small antigenic changes (antigenic drift), and less frequently, major alterations (antigenic shift) that gives rise to three HA and two NA types. Both antigenic drift and shift are due to RNA mutation, with the former due to small coding changes, and the latter probably due to a major reassortment of the eight RNA segments of the genome (2, 8). This allows the virus to avoid host immunity generated to past exposures of influenza antigens, and leads to recurrence of epidemics and/or pandemics. Aside from the suffering and mortality caused by influenza, it is estimated that $300 million is expended in the U. S. on hospitalization alone due to one epidemic of this disease (1).

Because of the changing nature of the identifying H and N antigens, a uniform system of naming viral subtypes of Type A has been developed. The virus is therefore designated with information arranged as follows: Type/source (if not human)/geographical location of isolation/

strain number/year of isolation(HA-NA types). As examples, the strain you will be using in this exercise is A/PR/8/34(H1N1) (8). An early isolate of the Asian flu outbreak of 1957 responsible for a disease of pandemic proportions is designated A/Japan/305/57(H2N2), the first time this HA-NA combination had been isolated, arising from an antigenic shift (6, 11). During the 1989-90 influenza season, 98% of cases were caused by a strain of A/Shanghai/11/87(H3N2) (3). All of this has a practical laboratory impact since antibodies are specific for virus type and HA and NA subtypes necessitating the correct antiserum be available if proper identification is to be accomplished.

Laboratory identification of influenza virus is summarized in the Introduction to Virology. Cell cultures as Madin-Darby canine kidney cells are commonly used, but primary rhesus monkey kidney cells also can be employed. In these, both cytopathogenic effect and hemadsorption (due to HA expression on cell surfaces) will show the presence of virus, while FA and EIA may be used to detect and identify it (2, 12). The use of the shell vial method can reduce the time before virus is detected in culture (12). Furthermore, embryonated eggs can be used to cultivate the virus, a topic addressed more thoroughly below.

Viral identification also can be carried out by the hemagglutination inhibition (HI) test. Both viral type and HA subtype is determined in this variation of a virus neutralization test. HA, in the absence of antibodies or other inhibitors, attach to red cell surfaces producing a macroscopically visible aggregation of these cells from a physical linking together due to virus HA. If the homologous antibody is present (i.e. anti-H1 for H1 antigen, etc.), the HA is blocked from binding to its neuraminic acid site, and hemagglutination is inhibited.

Rapid tests have become available to detect the presence of influenza virus, some directly from the clinical specimen. An example of this is the Directigen® FLU-A, a solid-phase EIA test that detects virus in nasopharyngeal washes, aspirates, or from swabs in a 15 minute run time. This assay has a sensitivity of 90% with clinical nasopharyngeal washes, and also detects virus from avian and swine samples at a 75% and 86% sensitivity, respectively, compared to cell culture methods (10). In another study, it had a sensitivity of 100% compared to indirect fluorescent antibody on smears prepared from throat swabs, but 62% compared to culture (5). Fluorescent antibody also can be used directly on clinical respiratory specimens to detect the presence of several viruses, including Type A influenza, preferably as an adjunct with other established methods (9).

Detection and titration of patient anti-influenza response can also be important for certain purposes. Here, an increase in antibody titer of at least four times in paired serum samples is indicative of infection. While this information can be useful in conjunction with virus isolation methods, two factors lessen the impact of this in direct diagnosis. One of these is that an acute phase sample is frequently not obtained; the other is that the titer may not peak for four weeks or longer after onset. This means that the titer change needed to be of diagnostic significance will not become available until well after symptoms have abated, which in most cases of influenza is within a week after onset (4, 12). However, the virus neutralization, complement fixation, hemagglutination inhibition, or enzyme-linked immunoassay tests used to assay for anti-influenza antibodies have the advantage of being more economical than virus isolation. Also, such assays are useful in epidemiological studies (4).

The chick embryo, while rarely used in diagnostic virology, provides an effective procedure for cultivating a wide variety of animal viruses and rickettsia. It will be used here to culture *Influenzavirus* Type A. An embryonated egg is diagrammed in Figure 27-1 as it would appear at 11 days showing the important structures involved in virus culture. The area into which the embryo is inoculated depend on the virus. For example, the measles agent and first isolation attempt for influenza A and B viruses are inoculated into the amniotic cavity. Egg adapted influenza virus and other species are usually inoculated into the allantoic cavity of 10-12 day-old embryonated eggs. In both of these instances, the virus diffuses to the adjacent tissue where replication occurs. Vaccinia and herpes simplex viruses are obtained by inoculating the chorioallantoic membrane of 10-12 day-old embryos where they form visible pock lesions (4, 7).

In general, what will be done in this exercise is to inoculate dilutions of *Influenzavirus* Type A into groups of embryonated eggs. During the incubation period, virus enters the cells of the chorioallantoic membrane, replicate, then are released back into the chorioallantoic fluid. These new virions infect other cells, thus continuing the infection. After an appropriate time, the chorioallantoic fluid is harvested, and assayed for the presence of virus, as well as for its titer (i. e. relative amount).

To detect the presence and relative amounts of *Influenzavirus,* advantage can be taken of its capacity to agglutinate red cells. Furthermore, as pointed out above, this reaction can be specifically blocked by antibody. If the virus was of an unknown type, as would be true from a clinical specimen, the HI test offers a method of viral identification. Both of these procedures will be carried out in this exercise. Further details concerning the procedures used here can be found in Reference 4.

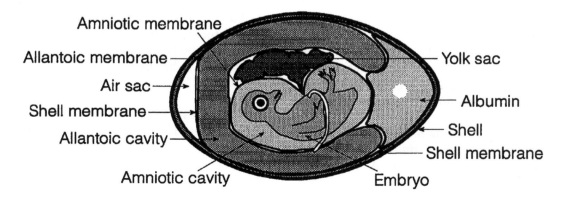

Figure 27-1: The embryonated chicken at 11 days of age.

MATERIALS

Part 1

A. Per pair of students:
Ten-twelve days before starting Exercise 27:

    2 fertile chicken eggs

On inoculation day

    1 jar sterile pledgets
       70% ethanol
       Egg holder
       Egg candler
       Egg punch

B. Per pair of students:

    1 1 ml syringe fitted with 26 gauge needle
    1 Dilution of influenza virus in phosphate buffered saline (pH 7.2) contained in vaccine vial or tube
    1 Swab
       Plastic tape or wax (as candle wax)
       70% ethanol

C. Per pair of students:

    1 pair of forceps
    1 Egg holder
    1 Sterile Pasteur pipette and bulb
    1 porcelain pan
    1 Sterile tube for containing harvested allantoic fluid
    2 petri dishes
       70% ethanol
       95% ethanol
    1 jar sterile pledgets

Part 2

A. Per pair of students

    10 Kahn (12 x 75 mm) tubes
    5 ml 0.5% chicken red cell suspension (in PBS)
    1 5 ml pipette
    3 ml plugged pipettes
    5 ml 0.01M, pH 7.2 phosphate buffered saline (PBS)
    1 pipette bulb or aid

B. Per pair of students:

    10 ml 0.5% chicken red cell suspension in PBS
    3 1 ml plugged pipettes
    11 Kahn tubes
    1 pipette bulb or pipette aid
    25 ml phosphate buffered saline, pH 7.2
    0.5 ml anti-influenza serum treated with receptor destroying enzyme

LABORATORY PROCEDURES

Part 1: Egg Preparation and Influenza Virus Culture

A. Each pair of students will carry out the following procedure:

1. Preparation of eggs: The class will be provided with fertile eggs (2 per pair). It is necessary that these are incubated at 38°C for 10-12 days in a humid atmosphere. Also, it is required that the eggs are turned at least once a day for proper embryo development. This will be done by individuals of the class by assignment.

2. After the needed incubation period candle the egg. Determine the viability of the embryo (does it move?) and the position of the air sac. Mark the position of the latter with a pencil.

3. Place the egg in an egg holder. Swab a small area immediately below the air sac with 70% alcohol, then gently puncture the egg shell with a punch or drill as shown. Be careful not to penetrate the chorioallantoic membrane (CAM). Also, swab another area over the air sac and again puncture the shell.

B. Inoculation (Caution: Do all open culture work within a containment hood):

1. In order to (i) obtain virus for subsequent work, and (ii) attempt to obtain an endpoint of infection, dilutions of influenza virus (Type A, Strain PR8) will be provided. The class will inoculate these as follows:

2. Working within a containment hood, draw 0.2 ml of virus solution into a 1 cc syringe fitted with a 26 gauge needle. Expel any air bubbles back into the vaccine-type tube or vial.

Dilution	Group
10^{-1}	1, 2
10^{-2}	3, 4
10^{-3}	5, 6
10^{-4}	7, 8
10^{-5}	9, 10

3. Carefully insert the needle through the hole in the shell below the air sac and through the CAM about ½ inch, angling it slightly toward the air sac.

4. Inject exactly 0.1 ml by twisting the barrel of the syringe inward.

5. Carefully remove the needle and seal the holes with small pieces of plastic tape or melted candle wax. Label each egg with your name or group number, date and virus dilution inoculated.

6. Place the eggs at 35°C and incubate for 24-48 hours.

C. Collection of sample and gross test for virus. Each pair of students:

1. Retrieve your eggs from the incubator. Chill by placing them in the refrigerator overnight (or for *at least* 2 hours before Step 2).

2. Place the egg in a holder contained in a porcelain pan.

3. Swab the top of the egg with 70% ethanol, then break the shell over the air sac by penetrating it with the point of a pair of forceps or scissors. Carefully peel or cut back the shell over the air sac.

4. Tear open the shell membrane over the allantoic cavity with sterile forceps flamed in 95% ethanol. Insert a sterile Pasteur pipette equipped with a rubber bulb into the allantoic cavity, being careful not to rupture blood vessels.

5. If the fluid is clear, aspirate 2-3 ml and transfer to a sterile tube. (If fluid is turbid, it is probably contaminated with bacteria, and the entire embryo should be discarded.)

6. Empty embryo and remaining allantoic fluid into a petri dish and further tear the allantoic membrane, now to encourage bleeding. Allow to sit at room temperature for 10 minutes then observe for clumping of erythrocytes. If virus is present a positive test may be observed.

7. Repeat the procedure with the remaining embryo inoculated with the same virus dilution and pool the samples. Use the pooled sample for the hemagglutination test in *Part 2*.

8. Discard the embryos into appropriate container.

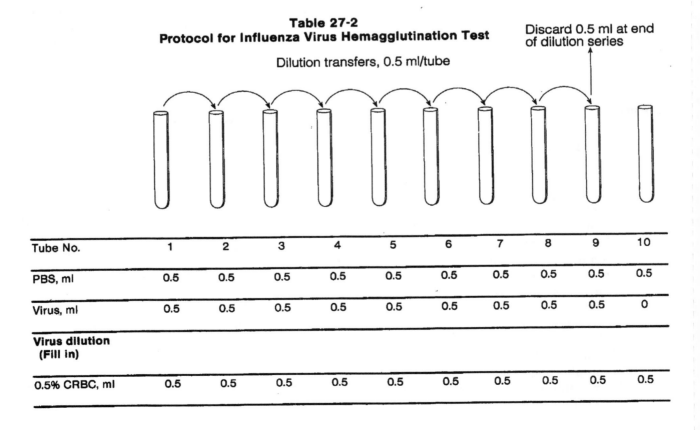

Table 27-2
Protocol for Influenza Virus Hemagglutination Test

Discard 0.5 ml at end of dilution series

Dilution transfers, 0.5 ml/tube

Tube No.	1	2	3	4	5	6	7	8	9	10
PBS, ml	0.5	0.5	0.5	0.5	0.5	0.5	0.5	0.5	0.5	0.5
Virus, ml	0.5	0.5	0.5	0.5	0.5	0.5	0.5	0.5	0.5	0
Virus dilution (Fill in)										
0.5% CRBC, ml	0.5	0.5	0.5	0.5	0.5	0.5	0.5	0.5	0.5	0.5

Part 2: Influenza Virus Assay—The Viral Hemagglutination and Hemagglutination Inhibition Tests

A. The Hemagglutination Test: Each pair of students carry out the hemagglutination test with the influenza virus harvested in *Part 1* C following the protocol shown in Table 27-2. Remember to prepare virus dilutions and additions within a containment hood.

1. After adding components to all tubes, shake and incubate *undisturbed* at room temperature for 1-2 hours until chicken red blood cells (CRBC) in Tube 10 settle to form a "button" of red cells at the bottom. Observe results. Non-hemagglutination, the button seen in the control tube (Tube 10), is to be compared to hemagglutination that is characterized by a "spread" pattern of CRBC on the bottom of the tube.

2. The highest dilution showing typical hemagglutination is called the "hemagglutination unit." If, for example, the end point occurred in Tube 7, this would be one unit in the dilution of virus in that tube. Four such units are used in the hemagglutination inhibition (HI) test.

3. Place your results on the board and compare with the remainder of the class. Discuss the significance of your results and that of the class as a whole. Was an infectious dose endpoint obtained by inoculation of varying dilutions into embryonated eggs? Does the original dilution of virus inoculated into the egg appear to influence the eventual titer of virus recovered as determined by the hemagglutination test?

Record all results on the data sheet provided at the end of this exercise.

B. The Hemagglutination Inhibition Test: This assay is carried out by first diluting the stock virus so as to contain 4 hemagglutinating units in 0.25 ml (enter the computation of this value into your notebook). Follow the protocol given in Table 27-3 using antiserum previously treated with receptor-destroying enzyme (RDE, a neuraminidase). The purpose of this treatment is to remove non-specific inhibitors that are frequently found in serum that react with viral hemagglutinins and would therefore inhibit binding to red cells (4, 6). Other methods are also employed to inactive these inhibitors.

**Table 27-3
Protocol for Influenza Virus Hemagglutination Inhibition Test**

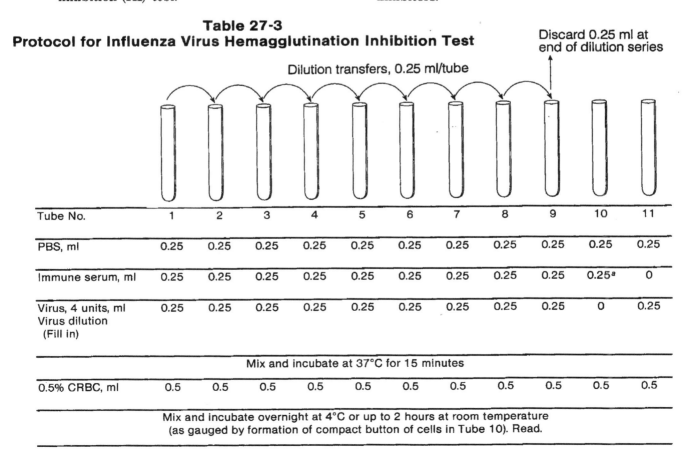

Discard 0.25 ml at end of dilution series

Dilution transfers, 0.25 ml/tube

Tube No.	1	2	3	4	5	6	7	8	9	10	11
PBS, ml	0.25	0.25	0.25	0.25	0.25	0.25	0.25	0.25	0.25	0.25	0.25
Immune serum, ml	0.25	0.25	0.25	0.25	0.25	0.25	0.25	0.25	0.25	0.25[a]	0
Virus, 4 units, ml Virus dilution (Fill in)	0.25	0.25	0.25	0.25	0.25	0.25	0.25	0.25	0.25	0	0.25
Mix and incubate at 37°C for 15 minutes											
0.5% CRBC, ml	0.5	0.5	0.5	0.5	0.5	0.5	0.5	0.5	0.5	0.5	0.5

Mix and incubate overnight at 4°C or up to 2 hours at room temperature (as gauged by formation of compact button of cells in Tube 10). Read.

[a]Same dilution as contained in Tube 1.

1. After addition of CRBC's to all tubes, mix and incubate overnight in the refrigerator, or, if time permits, allow to stand until cells have settled sufficiently to read their hemagglutination patterns. Read for the endpoint of hemagglutination inhibition. Be sure the controls (Tubes 10 and 11) give the proper reactions. (What are those reactions?)

2. Record your results in terms of the highest serum dilution giving inhibition of agglutination of CRBCs.

3. Discuss your results.

REFERENCES

1. Barker, W. H. 1986. Excess pneumoniae and influenza associated hospitalization during influenza epidemics in the United States, 1970-78. Am. J. Public Health **76**:761-765.

2. Betts, R. F., and R. G. Douglas, Jr. 1990. Influenza virus, p. 1306-1325. *In* G. L. Mandell, R. G. Douglas, Jr., and J. E. Bennett (ed.), Principles and practices of infectious diseases, 3rd ed. Churchill Livingstone, New York.

3. Chapman, L. E., M. A. Tipple, L. M. Schmeltz, S. E. Good, H. L. Regnery, A. P. Kendal, H. E. Gary, Jr., N. J. Cox, and L. B. Schonberger. 1992. Influenza - United States, 1989-90 and 1990-91 seasons. MMWR **41**(No. SS-3):35-46.

4. Harmon, M. W., and A. P. Kendal. 1991. Influenza viruses, p. 868-877. *In* A. Balows, W. J. Hausler, Jr., K. L. Herrmann, H. D. Isenberg, and H. J. Shadomy (ed.), Manual of clinical microbiology, 5th ed. American Society for Microbiology, Washington, D. C.

5. Johnston, S. L. G., and H. Bloy. 1993. Evaluation of a rapid enzyme immunoassay for detection of influenza A virus. J. Clin. Microbiol. **31**:142-143.

6. Kilbourne, E. D. 1987. Influenza. Plenum Medical Book Co., New York. p. 3-22, 219-228, 255-289.

7. Landry, M. L., and G. D. Hsiung. 1986. Primary isolation of viruses, p. 31-51. *In* S. Specter, and G. J. Lancz, Clinical virology manual. Elsevier Science Publishing Co., Inc., New York.

8. Levine, A. J. 1992. Viruses. Scientific American Library, New York. p. 155-175.

9. Minnich, L., and C. G. Ray. 1980. Comparison of direct immunofluorescent staining of clinical specimens for respiratory virus antigens with conventional isolation techniques. J. Clin. Microbiol. **12**:391-384.

10. Ryan-Poirier, K. A., J. M. Katz, R. G. Webster, and Y. Kawaoka. 1992. Application of Directigen FLU-A for the detection of influenza A virus in human and nonhuman specimens. J. Clin. Microbiol. **30**:1072-1075.

11. Stuart-Harris, C. H., G. C. Schild, and J. S. Oxford. 1985. Influenza: the virus and the disease, 2nd ed. Edward Arnold, Baltimore. p. 118-138.

12. Wiedbrauk, D. L., and S. L. G. Johnston. 1993. Manual of clinical virology. Raven Press, Ltd., New York, p. 11-17, 127-140.

Exercise 27: Influenza Virus Results

Part 1 C: Gross Test for The Presence of Influenza Virus in the Embryonated Egg:

Part 2 A: Class Data-Hemagglutination and Egg Infectivity

Group No.	PR8 Virus Dilution Inoculated	Virus Hemagglutination Titer

Results:
1. Virus Hemagglutination

   1 Hemagglutination unit = _____ in 0.5 ml

   4 Hemagglutination units = _____ in 0.25 ml

   Calculations:

2. Virus Infectivity Titer for Embryonated Egg:

   Infectivity titer of inoculated virus: _____

Part 2 B: Hemagglutination Inhibition Assay Results.

Antibody HI Titer: _____

Results of controls:

Tube No. 10: _____ Tube No. 11: _____

Other Laboratory Notes

EXERCISE 28
Poliomyelitis Virus and the Plaque Assay

I. Poliovirus and other Enteroviruses

Another member of the RNA viruses is poliovirus, belonging to the *Enterovirus* of the family *Picornaviridae* (*pico* = small, rna = type of nucleic acid). Also included in the genus are the following: (i) echoviruses (an acronym for "enteric cytopathic human orphan, so named because at the time of their discovery no disease could be attributed to them); (ii) coxsackievirus (named after the location in New York where it was first isolated); and (iii) enterovirus (3). All of these are grouped into serologic types such that now the genus consists of at least 68, including three types of poliovirus, Types P1, P2, and P3 (8). In this exercise, our focus will be primarily on this latter agent, its culture and enumeration.

All serologic types of poliovirus cause the same disease, poliomyelitis. The virus is transmitted by the oral-fecal route with initial replication occurring in both the pharynx and gastrointestinal tissue. In subclinical disease, which occurs in 95% of cases, the virus multiplies in the regional lymph nodes, then stops, resulting in mild gastrointestinal or no symptoms (9). Of course, the well recognized symptoms of paralytic poliomyelitis does occur, the rate estimated to be about 0.1 to 0.05% (3, 10) causing epidemics in the 1940's and 1950's in developed countries worldwide preceding the arrival of the vaccines. In the U. S. alone, from 15,000 to 20,000 cases per year were reported, as compared to the less than 10 cases/year that have occurred since 1970 (10). However, outbreaks still occur as evidenced by one in the Netherlands where 54 cases were reported among unvaccinated persons in the last half of 1992. Of these, 76% had manifestations of paralysis, 22% aseptic meningitis, and one neonate died (2). Protection against this infection is achieved through immunization, either by administration of attenuated oral (Sabin) or inactivated (Salk) vaccine. Total protection can only be obtained by receiving all three virus types in the vaccine.

Clinical samples for poliomyelitis, as suggested by the foregoing description, are primarily throat or rectal swabs, stool specimens, and throat washings (8, 13). Virus isolation may be done through either animals or cell cultures, but the latter is preferred, especially since live monkeys are the only non-human host susceptible to all types (13). Many kinds of cell culture support virus replication, however, including, for example, primary monkey kidney (PMK) cells, RD cell line (derived from human embryo rhabdosarcoma), and HeLa cell line (derived from human cervical carcinoma). RD cells, in particular, are supportive of all except three coxsackie types within the enteroviruses (12). In culture poliovirus quickly produces cytopathic effects (CPE) followed by cell death, usually within three days, providing an important clue as to its presence. Many other enteroviruses also produce CPE on primary isolation, though less rapidly (8, 12).

Because of the large number of enterovirus types, equine serum pools of antibodies (the Lim and Benyesch-Melnick, or LBM pools) have been developed. In principle, these pools are used similarly to *Salmonella* antisera to group serovars discussed in Exercise 9 (p. 143). With the enteroviruses, all 42 types that can grow in tissue culture can be identified with the LBM pool. For poliovirus alone, however, a pool containing only anti-Types P1, P2, and P3 would identify its presence by a neutralization assay using cells cultures, the most common method for identifying it. Individual typing serum is then used to establish its precise type, again using the neutralization assay (8, 12, 13).

Analysis of patient antibody response to enteroviruses in general is limited by the large number of serotypes. However, the neutralization and complement fixation (CF) tests have been most commonly used. A four-fold increase in patient's antibody titer in paired serum samples taken two to three weeks apart implicates the virus as the vehicle of infection (8). Of course, if the clinical indications of poliomyelitis are present, serodiagnosis could be made more readily because of the limited number of serotypes, and would have significant importance in diagnosis.

While enteroviruses are important, the nature of this exercise is focussed equally on the use of cell cultures for their detection. Toward this end, a brief introduction to this topic is instructive.

II. Cell Culture.

In animal virology cell cultures (also frequently referred to as tissue cultures) can be found in a myriad of types derived from many organs of humans and lower animals. Overall, irrespective of the tissue source, they can be categorized into one of three types. Primary cell cultures, as MKC, are those that grow *in vitro* following isolation from intact tissue, and for a limited number of transfers after that. When subculture can be extended over many *in vitro* transfers (usually about 50 for human cells), these are then frequently referred to as diploid cell lines, including WI-38, MRC-5, both derived from human embryonic lung. These also represent secondary cell cultures (relating to that following "primary culture") of these cells. Most of these will eventually die out in a phenomenon of senescence. However, some will undergo transformation, losing their diploid character, but allowing immortality where they can now be grown and transferred indefinitely. These are continuous cell lines (11), and include HeLa and RD cells. Most common cell lines are available from American *Type Culture* Collection, Rockville, MD.

Primary culture of mammalian cells involves freeing individual cells from minced tissue, commonly by treatment with a protease, as trypsin. Gross material is removed, the cell suspension washed, then enumerated. After diluting cells to a desired concentration with an appropriate cell culture medium, these are added to glass or plastic containers. For most viral assays in clinical diagnosis, cells are allowed to settle onto a flat surface, where they attach and begin to multiply. When confluent growth (a monolayer of cells or a cell sheet) has occurred, they must be transferred. This process is similar to that done in the laboratory work of this exercise, and will be described in detail there.

The reagents, media, and distilled water used for cell cultures must be of high quality and purity since mammalian cells are highly susceptible to small amounts of toxic trace metals and other contaminants. The media used for their growth are very different from that used for bacteria and fungi, requiring similar nutrients as supplied to them within the living animal. There are several formulations of tissue culture media, many of which are chemically defined. Eagle's minimum essential medium (MEM), which is chemically defined, with added 2% (for maintenance of cultures) up to 10% (for culture growth) animal serum, that makes the total an undefined medium, is one of the most commonly used. MEM contains Hank's or Earle's balanced salt solution (BSS), a combination of inorganic salts, glucose, and phenol red; and vitamins, nucleosides, and amino acids (4). Serum supplies unspecified factors that are required for cell growth. Antimicrobial compounds are added to the culture medium to inhibit stray bacteria and fungi that otherwise readily grow in these media.

For the growth of mammalian cells pH is optimal at 7.2-7.4, maintained, at least for many cell culture media, with a 5% CO_2-bicarbonate buffering system. As growth occurs, lactic acid produced through cell metabolism will overcome the weak bicarbonate or other buffering system commonly used, and the pH will decrease. When it reaches a level of pH 6.5 to 6.8, the acid must be neutralized or the cell medium refreshed to allow cells to remain viable. Phenol red, the usual pH indicator, allows a visual cue for the amount of acidity present. A yellow color of the medium indicates a pH of 6.8 or less; orange a pH of 7.0; red is pH 7.4; and cerise for 7.6 or above (12). The latter is important since its occurrance is indicative of cell death, loss of CO_2, or other undesirable conditions.

This exercise will demonstrate cell culture methods using the HeLa "continuous" cell line. After these have been established following transfer they will be infected with poliomyelitis virus. The result of virus-cell interaction will finally be shown by formation of plaques using the agar overlay method. (Note: All individuals using poliovirus *must* have had immunizations against it well before doing this exercise.)

MATERIALS

Part 1

Per pair of students:
    1 Bottle culture of HeLa cells (75 cm² bottle size)
    2 sterile 10 ml pipettes
    4 sterile 60 mm culture dishes
    5 ml 0.25% trypsin-0.02% EDTA in phosphate buffered saline (PBS, without Ca⁺⁺ and Mg⁺⁺)
  30ml Eagle's MEM with 5% fetal bovine serum (FBS)
    Fluid discard container

Part 2

Per pair of students:
  1 dilution of poliovirus Type 2 in Eagle's MEM with 2% FBS, 4 ml/tube
  2 sterile 1 ml pipette
  1 sterile 5 ml pipette
  2 ml Eagle's MEM with 2% FBS
  25ml Hank's BSS
  15ml melted 0.6% agarose overlay medium held in a 50°C waterbath
  Fluid discard container

LABORATORY PROCEDURES
(Also see Figure 28-1)

Part 1: Cell Culture (4, 5, 12):

For each pair of students:

Preliminary steps: Cell culture transfer steps should be done in an area free of dust and foot traffic. Work within a dust-free cabinet or hood, especially a laminar flow hood, will increase chances for your cultures being free from contaminants. Thoroughly wipe the work area with 0.5% hypochlorite or other disinfectant before starting and after completing your work. Plan your work so as to have all needed materials at hand within the hood before starting.

1. Obtain one 75 cm² bottle containing approximately 2 x 10⁷ HeLa cells. Grossly examine the culture to learn the condition of the cells. Does the phenol red indicate cell growth and metabolism shown by an orange to yellow color? Or is the medium alkaline suggesting cell death and deterioration? Furthermore, are the cells attached to the bottom surface and the medium clear? This is also an indication of cell viability; turbidity suggests microbial contamination.

2. Microscopically examine cell culture with the low power objective. Note the cell arrangement and morphology. Monolayer cultures form either fibroblastic (spindle-like) or epithelioid (polygonal) shapes. Which form are HeLa cells? Are they in a relatively continuous sheet? Sketch.

3. If the cells are viable and appear healthy, remove the culture medium with a 10 ml plugged pipette and place into a disposal container. Rinse with 10 ml Dulbecco's phosphate buffered saline *without* Mg^{++} and Ca^{++} (PBS). Do so by running the wash solution down the side of the flask, gently covering surface of the cells. (Note: You should not add any solution directly to surface of monolayer.) Rock flask back and forth, then aspirate to remove wash solution. Replace with sufficient trypsin-ethylenediametetraacetic acid (EDTA) solution warmed to 37°C to cover completely the cells (about 3 ml), and allow to remain in contact for 1 to 5 minutes, when it should be removed by aspiration. Continue to incubate the cells at 37°C until the cell sheet becomes detached from the glass. Because it is important not to overexpose cells to enzyme treatment, observe the cultures closely. When cells begin to detach as seen by tilting the container, (probably within 15 minutes of addition of enzyme-EDTA solution) jar the latter with your hand to free the remainder of the sheet.

4. Add 10 ml Eagle's MEM with 5% fetal bovine serum (complete growth medium) to the cells.

5. *Gently* aspirate the cell suspension with a sterile 10 ml pipette to obtain a single cell suspension.

6. Swirl the container to mix the cells, then, with the same 10 ml pipette, transfer 1.2 ml to each of four 60mm culture dishes provided. (Approximately how many HeLa cells are being added to each dish?) Add sufficient complete growth medium to give a total volume of 4 ml/dish.

7. Place all newly prepared cultures at 37°C in a CO_2 incubator. It is important that a 5% CO_2 concentration is maintained during incubation to keep the pH of the medium in the correct range.

8. After 24 hours observe your cultures to assess their progress, and whether contamination has occurred. Discard any that show signs of microbial growth.

9. After 48 hours of incubation, again observe your cultures. Determine whether cells have formed a confluent monolayer sheet; if so, they may be used for *Part 2*. If not, continue to incubate cells until this is obtained. If the pH of the growth medium drops to 6.8, the cells should be refed by replacing 2 ml of spent medium with prewarmed complete growth medium.

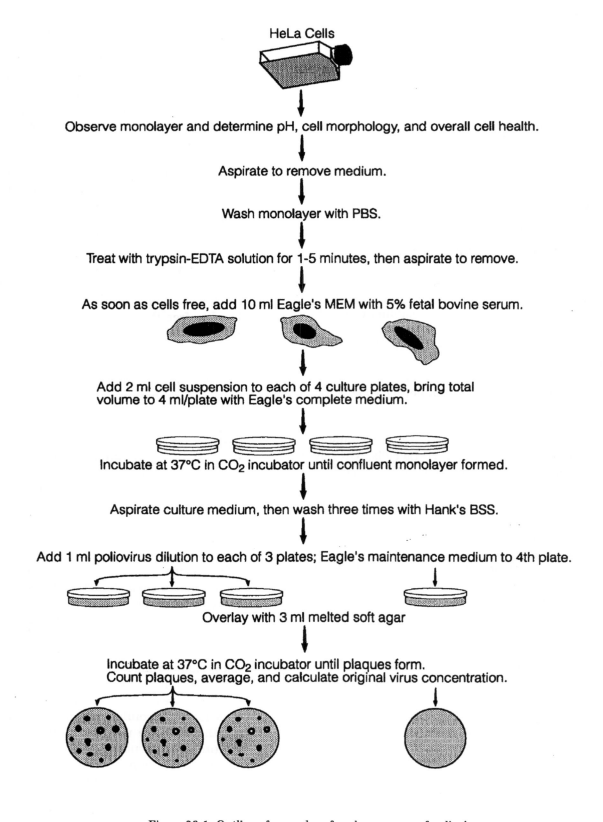

HeLa Cells

Observe monolayer and determine pH, cell morphology, and overall cell health.

Aspirate to remove medium.

Wash monolayer with PBS.

Treat with trypsin-EDTA solution for 1-5 minutes, then aspirate to remove.

As soon as cells free, add 10 ml Eagle's MEM with 5% fetal bovine serum.

Add 2 ml cell suspension to each of 4 culture plates, bring total
volume to 4 ml/plate with Eagle's complete medium.

Incubate at 37°C in CO_2 incubator until confluent monolayer formed.

Aspirate culture medium, then wash three times with Hank's BSS.

Add 1 ml poliovirus dilution to each of 3 plates; Eagle's maintenance medium to 4th plate.

Overlay with 3 ml melted soft agar

Incubate at 37°C in CO_2 incubator until plaques form.
Count plaques, average, and calculate original virus concentration.

Figure 28-1: Outline of procedure for plaque assay of poliovirus.

Part 2: **Poliomyelitis Virus Infection and the Plaque Assay (1, 6, 7)**

For each pair of students:

1. Obtain one tube containing a dilution of poliomyelitis virus, type 2, as follows:

Group	Dilution
1, 2	10^{-3}
3, 4	10^{-4}
5, 6	10^{-5}
7, 8	10^{-6}
9, 10	10^{-7}

2. Retrieve your four cell cultures containing confluent cell growth set up in *Part 1*. Remove the medium by aspiration and wash the cell monolayers 3 times with Hank's BSS (containing Ca^{++} and Mg^{++}). Do this by adding 2 ml along the side of each dish, gently swirl, then aspirate to remove. Repeat 2 more times.

3. Add one milliliter of virus suspension (prepared in Eagle's MEM with 2% fetal bovine serum, a maintenance medium) to each of your three cell cultures and 1 ml of maintenance medium to the fourth, which now serves as an uninoculated control. Incubate at 37°C for one hour in the CO_2 incubator, agitating every 15 minutes through this period to distribute evenly unabsorbed virus.

4. To each dish now add 3 ml of melted soft agar overlay medium using a pre-warmed 5 ml pipette. Allow the agar to flow over the monolayer from the side of the dish, then spread it across the monolayer of cells and allow to solidify. Do this quickly so that a smooth overlay is obtained.

5. Continue incubation of cultures at 37°C. Examine daily for plaque formation, foci of dead of dying cells seen as vacant spots in the monolayer of cells.

6. Count the number of plaques on each plate when they become readily visible and average these. Make your data available to other students. Find the number of plaque-forming poliovirus particles in the original undiluted suspension based upon the class data. Discuss.

QUESTIONS

1. Describe two other types of cell culture lines than HeLa. Indicate their source and whether they are: (i) primary or continuous cell lines; (ii) fibroblasts or epithelioid; and (iii) diploid or heteroploid.

2. What is the purpose of EDTA used with trypsin for the freeing of cell monolayers from solid surfaces? Of the agar overlay following virus attachment to HeLa cells?

3. The plaque assay outlined in this exercise detects the presence of poliomyelitis virus. How can this same assay now be used to identify it and its serotype?

4. The plaque assay is one method of detecting the presence and enumeration of viruses. Give at least 2 other methods as to how this information may be obtained using cell cultures.

REFERENCES

1. Aarnaes, S., and B. J. Daidone. 1992. Observation and maintenance of inoculated cell cultures, p. 8.7.1-8.7.16. *In* H. D. Isenberg (ed.), Clinical microbiology procedures handbook, Vol. 2: L. M. Clarke (Sect. ed.), Viruses, rickettsiae, chlamydiae, and mycoplasmas. American Society for Microbiology, Washington, DC.

2. Centers for Disease Control. 1992. Update: Poliomyelitis outbreak - Netherlands, 1992. MMWR **41**:917-919.

3. Davis, B. D., R. Dulbecco, H. N. Eisen, and H. S. Ginsberg. 1990. Microbiology, 4th ed. J. B. Lippincott Co., Philadelphia. p. 961-984.

4. Hodinka, R. L. 1992. Cell culture techniques: preparation of cell culture medium and reagents. p. 8.19.1-8.19-15. *In* H. D. Isenberg (ed.), Clinical microbiology procedures handbook, Vol. 2: L. M. Clarke (Sect. ed.), Viruses, rickettsiae, chlamydiae, and mycoplasmas. American Society for Microbiology, Washington, DC.

5. Hodinka, R. L. 1992. Cell culture techniques: Serial propagation and maintenance of monloyer cell cultures. p. 8.20.1-8.20-14. *In* H. D. Isenberg (ed.), Clinical microbiology procedures handbook, Vol. 2: L. M. Clarke (Sect. ed.), Viruses, rickettsiae, chlamydiae, and mycoplasmas. American Society for Microbiology, Washington, DC.

6. Landry, M. L., and G. D. Hsiung. 1986. Primary isolation of viruses, p. 31-51. *In* S. Specter, and G. J. Lancz, Clinical virology manual. Elsevier Science Publishing Co., Inc., New York.

7. Lipson, S. M. 1992. Neutralization test for the identification and typing of viral isolates, p. 8.14.1-8.14.8. *In* H. D. Isenberg (ed.), Clinical microbiology procedures handbook, Vol. 2: L. M. Clarke (Sect. ed.), Viruses, rickettsiae, chlamydiae, and mycoplasmas. American Society for Microbiology, Washington, DC.

8. Menegus, M. A. 1991. Enteroviruses, p. 943-949. *In* A. Balows, W. J. Hausler, Jr., K. L. Herrmann, H. D. Isenberg, and H. J. Shadomy (ed.), Manual of clinical microbiology, 5th ed. American Society for Microbiology, Washington, D. C.

9.   Modlin, J. F. 1990. Picornaviridae. Introduction, p. 1352-1359. *In* G. L. Mandell, R. G. Douglas, Jr., and J. E. Bennett (ed.), Principles and practices of infectious diseases, 3rd ed. Churchill Livingstone, New York.

10. Modlin, J. F. 1990. Poliovirus, p. 1359-1367. *In* G. L. Mandell, R. G. Douglas, Jr., and J. E. Bennett (ed.), Principles and practices of infectious diseases, 3rd ed. Churchill Livingstone, New York.

11. White, D. O., and F. Fenner. 1986. Medical virology, 3rd ed. Academic Press, Inc., Orland, FA., p. 35-51.

12. Wiedbrauk, D. L., and S. L. G. Johnston. 1993. Manual of clinical virology. Raven Press, Ltd., New York, p. 11-17, 33-44, 92-97.

13. Zeichhardt, H. 1986. Enteroviruses, p. 283-299. *In* S. Specter, and G. J. Lancz, Clinical virology manual. Elsevier Science Publishing Co., Inc., New York.

Exercise 28: Poliomyelitis Virus and the Plague Assay Results

Part 1-1: **Macroscopic and Microscopic Observation of HeLa Cells.**

General description of stock HeLa cell culture:

Culture age: _____

Color of phenol red and approximate pH: _____

Clarity of medium: _____

Cells attached to surface of container: _____

Other observations:

Macroscopic:

Microscopic:

Sketch of microscopic morphology:

Part 2: **Plaque Assay.**

Date: _____

Your Data:

Incubation period (hrs) for virus: _____

Poliovirus Dilution: _____

Plaque Count:

Dish 1: _____ Dish 2: _____ Dish 3: _____

Average for Dishes 1, 2, and 3: _____

Control: _____

Class Data:

Group No.	Virus Dilution Inoculated	No. Plaques (Average)	No. Plaques/ml Undiluted

Other Laboratory Notes

SECTION IV
APPENDICES

APPENDIX 1
Glossary of Descriptive Terms for Bacterial Colony Form

Surface Colonies (plate cultures)

Form
  punctiform - very small, but visible to naked eye; under 1 mm in diameter.
  circular.
  irregular.
  filamentous - growth composed of long, irregularly placed or interwoven threads.
  rhizoid - growth of an irregular branched or root-like character, as *B. mycoides.*

Elevation
  effuse - growth thin, veily, unusually spreading.
  flat.
  raised - growth thick, with abrupt or terraced edges.
  convex - surface of the segment of a circle. but flattened.
  pulvinate - in the form of a cushion, decidedly convex.

Surface
  smooth.
  rough.
  concentrically ringed - marked with rings, one inside the other.
  contoured - an irregular, smoothly undulating surface, like that of a relief map.
  radiately ridged - ridges radiating from the center, i. e., like spokes in a cartwheel.
  rugose - wrinkled.

Edge
  entire - smooth, having a margin destitute of teeth or notches.
  undulate - border wavy, with shallow sinuses.
  lobate - border deeply undulate, producing lobes (see undulate).
  erose - border irregularly toothed.
  filamentous - see definition above.
  curled - composed of parallel chains in wavy strands, as in anthrax colonies.

Optical Characters
  opaque - not allowing light to pass through.
  translucent - allowing light to pass through without allowing complete visibility of objects seen through the substance in question.
  opalescent - resembling the color of an opal.
  iridescent - exhibiting changing rainbow colors in reflected light.
  dull - not glossy or glistening.
  glistening - glossy, not dull.
  photogenic - glowing in the dark, phosphorescent.
  fluorescent - having one color by transmitted light and another by reflected light.

Consistency
   butyrous - growth of butterlike consistency.
   viscid - growth follows the needle when touched and withdrawn.
   membranous - growth thin, coherent, like a membrane.
   brittle - growth dry, friable under the platinum needle.

Streak (agar slant)

Form
   filiform - in stroke or stab cultures, a uniform growth along the line of inoculation.
   echinulate - a growth along line of inoculation with toothed or pointed margins.
   beaded (in stab or stroke culture) - separate or semi-confluent colonies along the line of inoculation.
   spreading - growth extending much beyond the line of inoculation, i.e., several millimeters or more.
   arborescent - branched treelike growth.
   rhizoid - see definition above.

Stab (gelatin)

Form
Non-liquifaction
   filiform - see definition above.
   beaded - see definition above.
   papillate - growth beset with small nipple-like processes.
   villous - having short, thick, hair-like processes on the surface, intermediate in meaning between papillate and filamentous.
   arborescent - see definition above.
Liquifaction
   crateriform - a saucer-shaped liquifaction of the medium.
   infundibuliform - in the form of a funnel or inverted cone.
   napiform - liquifaction in the form of a turnip.
   saccate - liquifaction in the form of an elongated sac, tubular, cylindrical.
   stratiform - liquifying to the walls of the tube at the top and then proceeding downward horizontally.

Liquid Cultures (nutrient broth)

Surface Growth
   ring - growth at the upper margin of a liquid culture, adhering to the glass.
   pellicle - bacterial growth forming either a continuous or an interrupted sheet over the culture fluid.
   flocculent - containing small adherent masses of bacteria of various shapes floating in the culture fluid.
   membranous - see definition above.

Sediment
   compact - refers to sediment in the form of a single, fairly tenacious mass.
   flocculent - see definition above.
   granular - composed of small granules.
   flaky - refers to sediment in the form of numerous separate flakes.
   viscid - sediment on shaking rises as a coherent swirl.

Surface colonies

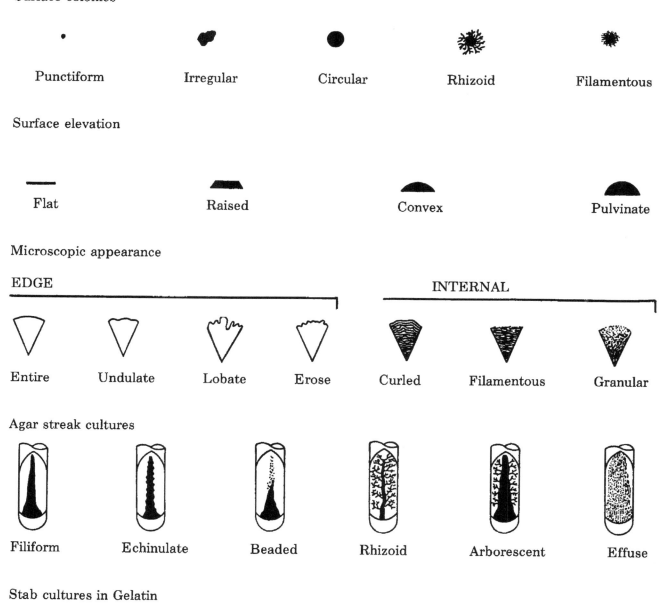

Surface elevation

Microscopic appearance

EDGE   INTERNAL

Agar streak cultures

Stab cultures in Gelatin

NON-LIQUIFYING   LIQUIFYING

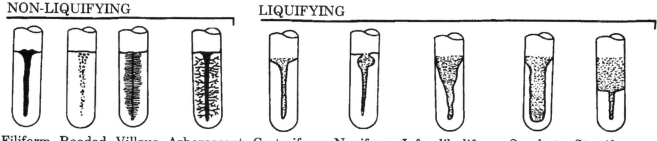

Illustrations of Some of the Terms Used in Describing Forms of Bacterial Growth. (From: G. L. Peltier, C. E. Georgi, and L. F. Lindgren. Laboratory Manual for General Bacteriology, 4th ed. Copyright© 1952 by authors. Reprinted by permission of John Wiley and Sons, Inc., and the American Society for Microbiology.)

APPENDIX 2
Stains

1. Auramine-Rhodamine Fluorochrome Stain for Mycobacteria (3):

Staining Solution:

Auramine O .... 1.5 g
Rhodamine B .... 0.75 g
Phenol .... 10 ml
Glycerol .... 75 ml
Distilled water .... 50 ml

Warm, then vigorously mix for five minutes. Pass through glass wool to filter, then store in a glass-stoppered bottle. Solution is stable for several months at refrigeration temperatures.

Decolorizing solution:

HCl, concentrated .... 0.5 ml
Ethanol, 70% .... 99.5 ml

Non-fluorescing counterstain:

Potassium permanganate .... 0.5 g
Distilled water .... 99.5 ml

Dissolve, then filter. Store in dark bottle.

See Exercise 21, *Part 1*-2 for staining procedure.

2. Calcofluor White Staining Reagents (5):

Formulations:

Calcofluor White Solution, 0.1%:

Fluorescent brightener .... 1 g
(Sigma Chemical Co., St. Louis)
Distilled water .... 100 ml

Filter if preciptate forms, and store at room temperature in dark.

Glycerinated KOH solution:

Glycerol .... 20 g
KOH .... 15 g
Distilled water .... 80 ml

Store at room temperature. Discard when precipitate is seen.

See Exercise 23, *Part* 2B-12 for calcofluor white staining procedure of fungi.

3. Flagella stain using Rhu staining solution (4):

Solution 1:

Carbolic acid, 5% solution .... 10 ml
Tannic acid, powdered .... 2 g
Aluminum potassium sulfate.12 H_2O,
    saturated solution .... 10 ml

Solution 2:

Crystal violet in ethanol, saturated
    solution .... 12 g/100 ml

Final stain:

Solution 1 .... 10 parts
Solution 2 .... 1 part

The final stain can be stored indefinitely at room temperature in a plastic wash bottle. See Exercise 10, *Part 2*A-6 ,page 000 for procedure.

4. Giemsa Stain (Exercise 7) (2):

Solution 1: Giemsa stain.

Giemsa stain, powdered, certified.... 0.75 g
Methanol, absolute .... 65 ml
Glycerol .... 35 ml

Dissolve stain in methanol, then mix with glycerol in container with glass beads. Filter if needed.

Solution 2: Phosphate buffer, pH 6.4.

KH_2PO_4 .... 6.63 g
Na_2HPO_4 .... 2.56 g
Distilled water .... 1000 ml

Working solution:

Solution 1 .... 1 part
Solution 2 .... 50 parts

Procedure:

1. Fix smear in absolute methanol, then allow to dry.
2. Stain for 30 to 60 minutes by flooding smear with Giemsa working solution.
3. Wash away stain with phosphate buffer.
4. Dry slide and examine.

5. Gram's stain for bacterial smears (3):

Formulation:

a. Modified Hucker's crystal violet

Solution A:

Crystal violet (certified) .... 2 g
Ethanol, 95% .... 20 ml

Solution B:

Ammonium oxalate .... 0.8 g
Distilled water .... 80.0 ml

Mix solution A and B and allow to stand at least 24 hours then filter before use.

b. Gram's iodine

Potassium iodide .... 2 g
Iodine .... 1 g
Distilled water .... 300 ml

Dissolve potassium iodide and iodine by grinding into a powder, then adding aliquots of water. Grinding is continued until chemicals are dissolved. Final solution is stored in an amber glass bottle.

c. Counterstain

Stock solution:

    Safranine O (certified) .... 2.5 g

    Ethanol, 95% .... 100 ml

Working solution:

    Stock solution Safranine O .... 10 ml

    Distilled water .... 90 ml

Procedure:

a. Gently heat-fix a dried smear of bacteria.

b. Flood smear with solution of crystal violet for one minute.

c. Briefly wash off crystal violet with *gentle* stream of tap water, then drain off excess.

d. Apply Gram's iodine for one minute and repeat washing procedure.

e. Decolorize with acetone. (This reagent quickly removes crystal violet, therefore use care not to overdecolorize.) Briefly wash in tap water as in Step c.

f. Counterstain with safranine for 10 seconds, then wash in tap water, blot dry, and observe. Observation: Gram-positive organisms will appear blue, Gram-negative red.

6. Kinyoun acid-fast stain for actinomycetes (3):

Formulation:

Kinyoun's carbol fuchsin solution:

    Basic fuchsin .... 4 g

    Ethanol, 95% .... 20 ml

    Phenol crystals .... 8 g

    Distilled water .... 100 ml

Acid alcohol:

    HCl, concentrated .... 3 ml

    Ethanol, 95% .... 97 ml

Methylene blue counterstain solution:

    Methylene blue .... 2.5 g

    Ethanol, 95% .... .100 ml

See Exercise 22, *Part 1*A-1 (p. 000) for procedure and interpretation of results for this stain.

7. Lactophenol cotton blue mounting medium (3):

Formulation:

    Phenol crystals .... 20 g

    Glycerol .... 40 ml

    Lactic acid .... 20 ml

    Distilled water .... 20 ml

Ingredients are dissolved by heating over a steam bath, after which 0.05 g cotton blue dye

(Poittier's blue) is added. See Exercise 23, *Part 2*A-2b, 2c (p. 343) for procedure and purpose of this mounting medium.

8. Loeffler's Methylene blue stain (1, 3):

Formulation:

    Methylene blue .... 0.3 g

    Ethanol, 95% .... 30 ml

After methylene blue is dissolved, add 100 ml distilled water. Method and interpretation for this stain is given in Exercise 20, *Part 1*A-1.

9. Wirtz-Conklin spore stain (1, 3):

Formulations:

Malachite green:

    Malachite green .... 5 g

    Distilled water .... 100 ml

Safranine counterstain (See Gram's stain formulation)

Procedure for use of this stain is given in Exercise 17, *Part 1*A-1 (p. 260).

10. Ziehl Neelsen acid-fast stain (3):

Formulation:

Carbol fuchsin stain:

    Basic fuchsin .... 0.3 g

    Ethanol, 95% .... 10 ml

Dissolve stain, then mix with solution of:

    Phenol, melted crystals .... 5 ml

    Distilled water .... 95 ml

Allow to stand for a few days before using.

Acid-alcohol solution:

    HCl, concentrated .... 3 ml

    Ethanol, 95% .... 97 ml

Methylene blue stain:

    Methylene blue .... 0.3 g

    Distilled water .... 100 ml

Procedure for this stain given in Exercise 21, *Part 1*-2 (p. 000).

REFERENCES

1. Baron, E. J., and S. M. Finegold. 1990. *Bailey & Scott's diagnostic microbiology*, 8th ed. The C. V. Mosby Co., St. Louis. p. A-35 - A-49.

2. Bell, R. H. 1987. Media, reagents and stains, p. 773-835. *In* B. B. Wentworth (ed.), *Diagnostic procedures for bacterial infections*, 7th ed. American Public Health Association, Inc., Washington, D. C.

3. Hendrickson, D. A., and M. M. Krenz. 1991. Reagents and stains, p. 1289-1314. *In* A. Balows, W. J. Hausler, Jr., K. L. Herrmann, H. D. Isenberg, and H. J. Shadomy (ed.), *Manual of clinical microbiology*, 5th ed. American Society for Microbiology, Washington, D. C.

4. Kodaka, H., A. Y. Armfield, G. L. Lombard, and V. R. Dowell, Jr. 1982. Practical procedure for demonstrating bacterial flagella. *J. Clin. Microbiol.* 16:948-952.

5. Pasarell, L., and W. A. Schell. 1992. Potassium hydroxide-calcofluor white procedure, p. 6.4.1-6.4.2. *In* H. D. Isenberg (ed.), Clinical microbiology procedures handbook, Vol. 1: M. R. McGinnis (sect. ed.), Mycology. American Society for Microbiology, Washington, DC.

APPENDIX 3
Reagent Formulation

1. Barium sulfate standard for antimicrobial sensitivity assay (2):

(Exercise 2, Section 3, *Part 1*B-2, p. 42):

BaCl$_2$ solution .... 0.048M (1.75% w/v BaCl$_2$.2H$_2$O)

H$_2$SO$_4$ .... 0.36N (1% v/v)

Mix 0.5 ml of BaCl$_2$ solution with 99.5 ml H$_2$SO$_4$ solution to give BaSO$_4$ precipitate equivalent to a McFarland 0.5 standard (see McFarland Turbidity Standards).

Notes: Dispense and tightly seal turbidity standard in tubes of equal size to that used to prepare bacterial cultures. It should be stored at room temperature in the dark. Shake vigorously (as with Vortex mixer) before use.

2. Bile reagent:

2% Solution:

Sodium desoxycholate .... 0.2 g

Distilled water .... 9.8 ml

For use, see Ex. 2, Section 1, *Part 3*A-3, page 33.

10% Solution (5):

Sodium desoxycholate .... 1 g

Distilled water .... 9 ml

3. Catalase reagent:

Hydrogen peroxide, 3% (Store in the refrigerator.) For use, see Ex. 1, *Part 2*A-7, page 11.

4. Catalase reagent with Tween 80 (for mycobacteria) (11):

a. Hydrogen peroxide, 30% (Store in refrigerator.)

b. Tween 80 solution.

Tween 80 .... 10 ml

Distilled water .... 90 ml

Autoclave at 121° for 10 minutes, then store in the refrigerator. Mix just before using.

For use mix equal parts of H$_2$O$_2$ and Tween 80 solutions. Note: Use as described in Ex. 21, *Part 2*B-6, **page 314.**

5. δ-aminolevulinic acid HCl solution (6):

δ-aminolevulinic acid HCl solution ... 2 mM

MgSO$_4$ .... 0.8 mM

Dissolve reagents in pH 6.9 phosphate buffer, 0.1M, dispense into tubes in 0.5 ml volumes, and store in refrigerator. Use and interpretation of results using this reagent are given in Exercise 5, *Part 1*A-3 and *Part 2*-5.

6. Digestant for mycobacteria-containing sputum samples (10):

Solution 1:

Trisodium citrate.3 H$_2$O (0.1M) ...... 2.94 g

Distilled water .... 100 ml

Solution 2:

Sodium hydroxide .... 4 ml

Distilled water .... 96 ml

To use, mix 50 ml of Solution 1 with an equal volume of Solution 2, and add 0.5 g powdered N-acetyl-L-cysteine. Discard solution after 48 hours.

Use as described in Ex. 21, *Part 2*A, **page 313.**

7. Hippurate test for *Legionella* (4):

Hippurate solution:

Sodium hippurate .... 1 g

Distilled water .... 100 ml

Dispense in 0.4 ml amounts into 13 x 100 mm screw-capped tubes. Store frozen at -20°C. Thaw as needed.

See Exercise 13, *Part 1*-4, p. 205 for use.

8. Sodium hippurate hydrolysis test reagent (5):

Acetone .... 50 ml

Butanol .... 50 ml

Ninhydrin .... 3.5 g

Mix acetone and butanol, then dissolve ninhydrin in mixed solution. Store in dark at room temperature.

Note: See Ex. 13, *Part 2*-5, page 207 for use and interpretation.

9. Indole spot test for anaerobic bacteria (7):

Reagent formulation:

p-dimethylaminocinnameldahyde .... 1 g

10% aqueous HCl .... 99 ml

Store at 4°C in brown bottle. See Exercise 16, *Part 2*A-4, p. 246.

10. Indoxyl acetate test disks (8, 9):

Prepare following solution:

Indoxyl acetate (Sigma Chemical Co, St. Louis, MO) .... 1 g

Acetone .... 10 ml

Place 25 μl of solution onto 0.25-inch diameter filter paper disks (Difco Laboratories, Detroit, MI). Allow to air-dry, then store in amber bottle containing drying agent at 4°C. (See Exercise 11, *Part 2*B-2, p. 189)

11. Kovacs' reagent for indole test (5):

p-dimethylaminobenzaldehyde .... 10 g
Pure amyl or isoamyl alcohol .... 150 ml
HCl, concentrated .... 50 ml
Aldehyde is first dissolved in the alcohol, then HCl is slowly added. Prepare in small quantities.
Note: Store in refrigerator. See Ex 5, *Part 2*-5 (p. 100) and Ex. 8, *Part 2*A-2, page 134 for applications and interpretations of the use of this reagent.

12. Lead acetate strips:

Soak filter paper in 10% neutral solution of lead acetate, remove, and allow to dry, Cut into strips about 1 X 6 cm. For use, hang into top of tube of appropriate medium. (See Exercise 6, *Part 1*A-2, p. 108):

13. Mcfarland Turbidity Standards (5):

H_2SO_4, concentrated ...... 1.0 ml in 99 ml distilled H_2O (1% solution)
$BaCl_2$ ... 0.1 g dissolved in 10 ml water (1% solution)
To prepare a set of 10 standards, select desired size test tubes, and label from "1" to "10." Make additions as shown below.

McFarland No. (and Tube No.)	1% H_2SO_4	1% $BaCl_2$	Bacterial Equivalency, $\times 10^8$/ml
	Additions of:		
1	9.9	0.1	3
2	9.8	0.2	6
3	9.7	0.3	9
4	9.6	0.4	12
5	9.5	0.5	15
6	9.4	0.6	18
7	9.3	0.7	21
8	9.2	0.8	24
9	9.1	0.9	27
10	9.0	1.0	30

Store sealed tubes in refrigerator. Mix vigorously before use. Turbidity in each tube approximates a bacterial concentration shown in the right column. (See Exercise 2, Section 3, *Part 1*B-2, p. 42)

14. Methyl red reagent (5):

Methyl red .... 0.1 g
Ethanol, 95% .... 300 ml
Distilled water .... 200 ml
Dissolve dye in ethanol, then add water.
Note: Use and interpretation of methyl red test given in Ex. 9, *Part 2*A-2d, page 146.

15. Ninhydrin reagent for *Legionella* hippurate test (5):

Ninhydrin .... 3.5 g
Acetone-butanol (1:1 mixture) ...... 100 ml
Dissolve ninhydrin and store at room temperature in the dark.
(See Exercise 13, *Part 2*-5, p. 207.)

16. Nitrate test reagent (5):

Reagent I:
Sulfanilic acid .... 8 g
Acetic acid, 5 N .... 1000 ml
Reagent II:
N,N-dimethyl-l-naphthylamine .... 6 ml
Acetic acid, 5 N .... 1000 ml
Note: See Exercise 1, *Part 2*A-5, page 11 for use and interpretation of nitrate reduction test.

17. Nitrate test reagent for mycobacteria (11):

A. Test reagents.
Substrate solution:
$NaNO_3$ .... 0.085 g
KH_2PO_4 .... 0.117 g
$Na_2HPO_4.12H_2O$ .... 0.485 g
Distilled water .... 100 ml
Adjust pH to 7.0.
MNRR-A:
HCl, concentrated .... 10 ml
Distilled water .... 10 ml
MNRR-B:
Sulfanilamide .... 0.2 g
Distilled water .... 100 ml
MNRR-C
n-napthylethylenediamine
dihydrochloride .... 0.1 g
Distilled water .... 100 ml
Note: Store reagents in the dark brown bottle in a refrigerator. Discard any solution if precipitate occurs, or MNRR-B and -C when color changes. See Ex 21, *Part 1*-7, page 312 for use and interpretation of results obtained from use of this reagent.
B. Preparation of Standards:
   1. Stock Solutions:

Na$_2$HPO$_4$ M/15
KH$_2$PO$_4$ M/15
Na$_3$PO$_4$ M/15
Phenolphthalein (1%) ... 1 g in 100 ml 95% ethanol
Bromthymol Blue (BTB, 1%) ... 1 g in 100 ml 95% ethanol
From 1% BTB, dilute 1 ml in 100 ml distilled water (0.01%)

2. Buffer solution:
Prepare buffer solution by mixing 35 ml M/15 Na$_2$HPO$_4$, 5 ml M/15 KH$_2$PO$_4$, and 100 ml Na$_3$PO$_4$.

3. Standards:
   a. Set up 8 tubes of the size to be used in the actual test.
   b. To Tubes 2-8, add 2 ml buffer solution.
   c. Prepare color solutions by mixing 10 ml buffer solution, 0.1 ml 1% phenolphthalein, and 0.2 ml 0.01% BTB. Mix and place 2 ml into tube 1, and 2 ml into Tube 2. Mix contents of Tube 2, then transfer 2 ml to Tube 3. Continue serial transfer of 2 ml from Tube 3 through Tube 8. Finally, discard 2 ml from Tube 8.
   d. Store capped tubes in refrigerator after autoclaving.
   e. The color equivalencies of the standards are as follows:

| Tube | Color | |
	Intensity	Shade
1	+5	Purple-red
2	+4	
3	+3	
5	+2	
6	+1	
8	±	Pink

18. Nitrate Reductase Disk Test for Anaerobes (13):

Prepare the following solution:
KNO$_3$ .... 3 g
Na$_2$MoO$_4$.2H$_2$O .... 10 mg
Water .... 10 ml
Completely dissolve ingredients, then filter sterilize. Autoclave filter paper disks (¼ inch diameter) in a glass petri dish. Aseptically apply 20 μl of sterile solution to each disk. Replace dish cover and allow disks to dry. (See Exercise 16, *Part 1*C, *Part 2*A-5, p. 246.)

Nitrate Reductase Disk Test Reagents:
Solution A:
   Sulfanilic acid .... 0.5 g
   Glacial acetic acid .... 30 ml
   Water .... 120 ml
Solution B:
   5-amino-2-naphthaline sulfonic acid ... 0.2 g
   Glacial acetic acid .... 30 ml
   Water .... 120 ml

19. Oxidase reagent (3):
Prepare the following solution:
   Tetramethyl-*p*-phenylenediamine
   dihydrochloride .... 0.5 g
   Distilled water .... 100 ml
Prepare solution at least 15 minutes before use, but discard after two hours. See Exercise 3 *Part 1*A-5, page 68, and Exercise 12, *Part 1*B-3 (p. 197) for procedure.

20. Phenyl pyruvic acid reagent (1):
   Ferric chloride .... 10 g
   Distilled water .... 100 ml
Note: Use described in Ex. 9, *Part 2*A-2g, page 147.

21. Pyrazinamidase test reagent (11):
Test reagent:
   Ferrous ammonium sulfate .... 1 g
   Distilled water .... 100 ml
Reagent is prepared fresh before use. (See Exercise 21, *Part 2*B-4, p. 313, and Appendix 4 for pyrazinamide test agar.)

22. 0.5% Sodium desoxycholate solution (Exercise 10, *Part 1*-5, p. 178):
   Sodium desoxycholate .... 0.25 g
   Distilled water .... 50 ml

23. Superoxol (30% H$_2$O$_2$):
   Hydrogen peroxide .... 15 ml
   Distilled water .... 35 ml
(See Exercise 3, *Part 1*A-6, p. 68.)

24. Vaspar
Melted paraffin (mp. 45°C) and white petrolatum mixed in equal parts. Autoclave at 121°C for 15 minutes to sterilize.

25. Voges-Proskauer reagent of Barritt (5):
Solution 1.
   Alpha naphthol .... 5 g
   Ethanol, absolute .... 100 ml

Solution 2.

    KOH .... 40 g

    Distilled water .... 100 ml

Note: See Ex. 9, *Part* 2A-2d, page **146**, for procedure and test interpretation.

REFERENCES

1. Baron, E. J., and S. M. Finegold. 1990. Bailey & Scott's diagnostic microbiology, 8th ed. The C. V. Mosby Co., St. Louis. p. A-1 - A-34.

2. Barry, A. L., and C. Thornsberry. 1992. Susceptibility testing: diffusion test procedures, p. 1117-1125. *In* A. Balows, W. J. Hausler, Jr., K. L. Herrmann, H. D. Isenberg, and H. J. Shadomy (ed.), Manual of clinical microbiology, 5th ed. American Society for Microbiology, Washington, D. C.

3. Bell, R. H. 1987. Media, reagents and stains, p. 773-835. *In* B. B. Wentworth (ed.), Diagnostic procedures for bacterial infections, 7th ed. American Public Health Association, Inc., Washington, D. C.

4. Hébert, G. A. 1991. Hippurate hydrolysis by *Legionella pneumophilia.* J. Clin. Microbiol. **13**:240-242.

5. Hendrickson, D. A., and M. M. Krenz. 1991. Reagents and stains, p. 1289-1314. *In* A. Balows, W. J. Hausler, Jr., K. L. Herrmann, H. D. Isenberg, and H. J. Shadomy (ed.), Manual of clinical microbiology, 5th ed. American Society for Microbiology, Washington, D. C.

6. Kilian, M. 1991. *Haemophilus,* p. 463-470. *In* A. Balows, W. J. Hausler, Jr., K. L. Herrmann, H. D. Isenberg, and H. J. Shadomy (ed.), Manual of clinical microbiology, 5th ed. American Society for Microbiology, Washington, D. C.

7. Lombard, G. L., and V. R. Dowell, Jr. 1983. Comparison of three reagents for detecting indole production by anaerobic bacteria in microtest systems. J. Clin. Microbiol. **18**:609-613.

8. Mills, C. K., and R. L. Gherna. 1987. Hydrolysis of indoxyl acetate by *Campylobacter* species. J. Clin. Microbiol. **25**:1560-1561.

9. On, S. L. W., and B. Holmes. 1992. Assessment of enzyme detection tests useful in identification of campylobacter. J. Clin. Microbiol. **30**:746-747.

10. Roberts, G. D., E. W. Koneman, and Y. K. Kim. 1991. *Mycobacterium,* p. 304-339. *In* A. Balows, W. J. Hausler, Jr., K. L. Herrmann, H. D. Isenberg, and H. J. Shadomy (ed.), Manual of clinical microbiology, 5th ed. American Society for Microbiology, Washington, D. C.

11. Vestal, A. L. 1975. Procedures for the isolation and identification of mycobacteria. HEW Pub. No. (CDC) 77-8230. U. S. Dept. of Health, Education, and Welfare, Atlanta, GA., 136 p.

12. Wayne, L. G. 1974. Simple pyrazinamidase and urea tests for routine identification of mycobacteria. Am. Rev. Respir. Dis. **109**: 147-151.

13. Wideman, P. A., D. M. Citrobaum, and V. L. Sutter. 1977. Simple disk technique for detection of nitrate reduction by anaerobic bacteria. J. Clin. Microbiol. **5**:315-319.

APPENDIX 4
Culture Media Formulation and Preparation

Only media used in this manual are described in this section. Generally, a single reference source number is given with each formulation, although many are usually available. In most cases, if further information is needed concerning a medium, the reference given will either provide the desired information or it will lead you to a more complete source. While not always given as references in the following media list, manuals from manufacturers are helpful, particularly the *BBL Manual of Products and Laboratory Procedures* (6th edition, 14), the *Difco Manual* (10th edition, 5) and *The Oxoid Manual* (6th edition, 3).

Culture media sources indicated here are not exhaustive, nor are they given as recommended sources; they are provided to assist in the use of this manual. It should be noted that if more than one source is given, media formulation may vary between them. Most media are commercially available in both dehydrated and in ready-to use plate and tube forms. Sources of the former are indicated below and keyed by a capital letter to a manufacturer listed at the end of this section. Vendors of ready-to-use media (especially if preparation of the medium is particularly complex) are found in the text of the Manual, commonly in the materials list of the appropriate exercise. Address of all companies can be found in Appendix 6.

Unless otherwise indicated, all media listed below are sterilized by autoclaving at 121°C for 15 minutes. Prepared media should be stored in at refrigeration temperatures until used, unless otherwise specified.

1. Ascospore medium (Exercise 24) (12)

Potassium acetate .... 10 g
Yeast extract .... 2.5 g
Dextrose .... 1 g
Agar .... 30 g

Dissolve in 1000 ml distilled water, dispense into tubes, and autoclave to sterilize.

2. Bacteroides Bile Esculin Agar (BBE, Exercise 16) (13)

Trypticase soy agar (B) .... 40.0 g
Oxgall .... 20.0 g
Esculin .... 1.0 g
Ferric ammonium citrate .... 0.5 g
Gentamicin solution (40 mg/ml) ..... 2.5 ml
Hemin solution (5 mg/ml) .... 2.0 ml
Distilled water .... 1.0 l

Agitate components in water and heat to dissolve. After adjusting pH to 7.0, sterilize at 15 lb/in² (121°C) for 15 minutes. Prepare plates after cooling to 50°C.

3. Basic fuchsin and thionin tryptose agar for brucellae

(Exercise 6): Tryptose agar base (D) (Trypticase soy agar (B) and tryptone soya agar (L) may also be used as the base) (4):

Tryptose .... 20 g
Dextrose .... 1 g
Sodium chloride .... 5 g
Thiamine hydrochloride .... 0.005 g
Agar .... 15 g
Distilled water .... 1000 ml

Thionin and basic fuchsin solutions:

Thionin, certified (F, J) .... 1% solution
Basic fuchsin (D, F) .... 1% solution

Store dye solutions in refrigerator. Heat in a boiling water bath for 20 minutes immediately before use

Final medium:

Autoclave tryptose agar, pH 7.2, cool to 50°C and add thionin to a final concentration of 1:25,000. Mix agar and dye, then pour plates. Allow surface of medium to dry before inoculating. It should be used within 48 hours. Repeat procedure for basic fuchsin, but add to tryptose agar to a final concentration of 1:50,000.

4. Bile esculin agar for enterococci

(Exercise 2) (13) (A, D):

Beef extract .... 3 g
Peptone .... 5 g

Agar .... 15 g
Distilled water .... 400 ml
Heat to dissolve.
Oxgall .... 40 g
Distilled water .... 400 ml
Heat to dissolve.
Ferric citrate .... 0.5 g
Distilled water .... 100 ml

Mix solutions and heat medium to boiling to dissolve ingredients. Autoclave. pH is 6.6 at 25°C. After cooling to 55°C add 1 g esculin in 100 ml distilled water that has been filter-sterilized. Sterile horse serum, if desired, is added to a final concentration of 5%, then the mixed solution dispense into sterile tubes.

5. Bismuth sulfite agar (Introduction to Exercises 8 and 9; Exercise 9) (13) (B, D, L):
Beef extract .... 5 g
Peptone *or* polypeptone peptone ...... 10 g
Disodium phosphate .... 4 g
Ferrous sulfate .... 0.3 g
Dextrose .... 5 g
Bismuth sulfite indicator .... 8 g
Brilliant green .... 0.025 g
Agar .... 20 g
Distilled water .... 1000 ml
Final pH is 7.7

Ingredients are heated to boiling to dissolve. To avoid decreasing selective character of the medium, it should not be boiled longer than necessary (1-2 minutes) and should *not be autoclaved*. Dispense melted medium into plates. Store in a refrigerator.

6. Blood agar Exercise 1 and others (13):
Beef heart infusion agar base (D) consisting of:
Tryptose *or* peptic digest of animal
    tissue .... 10 g
Beef heart infusion .... 500 g
NaCl .... 5 g
Agar .... 15 g
Distilled water .... 1000 ml

Suspend components in distilled water and dissolve. Sterilize by autoclaving. Final pH is 7.4.

Complete medium: Cool medium to 45-50°C, then add preheated (45°C) sterile, defibrinated sheep, rabbit, or other whole blood (B, I) to the desired concentration (usually 5% for bacterial isolation). Mix, but avoid air bubbles. Pour plates. Incubate overnight at 35-37°C to assess sterility.

Brucella agar is also used as a base for blood agar, as seen in Exercise 6, *Part 1* A-3 for growth of *Brucella* and Vitamin K₁ blood agar used for the growth of anaerobic bacteria (Exercises 16 and 17). Furthermore, brain heart infusion and other formulations may be used as base media. (B, D, L)

7. Blood agar supplemented with vitamin K₁ for anaerobic bacteria (See: An Introduction to Exercises 16 and 17, and Exercises 16, 17) (17):
Brucella agar base (A, B, D):
Pancreatic digest of casein .... 10 g
Peptic digest of animal tissue .... 10 g
Yeast autolysate .... 2 g
NaCl .... 5 g
Dextrose .... 1 g
Bismuth sulfite .... 0.1 g
Agar .... 15 g
Distilled water .... 1000 ml

Final pH is 7.0±0.2. Slowly heat medium to dissolve components and autoclave, cool to 50°C, and now add 10 mg Vitamin K₁ in 1 ml, 5 mg hemin in 1 ml, and 50 ml defibrinated sheep blood (B, I; or laked sheep blood lysed by freezing and thawing). Pour plates. (B, D, L)

(Note: Antimicrobial compounds are commonly added with laked blood, but should not be used in K₁BA for these exercises. If used, add 75 mg kanamycin in 0.75 ml, and 7.5 mg vancomycin in 1 ml antimicrobial supplements.)

8. Bordet-Gengou agar (Exercise 5) (1) (B, D, L)
Potato infusion .... 125 g
NaCl .... 5.5 g
Agar .... 20 g

Suspend mixture in 1000 ml of a 1% glycerol solution. Dissolve components by heating, then sterilize. After cooling to 45-50°C, aseptically add sterile defibrinated sheep or rabbit blood (B, I) to a final concentration of 15-20%. Dispense into desired containers.

9. Bovine serum albumin, 0.2% solution (Exercise 21) (18):
10-times concentrated stock:
Bovine serum albumin, Fraction V
    (F, J) .... 2 g
Physiological saline solution .... 100 ml

Working solution:
Dilute 10X concentrated stock solution 1:10 with sterile distilledwater. Dispense into tubes in desired volumes.

10. Brain heart infusion agar (Exercises 19, 24) (13) (A, D, L):

Calf brain infusion	200 g
Beef heart infusion	250 g
Peptone	10 g
Dextrose	2 g
NaCl	5 g
Disodium phosphate	2.5 g
Agar	15 g

Add 52 g of the above mixture to 1000 ml water and heat to dissolve components. Autoclave and dispense as desired. Final pH is 7.4.

11. Brain Heart Infusion (Supplemented)-Blood Agar (for *Histoplasma capsulatum* (*Ajellomyces capsulata*) conversion) (Exercise 26) (15)

Brain heart infusion agar	5.2 g
Cysteine	0.1 g
Glucose	1g
Distilled water	90 ml

Dissolve components and autoclave at 121°C for 15 minutes, cool to 50°C, then add 10 ml defibrinated sheep blood. Pour plates to double standard thickness (30-40 ml/15 x 100 mm plastic petri dish).

12. Buffered Charcoal Yeast Extract (BCYEα) agar (Exercise 13) (13) (D, L):

1. ACES (N-[2-Acetamidol]-2-aminoethane-sulfonic acid) buffer, pK 6.8 (F) .... 10.0 g
   Distilled water .... 900 ml
2. Dissolve ACES by heating solution 45-50°C then mix with: KOH, (85%, reagent grade pellets) .... 2.8 g
3. Add the following ingredients to the above buffer solution:

Activated charcoal (Norit A)	1.5 g
Yeast extract	10 g
α-ketoglutarate, monopotassium	1 g
Agar	17 g

   Use 80 ml distilled water to rinse components from side of container.
4. Autoclave mixture to sterilize, cool to 50°C, then add the following filter-sterilized solutions:

L-cysteine HCl in 10 ml distilled water	0.4 g
Ferric pyrophosphate in 10 ml distilled water	0.25 g

Adjust pH of final solution to 6.9±0.05. Dispense as desired and incubate at 35°C overnight to assure sterility.
5. If required, the following antimicrobial solutions (filter-sterilized) can be added to the completed medium following step 4:

Anisomycin	80 mg/ml
Cefamandole lithium	4 μM
Polymyxin B sulfate	80 units/ml

13. Caffeic acid agar (Exercise 24) (13):

Ammonium sulfate	5 g
Dextrose	5 g
Caffeic acid (J)	0.18 g
Yeast extract	2 g
Magnesium sulfate	0.7 g
Potassium phosphate	0.8 g
Ferric citrate (10 mg in 20 ml distilled water)	4 ml
Agar	20 g
Distilled water	1000 ml

Heat to dissolve ingredients, then autoclave to sterilize. Dispense as desired.

14. *Campylobacter* agar (Exercise 11) (13) (B, D, L):

Base medium:

Proteose peptone	15 g
Yeast extract	5 g
Digest of liver	2.5 g
NaCl	5 g
Agar	12 g

Dissolve base medium in 1000 ml distilled water, adjust pH to 7.4 at 25°C, then autoclave to sterilize. Cool to 45-50°C and add 10% sterile defibrinated sheep blood or 5-7% sterile lysed horse blood.

Add antimicrobic supplement B consisting of:

Amphotericin B	2 mg
Cephalothin	15 mg
Trimethoprim	5 mg
Polymyxin B	2500 units
Vancomycin	10 mg

Add antimicrobic supplement S consisting of:

Polymyxin B	2500 units
Trimethoprim	5 mg
Vancomycin	10 mg

Mix ingredients thoroughly, then pour into plates.

15. Cefsulodin-irgasan-novobiocin (CIN) agar (Exercise 8) (1) (A, B):

Basal medium:

Peptone	17 g
Proteose peptone	3 g

Yeast extract . . . . 2 g
Sodium pyruvate . . . . 2 g
Mannitol . . . . 20 g
Sodium desoxycholate . . . . 0.5 g
Sodium cholate . . . . 0.5 g
NaCl . . . . 1 g
Magnesium sulfate.7H$_2$O . . . . 10 mg
Neutral red . . . . 30 mg
Crystal violet . . . . 1 mg
Irgasan . . . . 4 mg
Agar . . . . 13.5 g
Dissolve in 1000 ml distilled water and boil to dissolve constituents, then autoclave for 15 minutes. After cooling to 50°C, add the following, preheated to 50°C:
Cefsulodin . . . . 4 mg
Novobiocin . . . . 2.5 mg
Mix solution well, but do not generate bubbles. Pour into petri dishes.

16. Charcoal yeast extract (CYE) (Exercise 13) (13):
Base medium:
Activated charcoal (Norit SG) (J) . . . . 2 g
Yeast extract . . . . 10.0 g
Agar . . . . 17 g
Dissolve ingredients in 980 ml distilled water by heating, then sterilize at 121°C for 15 minutes. Cool to 50°C.
Solubilize 0.25 g soluble ferric pyrophosphate in 10 ml water and filter sterilize. Also, dissolve 0.4 g L-cysteine HCl.H$_2$O in 10 ml distilled water and filter sterilize. Add the latter solution to the base medium followed by the ferric pyrophosphate solution. Final pH can be adjusted to 6.9 with 1 N KOH if required.

17. Christensen urea agar (Exercise 7 and others) (14) (B, D, L):
Urea . . . . 20 g
Monopotassium phosphate . . . . 2 g
NaCl . . . . 5 g
Dextrose . . . . 1 g
Peptone . . . . 1 g
Phenol red . . . . 0.012 g
Final pH is 6.8.
Suspend 29 grams of a mixture of the above components in 100 ml distilled water. Sterilize by filtration. Add this to 900 ml sterile agar solution (15 g agar/900 ml distilled water) cooled to 50-55°C. Mix and dispense into sterile tubes allowing to cool as slants.

18. Chocolate agar (Exercise 5) (2):
Solution 1:
GC Base (see modified Thayer-Martin medium) . . . . 7.2 g
Distilled water . . . . 100 ml
Heat to dissolve and autoclave at 121°C for 15 minutes.
Solution 2:
Hemoglobin . . . . 2 g
Distilled water . . . . 100 ml
Suspend and sterilize as above.
After cooling solutions to 50°C, mix and add 2 ml IsoVitaleX enrichment (see modified Thayer-Martin medium). Dispense into desired containers.
Alternatively, for neisseriae and haemophilae use GC base and 1% IsoVitaleX followed by 5-10% sterile defibrinated blood (B, I). This is maintain at 80°C for 15 minutes or until blood turns chocolate color. Cool to 50°C and dispense into appropriate containers. For other organisms, base medium such as those described for blood agar can be used (13).

19. Cooked meat medium (Exercise 17) (B, D, L):
Beef heart . . . . 454 g
Peptone . . . . 20 g
NaCl . . . . 5 g
Dextrose . . . . 2 g
Place 125 g medium into 1000 ml distilled water, and allow to stand for 15 minutes to wet particles. Suspend particles and dispense into tubes. Autoclave to sterilize. If not used for culture of anaerobic bacteria on the day prepared, the medium should be placed in a boiling water bath for a few minutes to drive off dissolved oxygen. Final pH is 7.2.

20. Corn meal Tween 80 agar for *Candida* (Exercise 24) (12) (B, D):
Corn meal infusion . . . . 50 g
Agar . . . . .15 g
Add 17 g of medium to 1000 ml distilled water and heat to dissolve. Add Tween 80 to a 1% final concentration. Autoclave to sterilize, then dispense into plates.

21. CTA carbohydrate medium (Exercise 3) (1) (B):
Trypticase peptone . . . . 20 g
NaCl . . . . 5 g
Sodium sulfite . . . . 0.5 g

Cystine .... 0.5 g
Phenol red .... 0.017 g
Agar .... 3.5 g
Water .... 1000 ml

Dissolve and sterilize CTA base media at a temperature of 115-118°C and not more than 12 lb. pressure for 15 minutes. Filter-sterilize desired 20% carbohydrate solutions, and aseptically add to give a 2% final concentration. Dispense into tubes to at least half full or to a depth of about 3 inches.

22. Cystine heart blood agar for culture of *Francisella tularensis* (Exercise 6) (13) (D):

Beef heart infusion .... 500 g
Proteose peptone *or* polypeptone peptone .. 10 g
Dextrose .... 10 g
L-cystine .... 1 g
NaCl .... 5 g
Agar .... 15 g
Final pH is 6.8

Add 10.2 g of the above mixture to 100 ml distilled water and heat to dissolve ingredients. Enrich by cooling to 60°C and adding 5-10 ml defibrinated rabbit blood (B, I), and maintaining temperature for 60 minutes. Cool to 45-50°C and pour into desired containers. (D)

23. Cystine tellurite blood agar (Exercise 20) (13):

Blood agar base (see blood agar) ...... 20 g
Distilled water .... 1000 ml

Dissolve blood agar base in water (final pH is 7.3) and sterilize by autoclaving. Cool and aseptically add 150 ml sterile 0.3% potassium tellurite solution (B, D) and 50 ml sterile sheep blood (B, I). After mixing, add 50 mg powdered L-cystine (need not be sterilized). After again mixing, pour into petri dishes. Swirl flask to mix contents while plates are being poured. This medium has a 1 month shelf life at refrigerator temperatures.

24. Decarboxylase medium of Moeller (Exercise 9, 12) (2) (B, D, L):

Peptone .... 5 g
Beef extract .... 5 g
Dextrose .... 0.5 g
Brom cresol purple .... 0.01 g
Cresol red .... 0.005 g
Pyridoxal .... 0.005 g

To prepare final medium 10.5 g of base medium is added to 1000 ml distilled water and heated to dissolve components. To this 10 g of either L-lysine, L-ornithine, or L-arginine is added and agitated until dissolved. Adjust pH of ornithine medium by adding 4.6 ml 1N NaOH. Dispense final medium into tubes, then sterilize. After autoclaving, medium should be pH 6.0.

25. Dextrose semisolid agar for *Listeria* (Exercise 19) (B, D, L):

Tryptose .... 10 g
NaCl .... 5 g
Dextrose .... 1 g
Agar .... 5 g

Suspend base medium in 1000 ml distilled water. Heat to dissolve ingredients, then dispense into tubes and sterilize by autoclaving. pH is 7.2 at 25°C.

26. Eagle's minimum essential medium (MEM) (Exercise 28) (9) (E, G):

Hanks's BSS:
KCl .... 0.4 g
$CaCl_2$ .... 0.14 g
$MgSO_4.7H_2O$ .... 0.2 g
KH_2PO_4 .... 0.06 g
$NaHCO_3$ .... 0.35 g
NaCl .... 8 g
$Na_2HPO_4.7H_2O$ .... 0.09 g
Glucose .... 1 g
Phenol red .... 0.010 g

Amino acids:
L-Arginine HCl .... 126.4 mg
L-cystine .... 24 mg
L-Histidine $HCl.H_2O$ .... 41.9 mg
L-Isoleucine .... 52.5 mg
L-Leucine .... 52.5 mg
L-Lysine HCl .... 73.1 mg
L-Methionine .... 14.9 mg
L-Phenylalanine .... 33 mg
L-Threonine .... 47.6 mg
L-Tryptophan .... 10.2 mg
L-Tyrosine .... 36.2 mg
L-Valine .... 46.8 mg

Vitamins:
D-Calcium pantothenate .... 1 mg
Choline chloride .... 1 mg
Folic acid .... 1 mg
i-Inositol .... 2 mg
Nicotinamide .... 1 mg
Pyridoxine HCl .... 1 mg
Riboflavin .... 0.1 mg
Thiamine HCl .... 1 mg

All of the components are contained in one liter of water. Other components that may be added include 20 ml 1M HEPES solution; 7.5% sodium bicarbonate solution, 29.3 ml; and 10 ml 200 mM L-glutamine solution. Antimicrobial compounds can also be added to the following concentrations (other combinations are also used):

Gentamicin 10μg/ml
Nystatin .... 20 units/ml
Vancomycin .... 100 μg/ml

Fetal bovine serum (E, G), heat inactivated, is added to the desired concentration, usually between 2% and 10%.

27. Egg yolk agar for *Clostridium* (Exercise 17) (17):

Polypeptone peptone (B) *or* Proteose peptone
No. 2 (D) .... 40 g
Dextrose .... 2 g
NaCl .... 2 g
Disodium phosphate .... 5 g
Monosodium phosphate .... 1 g
Magnesium sulfate .... 0.1 g
Vitamin K$_1$ (1 mg/ml) .... 1 ml
Hemin solution, 5 mg/ ml .... 1 ml
Agar .... 20 g
Distilled water .... 1000 ml

Mix ingredients in water and adjust pH to 7.6, then heat to dissolve components. Autoclave for 15 minutes at 121°C, cool to 50°C, and add 50 ml (D) or 74 ml (L) egg yolk emulsion. Dispense into plates.

28. Eosin methylene blue agar of Levine
(Introduction to Exercises 8 and 9; Exercise 9 and others) (1, 5) (B, D, L):

Peptone .... 10 g
Lactose .... 10 g
Dipotassium phosphate .... 2 g
Eosin Y .... 0.4 g
Methylene blue .... 0.065 g
Agar .... 15 g
Final pH 7.1

Dissolve in 1000 ml distilled water and heat to completely solubilize. Sterilize by autoclaving and dispense into petri dishes.

29. Fermentation broth (Exercise 1 and many others) (1) (B, D, L):
Phenol red broth base:

Pancreatic digest of casein .... 10 g
NaCl .... 5 g
Phenol red .... 0.018 g
Distilled water .... 1000 ml

pH should be 7.4

Suspend components in water then add desired amount of proper carbohydrate, usually 0.5-1% concentration. (Note: Those sugars which are unable to withstand autoclaving as arabinose, lactose, rhamnose, salicin, sucrose, trehalose, and xylose, should be filter-sterilized and aseptically added after base medium has been sterilized.) Dissolve compounds, distribute medium to tubes, and autoclave for no more than 15 minutes at 121°C.

The general interpretation of reactions of phenol red is given in Exercise 1, *Part 2* A-4.

30. Fletcher's semisolid medium for *Leptospira* (Exercise 15) (13):
Base medium (D):

Peptone .... 0.3 g
Beef extract .... 0.2 g
NaCl .... 0.5 g
Agar .... 1.5 g

Dissolve base medium in 920 ml distilled water by heating. Autoclave to sterilize, cool to 56°C, then add 80 ml Leptospira enrichment (B, D) or filter-sterilized normal rabbit serum (E, H) to a final concentration of 8% and dispense into sterile screw-capped tubes. Further inactivate the medium by heating at 56°C for one hour on two successive days. Final pH is 7.8-8.0.

Prepare 5-fluorouracil (F, J) as follows:
5-fluorouracil .... 10 g
Distilled water .... 50 ml

Add 1-2 ml 2N NaOH and gently heat (56°C) up to 2 hours until 5-FU solubilized. After adjusting pH to 7.4-7.6 with 1N NaOH bring total volume to 100 ml. Sterilize by filtration and store in refrigerator.

Final medium: Add sterile 5-FU solution to give a final concentration of 200μg/ml Fletcher's medium.

31. GN broth of Hajna (Introduction to Exercises 8 and 9; Exercise 9) (1) (A, B, D):

Tryptose *or* Polypeptone peptone ..... 20 g
Dextrose .... 1 g
D-mannitol .... 2 g
Monopotassium phosphate .... 1.5 g
Dipotassium phosphate .... 4 g
Sodium citrate .... 5 g
Sodium desoxycholate .... 0.5 g
NaCl .... 5 g

Dissolve components in 1000 ml distilled water, and adjust pH to 7.0. Dispense into tubes and sterilize by autoclaving for 15 minutes at 10 lb (116°C) or steam at 100°C for 0.5 hour. Avoid overheating.

32. Gelatin for actinomycetes (Exercise 22) (6):

Heart infusion broth (see Esculin broth for formulation) .... 25 g
Casitone (D) .... 4 g
Yeast extract .... 5 g
Dextrose .... 5 g
Gelatin .... 100 g

Dissolve in 1000 ml distilled water and adjust pH to 7.0. Autoclave to sterilize, then dispense into tubes.

33. Hektoen enteric agar (Introduction to Exercises 8 and 9; Exercise 9) (1) (B, D, L):

Peptone, peptic digest of animal
tissue .... 12 g
Yeast extract .... 3 g
Lactose .... 12 g
Sucrose .... 12 g
Salicin .... 2 g
Bile salts .... 9 g
Ferric ammonium citrate .... 1.5 g
Sodium thiosulfate .... 5 g
NaCl .... 5 g
Bromthymol blue .... 0.065 g
Acid fuchsin .... 0.1 g
Agar .... 14 g

Add to 1000 ml distilled water and heat to dissolve ingredients. Do not autoclave. Cool to 55-56°C, then dispense into plates and allow surfaces to dry.

34. Inhibitory mold agar (Exercise 23) (13) (A, B):

Salt Solution 1:
Monobasic sodium phosphate .... 10 g
Dibasic sodium phosphate .... 10 g
Distilled water .... 100 ml
Salt solution 2:
NaCl .... 0.5 g
$FeSO_4.7H_2O$ .... 0.5 g
$MgSO_4.7H_2O$ .... 10 g
$MnSO_4.7H_2O$ .... 2 ml
Distilled water .... 250 ml
Medium:
Tryptone .... 3 g
Yeast extract .... 5 g
Beef extract .... 2 g
Soluble starch .... 2 g
Glucose .... 5 g

Dextrin .... 1 g
Salt solution 1 .... 10 ml
Salt solution 2 .... 20 ml
Agar .... 17 g
Distilled water .... 970 ml

Mix and heat solution to dissolve, make pH 6.7, then autoclave to sterilize. Add 0.125 g chloramphenicol (dissolved in 95% ethanol) to hot medium. Dispense as desired. Thick-poured plates contain 30-35 ml medium.

35. Litmus milk (Exercise 18) (14) (B, D, L):

Skim milk .... 100 g
Litmus .... 0.5 g
Sodium sulfite .... 0.5 g

Dissolve 100 g litmus milk in 1000 ml distilled water, dispense into tubes, than autoclave at 121°C for 15 minutes. Final pH is 6.5.

36. Loeffler's slants (Exercise 20) (2, 5) (B, D):

Beef serum .... 3 parts
Dextrose broth .... 1 part
Dextrose broth consists of:
Tryptose .... 10 g
Beef extract .... 3 g
Dextrose .... 5 g
NaCl .... 5 g
Distilled water .... 1000 ml
Final pH is 7.2.

To prepare slants, dispense medium into tubes that can be sealed with tight-fitting closures. Include no greater than three rows of tubes in a wire basket placed in a slanted position in an autoclave. Close all parts on the autoclave before turning on steam. Autoclave at 10 lb. pressure for 20 minutes to coagulate, then open lowest port to bleed out trapped air and replace it with steam. Sterilize at 121°C, then allow pressure to slowly decrease to atmospheric levels, being certain that all ports are closed.

Alternatively, the medium may be sterilized by heating in the autoclave to 76°C for two hours on each of three consecutive days (Tyndallization process). Between heat treatments hold tubes in a slanted position at room temperature until at least after the second cycle.

After sterilization incubate medium for 24-48 hours at 37° to assure sterility.

37. Lowenstein-Jensen slants for myco-bacteria (Exercise 21) (1) (B, L):

Base medium:
Potato flour .... 30 g
Asparagine .... 3.6 g

Monopotassium phosphate .... 2.4 g
Magnesium sulfate.7H$_2$O .... 0.24 g
Magnesium citrate .... 0.6 g

Heat to dissolve constituents of base medium in 600 ml of distilled water containing 12 g glycerol. Autoclave for 30 minutes at 121°C, cool to 45-60°C, then add 1000 ml of a whole egg suspension and 20 ml 2% aqueous malachite green solution. Mix thoroughly, then dispense completed mixture into sterile tubes, slant in a water bath, autoclave, or inspissator, then heat at 85°C for 50 minutes to coagulate the medium.

Eggs are prepared by scrubbing shells in a 5% soap solution, rinsing thoroughly, then soaking in 70% ethanol for 15 minutes. After this, aseptically place egg contents in a sterile container with glass beads. Shake to blend eggs, and pass through 4 layers of sterile cheesecloth. Check sterility of medium by incubating slants at 35°C for 48 hours, then store at refrigerator temperature.

38. MacConkey agar (Exercises 4 and others; also Introduction to Exercises 8 and 9) (1) (B, D, L):

Peptone .... 17 g
Proteose peptone or polypeptone .... 3 g
Lactose .... 10 g
NaCl .... 5 g
Bile salts mixture .... 1.5 g
Neutral red .... 0.03 g
Crystal violet .... 0.001 g
Agar .... 13.5 g

Add medium to 1000 ml distilled water and dissolve by heating. Autoclave, then distribute into plates. Final pH should be 7.1. To inhibit spreading of *Proteus* agar concentration can be increase from 1.35% to 5%.

39. Mannitol salt agar (Exercise 1) (1) (B, D, L):

Proteose peptone No. 3, Polypeptone, or blend of pancreatic digest of casein and peptic digest of animal tissue .... 10 g
Beef extract .... 1 g
NaCl .... 75 g
Mannitol .... 10 g
Phenol red .... 0.025 g
Agar .... 15 g
Distilled water .... 1000 ml

Suspend medium in distilled water and heat to dissolve. Autoclave to sterilize and dispense into plates. Final pH is 7.4.

40. Methyl red-Voges-Proskauer (MR-VP) broth (Exercise 9) (1) (B, D, L):

Polypeptone or buffered peptone .... 7 g
Dextrose .... 5 g
Dipotassium phosphate .... 5 g

Dissolve MR-VP medium components in 1000 ml water, dispense into tubes, and autoclave to sterilize. Final pH is 6.9.

41. Methylene blue milk (Exercise 2) (1) (B, D):

Skim milk, dehydrated .... 10 g
Methylene blue .... 0.1 g

Dissolve components in 90 ml distilled water, dispense into tubes, and sterilize by autoclaving.

42. Middlebrook 7H10 agar (Exercise 21) (1) (A, B, D):

Ammonium sulfate .... 0.5 g
Monopotassium phosphate .... 1.5 g
Dipotassium phosphate .... 1.5 g
Sodium citrate .... 0.4 g
Magnesium sulfate .... 0.05 g
Ferric ammonium sulfate .... 0.04 g
Calcium chloride .... 0.0005 g
Zinc sulfate .... 0.001 g
Copper sulfate .... 0.001 g
D-glutamic acid (sodium salt) .... 0.5 g
Pyridoxine .... 0.001 g
Biotin .... 0.0005 g
Malachite green .... 0.001 g
Agar .... 15 g

Add constituents to 900 ml distilled water containing 5 ml glycerol solution and heat to dissolve. Dispense in 180 ml amounts, and autoclave for 10-15 minutes at 121°C. Cool to 50-55°C, then add 100 ml Middlebrook's OADC enrichment (B, D) consisting of:

Bovine albumin, Fraction V .... 5 g
Dextrose .... 2 g
Oleic acid .... 0.05 g
Catalase (beef) .... 0.004 g
NaCl .... 0.85 g

Dissolve components in 100 ml distilled water and sterilize by filtration.

The completed medium is dispensed into tubes or plates. It must be kept in the dark before and after inoculation.

43. Modified Thayer-Martin medium for *Neisseria gonorrhoeae* (Exercise 3) (13):

GC base medium (B, D, L):
Proteose peptone No. 3 *or* Polypeptone

peptone .... 15 g
Cornstarch .... 1 g
Glucose .... 1.5 g
NaCl .... 5 g
Dipotassium phosphate .... 4 g
Monopotassium phosphate .... 1 g
Agar .... 15 g
Distilled water .... 500 ml
Final pH is 7.2.

Hemoglobin solution:
 Hemoglobin .... 10 g
 Distilled water .... 500 ml

IsoVitalex Enrichment (B):
 Vitamin B$_{12}$ .... 0.010 g
 L-glutamine .... 10 g
 Adenine .... 1 g
 Guanine hydrochloride .... 0.03 g
 p-aminobenzoic acid .... 0.013 g
 L-cystine .... 1.1 g
 Dextrose .... 100 g
 Diphosphopyridine nucleotide oxidized
 (Coenzyme 1) .... 0.25 g
 Cocarboxylase .... 0.1 g
 Ferric nitrate .... 0.02 g
 Thiamine hydrochloride .... 0.003 g
 Cysteine hydrochloride .... 25.9 g
 Distilled water .... 1000 ml

Antibiotics, per ml of final medium (D):
 Vancomycin .... 3 μg
 Colistin .... 7.5 μg
 Nystatin .... 12.5 units
 Trimethoprim lactate .... 5 μg

Final medium: Prepare GC base medium by dissolving in distilled water. Also separately suspend 10 g hemoglobin in 500 ml distilled water and thoroughly mix. Sterilize both solutions by autoclaving, cool to 50°C, and aseptically pour hemoglobin solution into base medium. Add 10 ml IsoVitalex Enrichment and the antibiotics to a final concentration shown above, mix well, and dispense into desired containers.

44. Motility medium (Exercise 8 and others) (1) (A, B, D):
 Pancreatic digest of gelatin .... 10 g
 Beef extract .... 3 g
 NaCl .... 5 g
 Agar .... 4 g

Add constituents to 1000 ml distilled water and heat to dissolve. Dispense into tubes, autoclave, then allow to solidify in an upright (not slanted) position and store at room temperature. Final pH is 7.3.

45. Motility-Indole-Ornithine (MIO) test medium (Exercise 8 and others; also Introduction to Exercises 8 and 9) (7) (B, D):
 Peptone .... 10 g
 Tryptone .... 10 g
 Yeast extract .... 3 g
 L-ornithine monohydrochloride .... 5 g
 Dextrose .... 1 g
 Bromcresyl purple .... 0.02 g
 Agar .... 2 g

Dissolve medium components in 1000 ml distilled water by heating while agitating. Dispense into tubes, 5 ml/tube, then sterilize by autoclaving. Final pH is 6.6±0.2.

46. Mucate broth (Exercise 9) (8):
Broth base:
 Peptone .... 5 g
 Bromthymol blue (0.2% solution) ...... 6 ml
 Distilled water .... 500 ml

Autoclave broth at 121°C for 15 minutes, then, while still hot, aseptically add mucic acid (F, J) to a 1% concentration. Now, slowly add 5-10N NaOH to bring pH to 7.4. Dispense in 3 ml amounts and incubate tubes at 35°C to assure sterility.

(Alternately, mucic acid can be added to base medium before sterilization if it is certain that it has completely solubilized. Dispense and autoclave at 121°C for 10 minutes.)

47. Mueller-Hinton agar (Exercise 2, and others) (13) (B, D, L):
 Beef infusion .... 300 g
 Casein, acid hydrolyzed .... 17.5 g
 Starch .... 1.5 g
 Agar .... 17 g
 Distilled water .... 1000 ml

Medium is suspended in distilled water and dissolved by heating. Autoclave at 121° for no longer than 15 minutes. Cool to 45-50°C and add sterile serum (E, H) or defibrinated blood (B, I) if required. Mix and pour plates or tubes.

48. 6.5% NaCl broth for enterococci (Exercise 2) (13):
 Heart infusion medium base (D): ...... 25 g
 (Consisting of:)
 Tryptose or peptic digest of animal
 tissue .... 10 g
 Beef heart infusion .... 500 g
 NaCl .... 5 g
 NaCl .... 60 g

Dissolve components and add distilled water to one liter, dispense into tubes, and autoclave to sterilize.

49. Nitrate broth (Exercise 1 and many others) (13) (A, B, D):

Peptone .... 5 g
Beef extract .... 3 g
Potassium nitrate .... 1 g

Dissolve components in 1000 ml distilled water, dispense into tubes, containing Durham tubes if desired, and autoclave to sterilize. Final pH is 7.0. See Appendix 3 for nitrate test reagent formulae; Exercise 1, *Part 2* A-5 for interpretation of results.

50. Nitrate and nitrite broth, enriched (Exercise 3)(13):

Heart infusion broth (see 6.5% NaCl
    medium) .... 25 g
KNO_3 or KNO_2 .... 2 g

Dissolve in 1000 ml distilled water, dispense 4 ml/tube containing Durham tubes. Autoclave to sterilize.

Nitrate test reagent for mycobacteria (See Appendix 3)

51. Nutrient agar (Exercise 2 and others) (1) (B, D, L):

Pancreatic digest of gelatin *or* peptone .... 5 g
Beef extract .... 3 g
Agar .... 15 g

Suspend constituents in 1000 ml distilled water and dissolve by heating. Autoclave to sterilize and dispense as desired. Final pH is 6.8. (Note: Nutrient broth has the same formulation, but does not have agar.)

52. Nutrient gelatin (Exercise 19) (1) (B, D, L):

Gelatin .... 120 g
Nutrient broth .... 1000 ml

Heat to dissolve, dispense as desired, and autoclave to sterilize.

53. Oxford Agar (Exercise 19) (13) (L):

Columbia blood agar base .... 39 g
Lithium chloride .... 15.0 g
Esculin .... 1.0 g
Ferric ammonium citrate .... 0.5 g
Distilled water .... 1 l

Agitate and boil to dissolve ingredients. Autoclave at 15 lb/in² (121°C) for 15 minutes, then cool to 50°C. Now add the following components:

Cycloheximide .... 400 mg
Colistin sulfate .... 20 mg
Fosfomycin .... 10 mg
Acriflavine .... 5 mg
Cefotetan .... 2 mg
Mix gently, and dispense.

54. Oxidation-Fermentation (O-F) broth (Exercise 4 and others) (1) (A, B, D):

Pancreatic digest of casein .... 2 g
NaCl .... 5 g
Dipotassium phosphate .... 0.3 g
Bromthymol blue .... 0.03 g
Agar .... 3 g

Place the above components in 1000 ml distilled water. If *Vibrio parahaemolyticus* is to be assayed, add 30 g NaCl. Autoclave to sterilize, cool to 50-60°C, then aseptically add 10 ml of a 10% filter-sterilized carbohydrate solution (final concentration is 1%). Dispense into tubes.

55. Peptone broth (Exercise 10) (D, L):

Peptone *or* Polypeptone peptone ...... 10 g

Dissolve peptone in 1000 ml distilled water and add NaCl to desired concentration. Dispense into tubes and autoclave to sterilize.

56. Peptone yeast extract (PY) broth for anaerobes, pre-reduced anaerobically sterilized, PRAS (See Introduction to Exercises 16 and 17) (11):

Basal medium:

Peptone .... 0.5 g
Trypticase .... 0.5 g
Yeast extract .... 1 g
Salts solution .... 4.0 ml
Resazurin solution .... 0.4 ml
Distilled water .... 100 ml

(Resazurin solution is prepared by dissolving approximately 11 mg in 44 ml distilled water.)

The salts solution is prepared as follows:

Sodium bicarbonate .... 10 g
NaCl .... 2 g
Monopotassium phosphate .... 1 g
Dipotassium phosphate .... 1 g
Magnesium sulfate ($7H_2O$) .... 0.48 g
Calcium chloride .... 0.2 g

Dissolve calcium chloride and magnesium sulfate in 300 ml distilled water. Add 500 ml more distilled water and dissolve other salts. Bring final volume to 1000 ml and store in refrigerator.

Final medium:

Boil base medium until it becomes colorless, then cool in an ice bath while gassing with a stream of oxygen-free CO_2. Add 1 ml hemin (from 50 mg dissolved in 1 N NaOH diluted to 100 ml with distilled water), 0.02 ml Vitamin K_1 (F, J) (from stock of 0.15 ml Vitamin K_1 in 30 ml 95% ethanol), and 0.05 g L-cysteine hydrochloride. Allow latter to dissolve, then adjust pH to 6.8 while continuing to gas the medium. Dispense into tubes while flushing these with gas, then close with recessed butyl rubber stoppers (C) and screw caps. (Alternately, dispensing may be done in an anaerobic chamber.) Autoclave at 118° (112 lb) for 15 minutes.

If glucose, lactose, or sucrose are to be employed, add to the medium to a concentration of 1% and adjust pH to 6.9 before dispensing into tubes.

For PY glucose containing 20% bile, add dehydrated oxgall to a 2% concentration (which gives the equivalent of 20% bile) and 0.1% sodium desoxycholate. Dissolve and dispense as described above.

57. Phenylalanine agar (Exercise 9) (1) (A, B, D):

Yeast extract	3 g
DL-phenylalanine	2 g
NaCl	5 g
Disodium phosphate	1 g
Agar	12 g

Add components to 1000 ml distilled water and heat to dissolve. Dispense into tubes, autoclave for 10 minutes at 121°C, and allow to solidify in slant form. Final pH is 7.3.

58. Phenylethanol agar (Exercise 18) (13) (A, B, D):

Pancreatic digest of casein	15 g
Papaic digest of soy meal	5 g
NaCl	5 g
b-phenylethanol	2.5 g
Agar	15 g

Suspend components in 1000 ml distilled water and heat to dissolve. Autoclave to sterilize and dispense as desired. Final pH is 7.3. Five percent defibrinated sheep blood can be added for enrichment. Also, for anaerobic bacteria supplement with 10 mg/ml vitamin K_1 (F, J) after autoclaving.

59. Phosphate buffered saline (PBS), pH 7.2, 0.01M (Exercise 27) (20)

Ten-times concentrated stock solution:

Solution 1 (0.1M Na_2HPO_4):

Disodium phosphate	14.2 g
Distilled water	1000 ml

Solution 2 (0.1M NaH_2PO_4)

Monosodium phosphate	12 g
Distilled water	1000 ml

Solution 3:

NaCl	8.5 g
Distilled water	100 ml

Final solution:

Solution 1	28.8 ml
Solution 2	72 ml
Solution 3	100 ml
Distilled water	800 ml

Dispense as required and autoclave to sterilize.

60. Physiological saline solution (PSS, 0.85% or 0.15M NaCl Solution) (Exercise 2):

NaCl	8.5 g
Distilled water	1000 ml

61. Pyrazinamide Test Agar (Exercise 21) (19):

Medium:

Dubos broth base (B, D)	6.5 g
Distilled water	1.0 l

After dissolving, add:

Sodium pyruvate	2.0 g
Pyrazinamide (F, J)	0.1 g
Agar	15 g

Heat to dissolve agar, then dispense into 16 X 125 mm screw-capped tubes, 5 ml/tube. Autoclave at 15 lb/in² (121°C) for 15 minutes. Allow agar to solidify while tubes are in an upright position.

Test Reagent (to be freshly prepared):

Ferrous ammonium sulfate	1 g
Distilled water	100 ml

Dubos broth base consists of the following:

Casitone	0.5 g
Asparagine	2 g
Tween 80	0.2 g
KH_2PO_4	1 g
Na_2HPO_4	2.5 g
Ferric ammonium citrate	0.05 g
Magnesium sulfate	0.01 g
Calcium chloride	0.005 g

Zinc sulfate .... 0.001 g
Copper sulfate .... 0.001 g

Dissolve 1.3 g in 180 ml, sterilize, cool to 50°C, and add Dubos medium albumin or Dubos medium serum (D).

62. Sabouraud dextrose agar for fungi
(Exercise 25) (1) (B, D, L)

Neopeptone *or* Polypeptone peptone .... 10 g
Dextrose .... 40 g
Agar .... 15 g

Add constituents to 1000 ml distilled water and heat to dissolve. Autoclave to sterilize and dispense into plates. Final pH should be 5.6 For thick-poured plates, add 30-35 ml/petri dish.

63. Simmons citrate agar (Exercise 9) (13)
(B, D, L)

NaCl .... 5 g
Sodium citrate .... 2 g
Dipotassium phosphate .... 1 g
Monoammonium phosphate .... 1 g
Magnesium sulfate .... 0.2 g
Bromthymol blue .... 0.08 g
Agar .... 15 g

Suspend mixture in 1000 ml distilled water and heat to dissolve. Autoclave to sterilize, dispense into tubes, and allow to solidify in slant form. Final pH is 6.9.

64. SS (Salmonella-Shigella) agar (Introduction to Exercises 8 and 9; Exercise 9) (1) (B, D, L):

Peptone *or* Polypeptone peptone .... 5 g
Beef extract .... 5 g
Lactose .... 10 g
Bile salts mixture .... 8.5 g
Sodium citrate .... 8.5 g
Sodium thiosulfate .... 8.5 g
Ferric citrate .... 1 g
Brilliant green .... 0.33 g
Neutral red .... 0.025 g
Agar .... 13.5 g

Suspend mixture in 1000 ml distilled water and heat to boiling while mixing to dissolve. Do not autoclave. Cool to 45°C and dispense into plates. Final pH is 7.0.

65. Skimmed milk medium (Exercise 17) (1) (B, D, L):

Skimmed milk .... 10 g
Distilled water .... 100 ml

Dispense milk into tubes and autoclave at 10 lbs pressure (113-115°C) for 10 minutes. Alter-

natively, flowing steam may be used to heat the milk for 30 minutes on each of 3 days, holding at room temperature between heat treatments (Tyndallization). Store in refrigerator.

66. Starch agar for actinomycetes
(Exercise 22) (13):

Heart infusion agar (see blood agar) ... 40 g
Soluble starch .... 20 g

Dissolve in 1000 ml distilled water and autoclave to sterilize. Dispense into plates.

67. Thioglycollate broth without indicator
(Exercise 16) (13, 17) (B):

Papaic digest of soya meal .... 3 g
Pancreatic digest of casein .... 17 g
NaCl .... 2.5 g
Dextrose .... 6 g
Agar .... 0.7 g
Sodium sulfite .... 0.1 g
L-cystine .... 0.25 g
Hemin .... 5 mg
Sodium thioglycollate .... 0.5 g
Final pH is 7.0.

Add the above ingredients to 1000 ml distilled water; heat, and mix to dissolve, then boil one minute. Place a small marble chip (K) into each of several tubes, then dispense broth into these to about ⅔ depth. Autoclave for not more than 15 minutes to sterilize.

For anaerobe culture, add 1 mg/ml sodium bicarbonate and 0.1 g/ml vitamin K_1 (both filter-sterilized) prior to dispensing into tubes. Just before use, place in a boiling water bath for 5 minutes, cool, then add rabbit or horse serum to a final concentration of 10% (v/v) or Fildes (peptic digest of sheep blood) enrichment to 5% (v/v).

Thionine agar (see Basic fuchsin agar)

68. Thiosulfate citrate bile salts sucrose (TCBS) agar (Exercise 10) (2) (B, D, L)

Yeast extract .... 5 g
Peptone *or* polypeptone peptone ...... 10 g
Sucrose .... 20 g
Sodium thiosulfate .... 10 g
Sodium citrate .... 10 g
Sodium cholate .... 3 g
Oxgall .... 8 g
NaCl .... 10 g
Ferric citrate .... 1 g
Thymol blue .... 0.04 g
Bromthymol blue .... 0.04 g
Agar .... 15 g

Suspend components in 1000 ml distilled water and heat to dissolve. Do not autoclave. Dispense into plates. Final pH is 8.6.

69. Triple sugar iron agar (TSI agar) (Exercise 4 and others; also see Introduction to Exercises 8 and 9) (1) (B, D, L):

Polypeptone peptone	20 g
Lactose	10 g
Sucrose	10 g
Dextrose	1 g
NaCl	5 g
Ferrous ammonium sulfate ($FeNH_4(SO_4)_2.12H_2O$)	0.2 g
Sodium thiosulfate	0.2 g
Phenol red	0.025 g
Agar	13 g

Suspend medium in 1000 ml distilled water and heat to dissolve and autoclave. Dispense into tubes and cool in slanted position. Final pH is 7.3. For use with *Vibrio parahaemolyticus*, add 25 g NaCl to the above recipe.

70. Trypsin-EDTA solution (Exercise 28) (10):

Trypsin (F, J)	0.25 g
Ethylenediamintetracetic acid (EDTA) (F, J)	0.02 g
Phosphate buffered saline, pH 7.2	100 ml

For use in dissociating cell monolayers, calcium and magnesium ions must not be present. Sterilize by filtration, dispense as desired and store at -20°C or less. Thaw amounts to be used and do not refreeze.

71. Trypticase soy broth and agar (Exercise 2 and others) (1) (A, B, D):
Broth:

Trypticase peptone	17 g
Papaic digest of soya meal	3 g
NaCl	5 g
Dipotassium phosphate	2.5 g
Dextrose	2.5 g

Add the above components to 1000 ml distilled water and heat slightly to dissolve. Dispense into tubes and autoclave to sterilize. Final pH is 7.3.

Agar:

Trypticase peptone	15 g
Papaic digest of soya meal	5 g
NaCl	5 g
Agar	15 g

Suspend components in 1000 ml distilled water and heat to dissolve. Autoclave to sterilize and dispense as desired. Final pH is 7.3.

72. Tryptose agar (Exercise 6) (D):

Tryptose	20 g
NaCl	5 g
Dextrose	1 g
Agar	15 g

Dissolve in 1000 ml distilled water and adjust pH to 7.2 Autoclave to sterilize and dispense as desired. (D, B)

73. Tween 80 medium (Exercise 21) (18):

Tween 80 (B, D)	0.5 ml
Phosphate buffer, pH 7.0, M/15	100 ml
Neutral red solution (D), 0.1% aqueous (adjusted to 100% dye concentration)	2 ml

Phosphate buffer is prepared as follows:
Stock solution 1 (M/15 Na_2PO_4):

Disodium phosphate, M/15	9.47 g
Distilled water	1000 ml

Stock solution 2 (M/15 KH_2PO_4):

Monopottasium phosphate	9.07 g
Distilled water	1000 ml

Final buffer:

Solution 1	61.1 ml
Solution 2	38.9 ml

Check final pH to assure it is 7.0.

Dispense mixture in 2 ml amounts in 16 X 125 mm screw capped tubes and autoclave at 121°C for 10 minutes.

74. Tyrosine agar (Exercise 22) (1):

Nutrient agar	23 g
Tyrosine (D, J)	5 g

Dissolve nutrient agar in 1000 ml distilled water, then add tyrosine. Adjust pH to 7, then autoclave to sterilize. Mix to distribute tyrosine evenly and dispense 20 ml/ plate.

75. Virulence test medium for *Corynebacterium diphtheriae* (Exercise 20) (13) (D):
Solution 1:

Maltose	3 g
Proteose peptone	15 g
Distilled water	500 ml

Solution 2:

NaCl	5 g
Agar	15 g
Distilled water	500 ml

Adjust pH to 7.8, then steam to dissolve ingredients. Mix solution 1 and 2 and dispense 10 ml/tube. Steam for 15 minutes on three consecutive days to sterilize. On the last day, cool to 40°C, then add 2-4 ml sterile bovine serum, mix, and pour into petri dishes. Before cooling, submerge antitoxin-containing strips as described in Exercise 20, *Part 3*B, page 291. (Note: Although the product from Difco Laboratories differs in formulation, its preparation is less complex.)

76. Wagatsuma agar for *Vibrio* (Exercise 10) (16):

Peptone (D)	10 g
Yeast extract	3 g
Mannitol	10 g
NaCl	70 g
Dipotassium phosphate	5 g
Crystal violet	0.001 g
Agar	15 g

Dissolve components in 1000 ml distilled water by heating. pH should be approximately 8.0. Do not autoclave. Cool to 50°C. Prepare a saline-washed (3 times) and packed suspension of rabbit red cells (B, I) and add to the medium to a final concentration of 5%. Mix and dispense into plates. Do not store for long periods and dry surface before use.

77. Wickerham medium, modified, for yeast carbohydrate assimilation tests (Exercise 24) (13):

Solution 1:

Yeast nitrogen base (B, D), 10-times concentrated, filter-sterilized	50 ml

Solution 2:

Bromcresyl purple, 1.6 %	1 ml
Distilled water	450 ml
NaOH, 0.1 N	5 ml
Agar	10 g

Heat components to dissolve.

Final preparation:

Cool Solution 2 to 45-50°C then mix with Solution 1 and add 5 g desired carbohydrate. Dispense into tubes and autoclave for 10 minutes at 115°C. Cool in a slanted position.

REFERENCES

1. Baron, E. J., and S. M. Finegold. 1990. Bailey & Scott's diagnostic microbiology, 8th ed. The C. V. Mosby Co., St. Louis. p. A-1 - A-34.
2. Bell, R. H. 1987. Media, reagents and stains, p. 773-835. *In* B. B. Wentworth (ed.), Diagnostic procedures for bacterial infections, 7th ed. American Public Health Association, Inc., Washington, D. C.
3. Bridson, E. Y. (compiler). 1990. The Oxoid manual, 6th edition. Unipath Ltd., Basingstoke, England
4. Corbel, M. J., and W. J. Brinley-Morgan. 1984. Genus *Brucella* Meyer and Shaw 1920, p. 377-388. *In* N. R. Krieg, and J. G. Holt (ed.), Bergey's manual of systematic bacteriology, Vol. 1. Williams & Wilkins, Baltimore.
5. Difco Laboratories. 1984. Difco Manual, 10th ed. Difco Laboratories, Inc., Detroit, MI. 1155 p.
6. Dowell, V. R., Jr., and A. C. Sonnenwirth. 1980. Gram-positive, anaerobic, non-sporeforming bacilli, p. 1914-1923. *In* A. C. Sonnenwirth, and L. Jarett, (ed.), Gradwohl's clinical laboratory methods and diagnosis, 8th ed., Vol. 2. The C. V. Mosby Co., St. Louis.
7. Ederer, G. M., and M. Clark. 1970. Motility-indole-ornithine medium. Appl. Microbiol. **20**:849-850.
8. Ewing, W. H. 1986. Edward and Ewing's identification of the *Enterobacteriaceae*, 4th ed. The C. V. Mosby Co., St. Louis.
9. Hodinka, R. L. 1992. Cell culture techniques: preparation of cell culture medium and reagents, p. 8.19.1-8.19.12. *In* H. D. Eisenberg (ed.), Clinical microbiology procedures handbook, Vol. 2; L. M. Clarke (sect. ed.), Viruses, rickettiae, chlamidae, and mycoplasmas. American Society for Microbiology, Washington, DC.
10. Hodinka, R. L. 1992. Cell culture techniques: serial propogation and maintenance of monolayer cell cultures, p. 8.20.1-8.20-14. *In* H. D. Eisenberg (ed.), Clinical microbiology procedures handbook, Vol. 2; L. M. Clarke (sect. ed.), Viruses, rickettiae, chlamidae, and mycoplasmas. American Society for Microbiology, Washington, DC.
11. Holdeman, L. V., E. P. Cato, and W. E. C. Moore (ed.). 1977. Anaerobe laboratory manual, 4th ed. The Virginia Polytechnic Institute and State University Anaerobe Laboratory, Blacksburg, VA. p. 137-149.
12. Larone, D. H. 1987. Medically important fungi: a guide to identification. Elsevier Science Publishing Co., Inc., New York, NY. p. 193-211.
13. Nash, P., and M. M. Krenz. 1991. Culture media, p. 1226-1288. *In* A. Balows, W. J. Hausler, Jr., K. L. Herrmann, H. D. Isenberg, and H. J. Shadomy (ed.), Manual of clinical microbiology, 5th ed. American Society for Microbiology, Washington, D. C.
14. Power, D. A. (ed.), and P. J. McCuen. 1988. Manual of BBL products and laboratory procedures, 6th ed. Becton Dickinson Microbiology Systems, Cockeysville, MD. 389 p.
15. Rhodes, J. C., and K. J. Kwon-Chung. 1989. Identification of agents of systemic mycoses, p. 141-170. *In* E. G. V. Evans, and M. D. Richardson (ed.), Medical mycology: a practical approach. IRL Press, Oxford
16. Sonnenwirth, A. C. 1980. Gram-negative bacilli, vibrios, and spirilla, p. 1731-1852. *In* A. C. Sonnenwirth, and L. Jarett, (ed.), Gradwohl's clinical laboratory methods and diagnosis, 8th ed., Vol. 2. The C. V. Mosby Co., St. Louis.
17. Summanen, P., E. J. Baron, D. M. Citron, C. A. Strong, H. M. Wexler, and S. M. Finegold. 1993. Wadsworth anaerobic bacteriology manual, 5th ed. Star Publishing Co., Belmont, CA. p. 161-181; 189-204.
18. Vestal, A. L. 1975. Procedures for the isolation and identification of mycobacteria. HEW Pub. No. (CDC) 77-8230. U. S. Dept. of Health, Education, and Welfare, Atlanta, GA., 136 p.
19. Wayne, L. G. 1974. Simple pyrazinamidase and urea tests for routine identification of mycobacteria. Am. Rev. Respir. Dis. **109**: 147-151.
20. Wold, A. D. 1992. Shell vial assay for the rapid detection of viral infections, p. 8.6.1-8.6.10. *In* H. D. Eisenberg (ed.), Clinical microbiology procedures handbook, Vol. 2; L. M. Clarke (sect. ed.), Viruses, rickettiae, chlamidae, and mycoplasmas. American Society for Microbiology, Washington, DC.

List of Manufacturers
(See Appendix 6 for addresses)
A. Acumedia
B. Becton Dickinson Microbiology Systems
C. Bellco Glass Inc.
D. Difco Laboratories
E. Gibco BRL
F. ICN Biochemicals, Inc.
G. Irvine Scientific
H. Pel-Freez
I. Remel
J. Sigma Chemical Co.
K. VWR Scientific
L. Unipath Co., Oxoid Div.

APPENDIX 5
Sources of Reagents, Media, Rapid Assays, and Other Supplies

(Note: Full names and addresses of suppliers given in Appendix 6. Listings in both Appendix 5 and 6 are provided only as as aid for the use of this manual. Neither supplies nor suppliers are necessarily recommended, and in many cases, are not the only available.)

Item	Source
Accuprobe™ DNA Probe Tests	Gen-Probe
Aladin™ System	Analytab
Anaerobic chamber	Shel-Lab
Anaerobe culturing device	Belco
Anaerobic jars, bags	Becton Dickinson, Difco, Marion, Unipath
Anaerobic transport system	Anaerobic Systems, Marion
An-Ident®	Analytab
Animals, Laboratory	Hilltop, Charles Rivers, Simonsen
Antigens, agglutinating:	
Brucellae	Difco, Remel, Unipath
Francisella tularensis	Becton Dickinson, Difco
Antimicrobial sensitivity testing:	
Automated or semi-automated	
Aladin™	Analytab
Autobact™	Organon Teknika
AutoSCAN®-WA	MicroScan
Esteem™ System	MSI/Micro Media
Sensititre® Microbiology Systems	Radiometer America
Vitek Systems	Vitek Systems
Antimicrobial sensitivity testing panels	Analytab, MSI/Micro Media
Antiserum for:	
Enteric serotyping and grouping	Becton Dickinson, Difco, Remel, Unipath
Haemophilus serogroups	Difco
Neisseria meningitidis serogroups	Difco, EY Laboratories
Streptococcus grouping	Difco, Remel
API® rapid tests	Analytab
AutoSCAN™	MicroScan
BACTEC® Systems	Becton Dickinson
Bacteroides bile esculin agar	Anaerobe Systems, Scott
Bacti-Cinerator® III	Thomas Scientific
Bactigen® tests	Wampole
Bacto™ products	Difco
Beta lysin disks	Remel
Birdseed agar	Becton Dickinson, Remel
BBL® products	Becton Dickinson
Bio-Bag™	Becton Dickinson
Biolog products	Biolog
Blood culture media	Becton Dickinson Diagnostic, Difco, Roche
Brucella agar	Becton Dickinson, Difco, Remel, Unipath
BSK-H medium	Sigma
Buffered charcoal yeast extract with α-ketoglutarate medium	Carr-Scarborough, Remel
Butzler medium	Difco
Campy-BAP	Becton Dickinson, Difco, Remel
Campyslide™	Becton Dickinson
Candida Bromcresol Green agar	Becton Dickinson, Difco, Remel
Cards Strep® A Test	Pacific Biotech
CDA® Clostridium difficile toxin A kit	bioMérieux
C. diff-CUBE™	Difco
Cefinase™ discs	Becton Dickinson
Cell culture lines	American Type Culture
Charcoal yeast extract agar	Remel
Clostridium difficile cyto-toxicity assay	Bartels
Clostridium difficile selective media	Remel, Unipath
Clostridium perfringens selective media	Unipath
CO₂-generating packets	Becton Dickinson, Difco
Coagulase plasma	Becton Dickinson, Difco
Colloidal gold-labeled antibodies	E-Y Laboratories
Columbia broth	Becton Dickinson, Difco
Complement fixation reagents for detection of anti-viral antibodies	Linmed, Virion
Culturette Brand CDT®	Becton Dickinson
Cystine heart blood agar	Difco, Remel
Cytoclone™ A+B EIA	Cambridge
Detect-A-Strep™	Antibodies Inc.
Directigen® tests	Becton Dickinson
E Test™	AB Biodisk
E. coli O157:H7 latex agglutination test	Pro-Lab
Egg candler	Carolina Biological
Egg yolk agar	Anaerobic Systems, Carr-Scarborough
Eggs, fertile chicken	Nasco West, Nebraska Scientific

ELISA-based kits for
detection of:
 Candida · · · · · · · · · · · · · · · Immuno-Mycologics
 Clostidium difficile · · · · · · · bioMérieux, Vitek, Meridian
  Toxin A
 Lyme disease antibody · · · · Access, bioMérieux,
                              Cambridge, Dako, General
                              Biometrics, 3M

EMJH medium · · · · · · · · · · · · Difco
Enteric enrichment broths · · · Becton Dickinson, Difco,
 (GN, Selenite, Tetra-   Remel
 thionate)
EnvironAmp™ Legionella kit · · Perkin Elmer Cetus
Equate® Legionella Urinary · · Binax
 Antigen RIA Kit
Exoantigen test kits · · · · · · · Immuno-Diagnostics,
                              Meridian

Fletcher's medium · · · · · · · · Difco
Fluorescent antibody
reagents for detection of:
 Bacteroides spp. · · · · · · · · · MicroScan, Organon Teknika
 Legionella · · · · · · · · · · · · · BioDx, MarDx, Meridian,
                              Pro-Lab, Sanofi

 Lyme Disease · · · · · · · · · · · Hillcrest, MarDx, Whittaker
 Neisseria gonorrhoeae · · · · Bartels, Syva
 Syphilis (FTA-ABS test) · · · Becton Dickinson, Difco,
                              Wampole
Fluorescent brightener · · · · · Sigma
 (Calcofluor White)
Fox Dual GNI Panel · · · · · · · Micro-Media Systems
Fungi-Fluor™ · · · · · · · · · · · · Polysciences

Gas liquid chromatography · · Microbial ID
 system
Gonochek™ · · · · · · · · · · · · · E·Y Laboratories
GonoGen™ II · · · · · · · · · · · New Horizons
Gonozyme™ · · · · · · · · · · · · Abbott
Grouping kit DR 585 · · · · · · Unipath

Helicobacter latex aggluti- · · Meridian
 nation kit
Hemagglutination Trepone- · · Difco
 mal Test for Syphilis
 (HATTS)
Hippurate test disks · · · · · · · Becton Dickinson, Difco,
                              Remel

Identicult™ Neisseria · · · · · · Scott
Immunoblot diagnostic kits · · MarDx, Whittaker
 for Lyme disease
ImmunoScan™ tests · · · · · · · MicroScan
Inhibitory mold agar · · · · · · · Becton Dickinson, Remel
Isolator Microbial Tube · · · · · Wampole

KL Antitoxin strips, virulence · Difco
 test medium

Latex agglutination tests to
detect:
 Clostridium difficile antigen · Becton Dickinson, Meridian
 E. coli O157:H7 · · · · · · · · · Pro-Lab
 Fungal antigens · · · · · · · · · Baxter, Immuno-Mycologics,
                              Linmed

Helicobacter · · · · · · · · · · · · Meridian
Salmonella-Shigella · · · · · · · Wampole
Staphylococcus · · · · · · · · · · MicroScan, Remel, Scott
Lectins · · · · · · · · · · · · · · · E·Y Laboratories
Legionella differentiation · · · Remel
 disks
Leptospirosis indirect · · · · · · Hillcrest
 hemagglutination test
Listeria monocytogenes · · · · Becton Dickinson, Difco,
 selective broths   Unipath
Loeffler's medium · · · · · · · · Remel, Scott
Lowenstein-Jensen medium · · Becton Dickinson, Carr-
                              Scarborough, Difco, Remel,
                              Scott

Meritec™ assay kits · · · · · · · Meridian
MICRO-ID LISTERIA · · · · · · Organon Teknika
 system
MicroScan System · · · · · · · · Baxter
MIDI Microbial Identification · Microbial ID
 System, MIS
Middlebrook's 7H10, 7H11 · · Becton Dickinson, Difco,
                              Remel, Scott
Minitek® assay kits · · · · · · · Becton Dickinson

Niacin strips · · · · · · · · · · · · Difco, Remel
Ninhydrin reagent · · · · · · · · Remel

O/129 filter paper disks · · · · Unipath
OFPBL agar · · · · · · · · · · · · Remel
Oxford medium · · · · · · · · · · Unipath
Oxidase reagent in filter · · · · E·Y Laboratories, General
 paper or swabs   Diagnostics, Marion, Unipath
Oxidase reagent solution · · · · Carolina Biological, Difco,
                              Remel
Oxyrase™ Enzyme · · · · · · · · Oxyrase

PathoDX® Strep Grouping · · · Diagnostic Products
PC agar · · · · · · · · · · · · · · · Becton Dickinson, Remel
Petragnani medium · · · · · · · Becton Dickinson, Difco,
                              Remel
Phadebact® CoA tests · · · · · Boule Diagnostics
Pouch System · · · · · · · · · · · Difco
PRAS media · · · · · · · · · · · · Anaerobe Systems, Carr-
                              Scarborough, Scott
Premiere™ ELISA kits · · · · · Meridian
Pro-Lab LA Panel · · · · · · · · Pro-Lab
Pyloragen™ Helicobacter · · · Hycor
 pylori Test kit
PyloriFiax® · · · · · · · · · · · · · Whittaker
Pyloristat Rapid EIA · · · · · · Whittaker
PYR test swabs and · · · · · · · Diagnostic Products
 developing reagent
Pyrazinamide test agar · · · · · Remel

Rapid CH, Rapid CHB · · · · · Analytab
Rapid Plasma Reagin Card · · Becton Dickinson, Remel,
 Test   Seradyn
RapID™ tests · · · · · · · · · · · Innovative Diagnostic
                              Systems
Remel Staph Latex kit · · · · · Remel
RIM™ M · · · · · · · · · · · · · · · Austin

RPLA (Reverse Passive Latex Agglutination) for enterotoxins	Unipath
Sabouraud dextrose agar	Carr-Scarborough, Difco
Sabouraud dextrose-brain heart infusion (SABHI) agar	Carr-Scarborough, Remel, Unipath
Satellite test filter paper strip or disk reagent	Becton Dickinson, Difco, Unipath
Sensititre®	Radiometer America
Septi-chek™ Blood Culture Bottles	Roche
Skirrow's medium	Becton Dickinson, Difco
Smart™	New Horizons
SNAP® Culture Identification Diagnostic kit	Syngene
SOC™ Yeast Identification System	Wadley
Staphase® III	Analytab
Staph-Ident®, Staph-Trac™	Analytab
Steri-Loop® Bacteriology Incinerator	Baxter
Syphilis-M, Syphilis-G test kits	Diagnostic Chemicals
Thermonuclease test agar	Remel
Thiosulfate-citrate-bile salts-sucrose (TCBS) agar	Becton Dickinson, Difco
Thioglycollate broth	Becton Dickinson, Difco, Unipath
Tissue culture media	Gibco BRL, Irvine, Sigma
Transport media:	
Amies, Stuart's	Difco, Remel
Cary and Blair	Becton Dickinson, Remel, Unipath
Trypticase soy broth	Becton Dickinson, Difco
Unisept® dezine-er™ System	Analytab
Uni-Yeast Tek™ plate and tube system	Remel
VDRL antigen	Becton Dickinson, Difco, Remel
Ventrascreen® Strep A	Ventrex
Vet-RPLA	Unipath
Visuwell™ reagin	ADI
Vitek AMS®	Vitek Systems
Wellcogen™ Tests	Wellcome Diagnostics
X, V disks or strips	(See Satellite test)

APPENDIX 6
Name and Addresses of
Commercial Resources

Listed here are names, addresses, and, for most, telephone numbers of many suppliers of materials used in this manual. See Appendix 5 for products provided by these companies.

AB Biodisk
Pyramidvägen 7, S-171 36
Solna, Sweden
(E* Test Strips available
from Remel)

Abbott Laboratories   1-800-323-9100
Diagnostic Division
Abbott Park
North Chicago, Illinois 60064
(For diagnostics)

Abbott Laboratories
Analytical Systems
P. O. Box 152020
Irving, TX 75015
(For MD-2)

Abbott Laboratories
Pharmaceutical Products Div.
N. Chicago, IL 60064 (For
Nembutal solution)

Access Medical System, Inc.   1-800-321-0207
21 Business Park Drive   1-481-3073 (In Connecticut)
Branford, CT 06405

Acumedia Mfrs. Inc.   (301) 467-3200
3651 Clipper Mill Road
Baltimore, MD 21211

ADI Diagnostics
30 Meridian Road
Rexdale, Ontario M9W 4Z7
(Visuwell™ Reagin Kit avail-
able from Organon Teknika
Corp.)

American Society for   (202) 737-3600
Microbiology
Board of Education and
Training
1325 Massachusetts Ave.,
N.W.
Washington, DC 20005

American *Type Culture*   1-800-638-6597
Collection
12301 Parklawn Drive
Rockville, MD 20852-1776

Anaerobe Systems   1-800-443-3108
15906 Concorde Circle
Morgan Hill, CA 95036

API Analytab Products   1-800-645-0666
200 Express St.   1-800-632-3101
Plainview, NY 11803-2469   (In New York)

Antibodies, Inc.   1-800-824-8540
P. O. Box 1560
Davis, CA 95617

Austin Biological   1-800-531-5106
Laboratories   1-800-252-9280 (In Texas)
6620 Manor Road
Austin, Texas 78723

Baxter Diagnostics, Inc.   1-800-227-8357
Bartels Diagnostics
2005 NW Sammamish Road
Issaquah, WA 98027

Baxter Diagnostics Inc.   1-800-631-7216
Scientific Products Div.
1430 Waukegan Road
McGaw Park, IL 60085-6787
(and other locations)

Becton Dickinson   1-800-638-8663
Microbiology Systems
P. O. Box 243
Cockeysville, MD 21030

Becton Dickinson Diagnostic
Instrument Systems   1-800-638-8656
383 Hillen Road
Towsen, MD 21204

Bellco Glass Inc.   1-800-257-7043
340 Edrudo Road   1-800-222-0227
P. O. Box B   (In New Jersey)
Vineland, NJ 08360

Binax Inc.   1-800-323-3199
95 Darling Ave.
South Portland, ME 04106

The Binding Site   1-800-633-4484
5889 Oberlin Dr., Suite 101
San Diego, CA. 92121

Biolog, Inc.   1-800-284-4949
3938 Trust Way
Hayward, CA 94545

bioMérieux Vitek, Inc.
(See Vitek Systems)

Boule Diagnostics AB
Lunastigen 3
S-14144 Huddinge
Sweden
(Phadebact available
through Remel)

Cambridge Biotech   1-800-637-8376
365 Plantation St.   1-800-439-5667 (In Mass.)
Worchester, MA 01605

Cappel Research Products   1-800-523-7620
Organon Teknika Corp.
100 Akzo Ave.
Durham, NC 27704

Carolina Biological   1-800-334-5551
Supply Co.
2700 York Road
Burlington, NC 27215

Carr-Scarborough   1-800-241-0998
Microbiologicals, Inc.
P. O. Box 1328
Stone Mountain, GA 30086

Charles Rivers   1-800-522-7287
250 Ballardvale St.
Wilmington, MA 01887

Dako Corporation   1-800-235-5763
6392 Via Real
Carpinteria, CA. 93013

Diagnostics Chemicals Ltd   1-800-225-5325
160 Christian St.
Oxford, CT 06483

Diagnostic Products Corp.   1-800-678-6699
5700 W. 96th St.
Los Angeles, CA. 90045

Difco Laboratories   1-800-521-0851
P. O. Box 331058
Detroit, MI 48232-7058

dms Laboratories, Inc.   1-800-526-5917
Darts Mill
Flemington, NJ 08822

Du Pont Company   1-800-551-2121
Biotechnology Systems
Division
Barley Mill Plaza
Wilmington, DE 19898

E·Y Laboratories   1-800-821-0044
127 N. Amphlett Blvd.   (650) 342-3296
San Mateo, CA 94401   (In California)

General Diagnostics
Division of Warner-Lambert
Co.
Morris Plains, NJ 07950

General Biometrics, Inc.   1-800-288-4368
15222 Avenue of Science,
Suite A
San Diego, CA 92128-9814

Gen-Probe Inc.   1-800-523-5001
9880 Campus Point Drive   1-800-342-7441
San Diego, CA 92121   (In California)

Gibco BRL   1-800-828-6686
P. O. Box 68
Grand Island, NY
14072-0068

The Gillette Co.
Stationery Products Group
Prudential Tower Building
Boston, MA 02199-3799

Hardy Media   **805 346-2766**
1430 West McCoy Lane   **fax 805 346-2760**
Santa Maria, CA 93455

Hillcrest Biologicals   1-800-445-0185
10703 Progess Way   1-800-233-7182
Cypress, CA 90630-4738   (In California)

Hilltop Lab Animals, Inc.   1-800-245-6921
Hilltop Drive
P. O. Box 183
Scottsdale, PA 15683

Hycor Biomedical Inc.   1-800-382-2527
7272 Chapman Ave.
Garden Grove, CA 92641

Hynson, Westcott,   1-800-638-1532
& Dunning   (301) 873-0890
Charles and Chase Streets
Baltimore, MD 21201

ICN Biochemicals, Inc.   1-800-854-0530
P. O. Box 19536
Irvine, CA 92713-9921

Immuno-Mycologics, Inc.   1-800-654-3639
P. O. Box 1151   (405) 288-2458
Norman, OK 73070   (in Oklahoma)

Innovative Diagnostic   1-800-225-5443
Systems, Inc.
3404 Oakcliff Road
Suite C-1
Atlanta, GA 30340

Irvine Scientific
2511 Daimler St.
Santa Ana, CA. 92705-5588

1-800-437-5706
(714) 261-7800
(In California)

Johnston Laboratories, Inc.
(See Becton Dickinson
Diagnostics Instrument
Systems)

Laboratory Consulting, Inc.
P. O. Box 1763
2702 International Lane
Madison, Wis. 53701

(608) 241-4151

Lee Laboratories
1475 Highway 78-SW
Grayson, GA 30221

1-800-732-9150

Linmed Biologics
2913 Saturn, Unit D
Brea, CA 92621

(714) 572-6011

Litton Bionetics Lab
Products
2020 Bridge View Dr.
Charlston, SC 29402

3M Diagnostic Systems,
Inc.
3380 Central Expressway
Santa Clara, CA. 95051

1-800-221-9765
(408) 739-2200
(In California)

MarDx Diagnostics, Inc.
847 Jerusalem Road
Scotch Plains, NJ 07076

1-800-331-2291

Meridian Diagnostics
3471 River Hills Drive
Cinncinnati OH 45244

1-800-534-1980 General
1-800-343-3850 Technical

Micro Media Systems (MSI)
2330 Denison Ave.
Cleveland, OH 44109

1-800-423-6496

MicroScan Div.
Baxter Healthcare Corp.
West Sacramento, CA. 95691

1-800-631-7216

MIDI
115 Barksdale Prof. Center
Newark, DE 19711-9918

(302) 737-4297

Molecular Biosystems, Inc.
11180-A Roselle Street
San Diego, CA 92121

(619) 452-0681

Murex Corporation
P. O. Box 2003
Norcross, GA 30091

1-800-826-8739

Nasco
1524 Princeton Ave.
P. O. Box 3837
Modesto, CA 95352-3837

1-800-558-9595

Nebraska Scientific
3823 Leavenworth St.
Omaha, NE 68105-1180

1-800-228-7117
(402) 346-7214
(Omaha area)

New Horizons Diagnostics
Corp.
Suite-B9110
Red Branch Road
Columbia, MD 21045

(301) 992-9357

Organon Teknika Corp.
100 Akzo Road
Durham, NC 27704

1-800-682-2666

Ortho Diagnostics Systems,
Inc.
Customer Service
Department
Route 202
Raritan, NJ. 08869

1-800-526-3875

Oxoid U. S. A.
See Unipath

Oxyrase, Inc.
P. O. Box 1345
Mansfield, OH 44901

(419) 589-8800

Pacific Biotech
9050 Camino Santa Fe
San Diego, CA. 92121

1-800-225-0730

Pel-Freez
P. O. Box 68
205 N. Arkansas St.
Rogers, AR 72757

1-800-643-3426

The Perkin Elmer Corp.
761 Main Ave.
Norwalk, CT 06859-0001

1-800-762-4002 (General)
1-800-762-4001 (Technical)

Pro-Lab Inc.
211 Sam Bass Road
P. O. Box 503
Round Rock, TX 78664

1-800-522-7740

Radiometer America Inc.
811 Sharon Drive
Westlake, OH 44145

1-800-736-0600

Remel
12076 Santa Fe Drive
Lenexa, Kansas 66215

1-800-255-6700
1-800-332-4377 (In Kansas)

Roche Diagnostic Systems
One Sunset Avenue
Montclair, NJ 07042-5199

1-800-526-1247

Scimedx Corp.
(Marketed through Linmed)
400 Ford Road
Denville, NJ 07834

Scott Laboratories, Inc.   1-800-556-6480
771 Main St.
Fiskville, RI   02823

Seradyne   1-800-428-9230
P. O. Box 1210   (317) 266-2992 (In Indiana)
Indianapolis, IN 46206

Shell-Lab   (503) 640-3000
300 N. 26th Ave.
Cornelius, OR 97113

Sigma Chemical Co.   1-800-325-8070
P. O. Box 14508
St. Louis, MO 63178-9916

Simonsen Laboratories, Inc.   (408) 847-2002
1180C Day Road
Gilroy, CA 95020

Syngene, Inc.   1-800-442-7627
10030 Barnes Canyon Road
San Diego, CA 92121

Syva Co.   1-800-227-9948
900 Arastradero Road   1-800-982-6135
Palo Alto, CA 94303-0847   (In California)

Thomas Scientific   1-800-345-2100
99 High Hill Road at I-295
P. O. Box 99
Swedesboro, NJ 08085-0099
(and other locations)

Triarch Incorporated   1-800-848-0810
P. O. Box 98   (414) 748-5125
Ripon, WI 54971   (In Wisconsin)

Unipath Co.   1-800-567-8378
Oxoid Div.
P. O. Box 691
Ogdensburg, NY 13669

Ventrex Laboratories Inc.   1-800-341-0463
P. O. Box 9731
217 Read St.
Portland, Maine 04103

Virion (U. S.) Inc.   1-800-524-2689
4 Upperfield Road
Morristown, NJ 07960

Vitek Systems   1-800-638-4835
595 Anglum Drive
Hazelwood, MO.
63042-2395

VWR Scientific   1-800-932-5000
P. O. Box 66929
O'Hare AMF
Chicago, IL 60666
(And locations throughout
U. S.)

Wadley Biosciences Corp.   1-800-762-0067
1720 Regal Row
Suite 215
Dallas, TX 75235

Ward's Natural Science   1-800-962-2660
Establishment, Inc.
5100 West Henrietta Road
P. O. Box 92912
Rochester, NY 14692-9012

Whittaker Bioproducts   1-800-638-3976
8830 Biggs Ford Road
Walkersville, MD
21793-0127

Wampole Laboratories   1-800-257-9525
P. O. Box 1001   (609) 655-6000
Cranbury, NJ 08512-0181   (In New Jersey)

Wellcome Diagnostics   1-800-334-8570
3030 Corwallis Road   (919) 248-4617
Research Triangle Park,   (In North Carolina)
NC 27709

APPENDIX 7
Notes on the Use and Care of the Microscope (1, 2)

Users of *Medical Microbiology, a Laboratory Manual* should have had previous exposure concerning the proper care and use of the compound microscope. For this reason, only a brief summary is presented here. For those not having adequate previous experience, more extensive information is given in references listed at the end of this section. These or others should be consulted. Everyone should read the instruction booklet for the particular make and model of microscope they are going to use if it is for the first time. Microscopes are expensive precision instruments built to last many years. With proper care and use each instrument will not only give maximum service, but provide the most information for which it was intended.

A. Use of the microscope:

1. Turn on the illuminator. If the light source is not built into the microscope adjust the distance of the light source and the plane surface of the reflecting mirror so that light fills the back lens of the objective. This is done by viewing down the tube after removing the eyepiece and opening the condenser iris diaphragm. After proper light adjustment, reinsert eyepiece and close the condenser diaphragm about half way.
2. Place slide with specimen to be observed on the stage.
3. Move proper low power objective, usually 10X for bacteria, into the optical pathway, if necessary. (Note: One should always leave the low power objective in this position when observations are completed. This objective cannot touch the empty stage, even when in its lowest position and is therefore not subject to impact damage by striking the stage.) Move to within a few millimeters of the specimen by using the coarse adjustment, then bring object into focus by moving the objective *upward* by use of the fine adjustment.
4. If higher magnification is required swing the high-dry (40X-45X) objective into the

optical path. (As a precautionary measure, always watch the objective while shifting it so that you are certain it will not strike the slide before reaching its final position.) Again bring the object into focus using the fine adjustment.
5. For maximum magnification use the oil immersion objective. Move the high-dry objective out of the optical path. Place a small drop of immersion oil on the slide, then move the oil immersion objective into the optical path. Bring object into focus by use of the fine adjustment.
6. After observations have been completed, raise the objective using the coarse adjustment, then return the low power objective into the optical path. If no further observations are to be made clean oil immersion objective as described below.

B. Kohler Illumination:

Kohler illumination is a procedure that provides optimal lighting for maximum resolution. These simple steps will aid in providing the clearest images and should be done each time the microscope is used.
1. Place the light source in a position described above in A-1, and focus on the specimen with the low power of the microscope.
2. Move the microscope condenser to its uppermost position, but do not hit the underside of the slide.
3. Set the condenser diaphragm at about one-half open, just providing full illumination of the field. Close the lamp diaphragm almost completely.
4. Looking through the eyepiece, focus the light spot (field stop image) by slightly lowering condenser.
5. Rotate the mirror to center the field stop image in the field of view. For built-in light sources the adjusting screws on the side of the condenser may be used.
6. Open the lamp diaphragm to give a fully illuminated field, then close the condenser

diaphragm to eliminate glare and give adequate contrast. Do not stop the latter down further than absolutely necessary nor change condenser height to change lighting intensity. Such manipulations reduce the resolving power. Light intensity is changed by lowering lamp voltage or by stopping down the lamp condenser.

7. Change objective to high dry and then to oil immersion. Repeat steps 1-6 with each.

C. Microscope and Illuminator Care:

1. When moving a microscope from one location to another hold it securely with *two* hands.

2. Always store the microscope with the low power objective in the optical path position.

3. Keep lenses clean.
   a. Dust with camel's hair brush and clean with lens paper.
   b. Remove oil from oil immersion lens by (i) wiping most of oil away with lens paper; (ii) removing the residual oil from lens using a *small* amount of xylene on a clean piece of lens paper; and (iii) thoroughly wiping lens with fresh lens paper to remove xylene. Do *not* soak lens in solvent since it can damage the lens mounting. Always use lens paper for cleaning, not tissue paper or cloth.
   c. Use care when switching from oil immersion to high dry objective if each is within its working distance. The latter can sweep through residual oil on the slide. The working distance of the high dry lens is such that it can touch the oil, and it is difficult to remove.

4. If your light source is equipped with a rheostat, always turn it to its lowest setting before storing. This will lengthen bulb life by avoiding high surges of current to it when switched on.

REFERENCES

1. Mollring, F. K. 1973. Microscopy from the very beginning. Carl Zeiss, Oberkochen, West Germany. 66 p.

2. Murray, R. G. E., and C. F. Robinow. 1981. Light microscopy, p. 6-16. *In* P. Gerhardt, R. G. E. Murray, R. N. Costilow, E. W. Nester, W. A. Wood, N. R. Krieg, and G. B. Phillips. (ed.), Manual of methods for general microbiology. American Society for Microbiology, Washington, DC.

Index